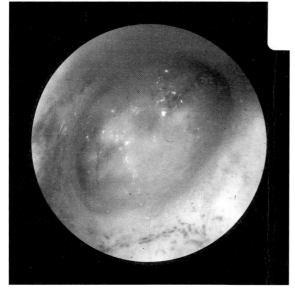

Plate 20.1   Panoramic hysteroscopy in a postmenstrual woman, illustrating the uterine cavity plus cornua. CO_2 distension

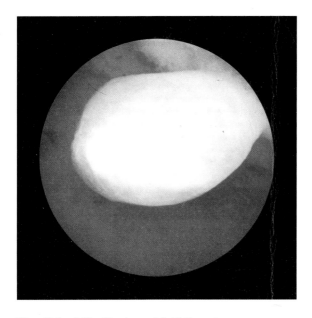

Plate 20.2   A fibroid polyp and fluid distension

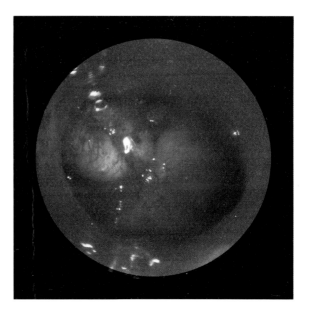

Plate 20.3   A submucous fibroid in a premenstrual woman, with CO_2 distension

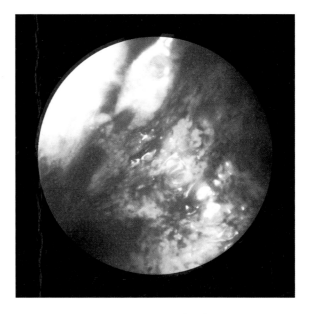

Plate 20.4   Postmenopausal endometritis and a panoramic view of the fundus and cornua to show vascular changes in the endometrium (in contrast with Plate 20.1)

PROGRESS IN OBSTETRICS AND GYNAECOLOGY

Contents of Volume 6

PROGRESS IN
OBSTETRICS AND
GYNAECOLOGY

PROGRESS IN OBSTETRICS AND GYNAECOLOGY

PROGRESS IN OBSTETRICS AND GYNAECOLOGY

Contents of Volume 6

PROGRESS IN OBSTETRICS AND GYNAECOLOGY
Volume Seven

EDITED BY

JOHN STUDD MD FRCOG
Consultant Obstetrician and Gynaecologist
King's College Hospital and Dulwich Hospital;
King's College Hospital Medical School, London

CHURCHILL LIVINGSTONE
EDINBURGH LONDON MELBOURNE AND NEW YORK 1989

CHURCHILL LIVINGSTONE
Medical Division of Longman Group UK Limited

Distributed in the United States of America by
Churchill Livingstone Inc., 1560 Broadway, New York,
N.Y. 10036, and by associated companies, branches
and representatives throughout the world

First published 1989
  Reprinted 1990

ISBN 0-443-03885-6

ISSN 0261-0140

British Library Cataloguing in Publication Data
Progress in obstetrics and gynaecology. Vol. 7
  1. Gynaecology—Periodicals 2. Obstetrics
  —Periodicals
  618.05   RG1

Library of Congress Cataloging in Publication Data
Progress in obstetrics and gynaecology. Vol. 7
  Includes indexes.
    1. Obstetrics—Collected works. 2. Gynecology—
Collected works. I. Studd, John [DNLM: 1. Gynecology—
Periodicals. 2. Obstetrics—Periodicals. WI PR675P]
RG39.P73   618   81–21699

Produced by Longman Singapore Publishers (Pte) Ltd.
Printed in Singapore

Preface

I write this Preface to Volume 7 during the 40th anniversary of one of this country's great achievements, the National Health Service, at a time when its defects are being emphasized from all directions. Certainly there are problems. One that should concern all in training is the question of future career prospects. It is hard to understand the co-existence of long waiting lists and middle-aged trainees waiting for jobs. Although this career bottleneck is worse in surgery and medicine than in our own specialty, our record is no cause for congratulation and our failure to promote married women is a waste of great talent. This enigma of unemployed doctors and untreated patients is even more incomprehensible because the UK has fewer doctors per unit population than any European country except Turkey. The response to this are plans to reduce the number of medical students and also limit the number of specialists in training!

There are many deficiencies, such as nurses' pay and equipment expenditure, in the National Health Service but the fundamental cause of these manpower anomalies is the fact that overwhelming health demands are supported by too few consultants. The promise of consultant expansion over the years has been a cruel political deception and simply has not happened. A 1986 report from the Royal College of Surgeons quantified this deficiency in terms of numbers of consultant surgeons. The 12 per hundred thousand population of West Germany, 11 in Belgium and the USA, 6 in Holland compare well to the miserable 2 in the United Kingdom. It is difficult to obtain comparable figures for obstetrics and gynaecology but it would appear to me that the 3000 ACOG Fellows in New York State and the 850 in rural North Carolina are examples of how the 900 consultants in England and Wales is a hopelessly inadequate number to do the job. This deficiency is the result of medicine being poorly funded by a monopoly employer.

The prolonged, even excessive, training for consultants in the United Kingdom creates highly trained and competent individuals but the result of the financial restrictions is that too few consultants chase around doing too many things. They have to cope with a busy NHS practice embracing all areas of our specialty from oncology to endocrinology. They will also have extensive undergraduate and postgraduate teaching commitments, occasionally a research interest and frequently a large private practice. The disheartened 'juniors' wait in the wings for a consultant post to appear at the average age of 38—sometimes 42 in many surgical specialties. All this is bad for the quality of patient care and for the recruitment of talented graduates into hospital medicine. It is my belief that greater use of the private sector can ease many of these problems.

Funding for health care in this country is believed to be inadequate because it compares unfavourably with the total health care budget of other Western countries. Comparable OECD figures for 1985 (Table 1) which are the latest available show

Table 1. Health expenditure in 1985 as a percentage of GNP (Gross National Product)

	Public %	Private %	Total %
Canada	6.5	2.1	8.6
Denmark	5.2	1.0	6.2
France	6.7	2.7	9.4
Germany	6.3	1.8	8.1
Greece	4.1	0.1	4.2
Italy	6.2	1.2	7.4
Netherlands	6.6	1.7	8.3
Spain	4.3	1.7	6.0
Sweden	8.4	0.9	9.3
United Kingdom	5.2	0.7	5.9
United States	4.4	6.4	10.8
OECD average	5.7	1.7	7.4

that the 5.9% of gross national product spent in the UK is almost the lowest with the USA, spending 10.8% of GNP, being the highest. However, the deficit is nearly all explained by the size of the contributions from the private sector (Table 1). The UK private health care expenditure is 12% of total health care expenditure compared to 20% for the Netherlands, 22% for Germany, 29% for France and 59% for the United States. The OECD average is 22%. If we can make this up we can have a properly funded health service.

The private sector is at last expanding with new hospitals being built and staffed. All this is for the good, but it must not become the privileged layer of a two-tier medical system. The challenge of the times is to use the revenue and skills from the private sector to increase the number of consultants by producing more posts for trainees, more choice for the patients and thus maintain high medical standards. We must recognize that this can only happen with little extra cost to the exchequer as no government of whatever hue has ever chosen to adequately fund the NHS or create the number of consultant posts necessary.

I have previously written (*Progress in Obstetrics & Gynaecology*, Volume 6) of the way in which excellent clinical research occurs using private funds. The private sector can also be used to support the NHS if consultants with busy private practice commitments give up sessions in order to create new consultant posts. This is already happening and one can only hope that the trend accelerates allowing many new and virtually cost-free five to eight session consultant posts to be created. The income will be made up by research sessions or from the greater amount of private work that will be available.

Would not our major hospital departments be better off without the senior registrar logjam but with 10 committed half-time consultants rather than five nearly whole-time consultants? At the same time it will remove the brutalizing effect of a perceived professional failure on the families of decent, able senior registrars. Such a formula will not work for all specialties, in all parts of the country but it is an option that could be offered to a London surgeon even if not to a Tyneside perinatal paediatrician.

There is no doubt that British medical standards are under siege and being eroded by crude financial controls. Fortunately alternative resources are available to correct this. We must forget our prejudices and allow the vast clinical, research and employment potential of private funding to be exploited for the general benefit of the nation's health care.

London, UK   J.S.
1989

Contributors

R H Asch MD
Professor of Obstetrics and Gynaecology, University of California at Irvine, UCI-AMI Centre for Reproductive Health, Garden Grove, California, USA

G H Barker FRCS MRCOG
Senior Clinical Medical Officer, Department of Obstetrics and Gynaecology, St George's Hospital, London, UK

S E Barton BSc MB BS MRCOG
Research Fellow in Gynaecology, Whittington Hospital, London, UK

Thomas F Baskett MB FRCS(Ed) FRCS(C) FRCOG
Professor of Obstetrics and Gynaecology, Dalhousie University, Halifax, Nova Scotia, Canada

Richard W Beard MD FRCOG
Professor and Head of the Department of Obstetrics and Gynaecology, St Mary's Hospital Medical School, London, UK

Diana Birch MB BS DCH MRCP MD
Director, 'Youth Support'; Principal Medical Officer, Camberwell Health Authority, London, UK

John Bonnar MA MD FRCOG
Professor and Head of Trinity College, Department of Obstetrics and Gynaecology, St James's Hospital, Dublin, Ireland

Mark I Boyd MD FRCS(C) FRCOG FACOG
Associate Professor, McGill University; Director of Gynecology, Royal Victoria Hospital, Montreal, Quebec, Canada

D J H Brock BA PhD MRCPath
Professor of Human Genetics, University of Edinburgh, Edinburgh, UK

Peter Bromwich MB ChB MRCOG
Medical Director, Midland Fertility Services, Little Aston Hospital, Sutton Coldfield, UK

Lex W Doyle MB BS FRACP
Senior Lecturer, Department of Obstetrics and Gynaecology, University of Melbourne, Melbourne, Australia

James Owen Drife MD FRCS(Ed) MRCOG
Senior Lecturer, Department of Obstetrics and Gynaecology, University of Leicester, Leicester, UK

David A Ellwood MA DPhil(Oxon), MRACOG
Senior Registrar, King George V Memorial Hospital for Mothers and Babies, Sydney, New South Wales, Australia

J R W Harris MB BCh DTM&H FRCP
Senior Consultant Physician, Department of Genito-urinary Medicine, St Mary's Hospital, London, UK

David James MA MD DCH MRCOG
Consultant Senior Lecturer in Feto-Maternal Medicine, Department of Obstetrics, University of Bristol, Bristol Maternity Hospital, Bristol, UK

William H Kitchen MD FRACP
First Assistant in Neonatal Paediatrics, Department of Obstetrics and Gynaecology, University of Melbourne, Melbourne, Australia

B Victor Lewis MD FRCS FRCOG
Consultant Obstetrician/Gynaecologist, District General Hospital, Watford, UK

M F Lowry MB ChB DCH FRCP
Sunderland District General Hospital; Clinical Lecturer in Child Health, University of Newcastle upon Tyne, Newcastle, UK

David Luesley MA MD MRCOG
Senior Lecturer and Honorary Consultant Obstetrician and Gynaecologist, University of Birmingham and Dudley Road Hospital, Birmingham, UK

Peter Milton MD(Lon) FRCOG
Consultant Gynaecologist, Cambridge Health District; Associate Lecturer, Cambridge University School of Clinical Medicine, Cambridge, UK

Camran Nezhat MD
Director, GYN Laser Workshop and Fertility and Endocrinology Center, Atlanta, Georgia, USA

N S Nicholas BSc MD MRCOG
Consultant in Obstetrics and Gynaecology, Hillingdon Hospital, Middlesex, UK

Kypios H Nicolaides BSc MRCOG
Senior Lecturer, Harris Birthright Research Centre for Fetal Medicine, Department of Obstetrics and Gynaecology, King's College Hospital, London UK

Michael C O'Connor MD DCH MRCOG FRACOG
Visiting Obstetrician and Gynaecologist, Drug and Alcohol Antenatal Clinic, King George V Memorial Hospital for Mothers and Babies, Sydney, New South Wales, Australia

Shirley Pearce PhD
Lecturer, Department of Psychology, University College London, London, UK

Roger J Pepperell MD FRCOG FRACOG

Dunbar Hooper Professor of Obstetrics and Gynaecology, University of Melbourne, Melbourne, Australia

Michael A Quinn MB ChB MGO MRCP MRCOG FRACOG

First Assistant, Department of Obstetrics and Gynaecology, University of Melbourne; Director, Oncology Unit, Royal Women's Hospital, Melbourne; Consultant Gynaecologist, Peter MacCallum Cancer Institute, Melbourne, Australia

Philip W Reginald MB BS MRCOG

Lecturer and Senior Registrar, Department of Obstetrics and Gynaecology, St Mary's Hospital Medical School, London, UK

Geoffrey D Reid MRACOG

Lecturer and Honorary Senior Registrar in Obstetrics and Gynaecology, University of Manchester, St Mary's Hospital, Manchester, UK

Brian L Sheppard MA MSc DPhil MRCPath

Associate Professor in Human Reproduction, Trinity College Department of Obstetrics and Gynaecology, Sir Patrick Dun Research Centre, St James's Hospital, Dublin, Ireland

Peter W Soothill BSc MB BS

Research Fellow, Harris Birthright Research Centre for Fetal Medicine, Department of Obstetrics and Gynaecology, King's College Hospital, London, UK

W P Soutter MD MSc MRCOG

Reader in Gynaecological Oncology, Institute of Obstetrics and Gynaecology, Royal Postgraduate Medical School, Hammersmith Hospital, London, UK

John A D Spencer BSc MB BS MRCOG

Senior Lecturer and Consultant, Royal Postgraduate Medical School, Institute of Obstetrics and Gynaecology, Queen Charlotte's Maternity Hospital, London, UK

Victor R Tindall MD MSc FRCS(Ed) FRCOG

Professor of Obstetrics and Gynaecology, University of Manchester, St Mary's Hospital, Manchester, UK

P C Wong MB BS (Malaya) MMed (OBGYN, Singapore) MRCOG FICS AM

Senior Lecturer and Consultant, Division of Reproductive Endocrinology, Department of Obstetrics & Gynaecology, National University of Singapore, Singapore

Contents

PART TWO: GYNAECOLOGY

Human fetal allograft survival

INTRODUCTION

The question of human fetal allograft survival and growth in a potentially hostile immunological environment constitutes the greatest paradox of all the laws of tissue transplantation. Rejection of foreign tissue by a host is known to be an immunological phenomenon, yet the human fetal allograft has the unique opportunity (under normal circumstances) to grow and develop for a limited period of time, prior to delivery. This perfect symbiotic relationship between mother and fetus has been alluded to as 'Nature's allograft' and an understanding of this phenomenon would be of prime importance to our understanding about cancer and transplantation immunology in general. One of the first pioneers in this field—Medawar (1953)—proposed some interesting explanations as to the success of Nature's allograft, some of which are shown in Table 1.1.

Table 1.1   Theories for the survival of the fetal allograft

Antigenic immaturity of the conceptus
Immunologically privileged uterine site
Placental barrier theory
Blocking antibodies
Altered maternal cellular immunity

Before discussing some of these theories further, a brief description of the components and function of the immune system is necessary.

IMMUNE SYSTEM

In recent years, important advances have been made due to new sophisticated methodology. Most of these discoveries have been carried out on inbred strains of mice and the results have been applied to humans. Care must be exercised in extrapolating results obtained in mice to humans.

The function of the immune system is to recognize and inactivate pathogenic organisms and their products. This relies upon the ability of the immune system to discriminate between 'self' and 'non-self' by detecting the presence of antigens on cell surfaces. Individual cells display self antigens which are genetically predetermined and unique to that individual. Hence, when cells are transferred from one genetically dissimilar individual into another, a rejection reaction occurs. Tissues transferred between individuals from the same species are referred to as 'allografts'. Genetically identical individuals, such as inbred strains of mice or uniovular twins, can thus accept grafts between each other freely. In man, the genes controlling antigens which provoke strong rejection reactions are situated on the short arm of chromosome 6 and are located within a region called the major histocompatibility complex (MHC). Within this complex are at least four major subregions or subloci called HLA-A, -B, -C and -D (also DR). Since these antigens were first isolated on leucocytes, they are also referred to as human leucocyte antigens (HLAs).

The products encoded by the HLA-A, -B, -C loci are known as class I MHC antigens, and the -D antigens are class II MHC antigens. At each locus there are many different alternative genes or alleles, which results in considerable genetic diversity or polymorphism. The HLA genotype of an individual consists of two haplotypes. A haplotype is a set of genes which occupy a given chromosome and which are inherited en bloc, one set from each parent.

The class I genes determine strong transplantation antigens by eliciting the development of cytotoxic T lymphocytes and then by serving as targets for T cell mediated cytolysis in allogeneic immune responses. Class I antigens are found on practically all cells of the body, especially on lymphoid organs. They are not detectable on erythrocytes. The normal physiological role of class I antigens may be in protection against viral infection.

Class II antigens have a restricted tissue distribution, being found on macrophages, activated T cells and B cells. T cells are apparently unable to recognize free conventional antigen and instead recognize antigen in the context of self MHC molecule, which is usually HLA-DR. Thus, if a tissue lacked class II MHC antigens, it would not be directly immunogenic to T lymphocytes, although it would act as a target for cytotoxic T cells, assuming class I antigens were expressed.

SOLUBLE FACTORS

Interleukin-1

Interleukin-1 (IL-1) is a macrophage-derived hormone-like factor having a molecular weight of 12–16 000. It is a genetically unrestricted and immunologically non-specific factor that is active at low concentrations. Resting monocytes or macrophages produce little IL-1, but when activated can be made to do so. IL-1 acts as an augmenting second signal.

Interleukin-2

Interleukin-2 (IL-2) is produced in response to IL-1 stimulating lymphocyte activation (Smith 1980). IL-2 is a lymphokine with a molecular weight of 15 000, and like IL-1 is genetically unrestricted and active at low concentration. IL-2 plays a key role in cellular and humoral T cell dependent immune responses by stimulating the clonal expansion of T cells by binding to specific receptors on their cell surface (Watson & Moschizuki 1980). It is thought that the IL-2 producing cell is a helper cell with the OKT4+ phenotype and that the responding cell bearing the IL-2 receptor is from a different group of cells, namely cytotoxic and suppressor cells having the OKT8+ phenotype.

Interferon-gamma (IFN-γ)

IFN-γ appears to play a key role in the cascade of lymphokines produced during an immune response. IFN-γ is produced during an immune response by antigen-specific T cells and probably also by natural killer (NK) cells recruited by IL-2. IFN-γ is a 20–25 KDa glycoprotein often seen as a 50 KDa dimer, and is coded for by a single gene on the long arm of chromosome 12 in man. IFN-γ enhances the expression of class II antigens on various cell types such as macrophages, Langerhans' cells, endothelial cells and tumour cells. The position of IFN-γ in the immunoregulatory pathway is different to that of IL-1 or IL-2. As an inducer of HLA-DR expression on antigen-presenting cells, it forms part of a positive feedback loop whereby activated T cells produce IFN-γ, thus inducing more HLA-DR and an augmented capacity to present antigen.

Little is known about the role of interferons in pregnancy, although they are thought to have immunoregulatory effects. Suppression of antibody activity and enhanced suppressor cell activity have been noted (Johnson et al 1977a,b). From both animal (Djeu et al 1979) and human studies (Santoli et al 1978) it now appears that NK cell function is promoted by interferons. Bizhan et al (1978) studied the production of endogenous interferons by T cells and found that in the first trimester there were elevated plasma levels and increased leucocyte interferon production, and that in the second trimester these levels dropped but rose again in the third trimester.

Clinical correlations between interferon production and disease susceptibility, such as cytomegalovirus (CMV) infection are only speculative. Stagno et al (1975) were able to show decreased susceptibility to CMV during the first part of pregnancy when interferon levels are greatest.

T cell activation and regulation

It appears that T cell proliferation occurs following a cascade of carefully orchestrated events. The resting T cell encounters a foreign antigen which it recognizes by its specific receptor structure in association with histocompatibility antigens on the antigen-presenting cell, i.e. the macrophage. In order to recognize both antigens, it is suggested that either the T lymphocyte has two receptors, one for foreign antigen and one for MHC-encoded self antigen (dual recognition theory), or that there is only one receptor on the T cell recognizing foreign antigen complexed to self antigen (modified self theory). Either model is difficult to prove or disprove. Within 6–12 hours the IL-2 receptor is expressed and has a high binding affinity to IL-2. In the second stage of the T cell response the same antigen stimulates the production of IL-2 predominantly by the T helper cell population. Since highly purified T lymphocytes free of macrophage contamination will respond to a T cell mitogen by expressing IL-2 receptors, but do not produce IL-2, it is generally assumed that macrophages or IL-1 are necessary for IL-2 production. Once IL-2 is produced it binds to the IL-2 receptor and DNA and cell mitosis occurs. In the absence of continued antigenic stimulation, there is re-expression of the surface T cell receptor and a reciprocal reduction of IL-2 receptors. This model of T cell proliferation was initially proposed by Meuer et al (1984). It does not necessarily follow that all T cells produce and respond to their own IL-2 (Fig. 1.1). In fact, failure of certain cells to proliferate to antigen

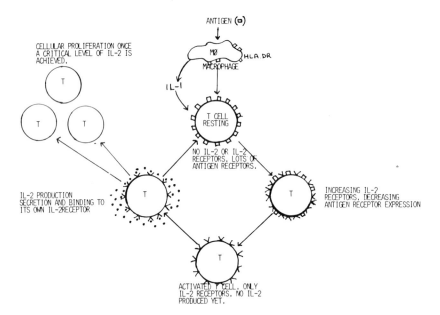

Fig. 1.1   Schematic representation of cellular activation

may occur as a result of their inability to produce sufficient IL-2, even though they may be triggered to express IL-2 receptors. The question of whether IL-2 receptor expression occurs on other cells, i.e. B and NK cells, has yet to be clearly answered. Certainly B cells taken from individuals with hairy cell leukaemias have been reported to express the receptor for IL-2 as defined by Tac antigen (Korsmeyer et al 1983).

FETAL ANTIGENICITY

The human conceptus is not antigenically immature for several reasons. The fertilized ovum is known to express both minor and major transplantation antigens very early on in embryogenesis (Seigler & Metzgar 1970). There is also strong evidence that the fetus plays an active role in its own protection by developing suppressor cells with functional activity by the eighth week of gestation (Unander & Olding 1981). Strong suppressor activity is one way that fetal lymphocytes are able to respond to the transplacental passage of maternal lymphocytes (Olding 1979). In vitro studies have shown that fetal lymphocytes can release soluble factors that inhibit both mixed lymphocyte reactivity and phytohaemagglutinin (PHA) response to adult lymphocytes (Olding et al 1977). Furthermore, as reported by Jacoby et al (1984), the identity of these factors is thought to be prostaglandins of the E series (namely PGE_1 and PGE_2 (Johnsen and Olding, unpublished observations).

PRIVILEGED UTERINE SITE

There are specialized sites in the body, such as the brain and anterior chamber of the eye, which display immunological privilege to transplanted tissues. The explanation is said to be due to the relative lack of lymphatic drainage in that region, thus delaying recognition of foreign antigen and subsequent attack (Billingham 1964). Current evidence indicates that the uterus is not immunologically privileged because it is adequately drained by pelvic and para-aortic lymph nodes (Park 1971). Tumour allograft transplanted into the uterine horn of pregnant, non-pregnant and pseudo-pregnant female rats are quickly rejected (Schlesinger 1962). Beer and Billingham (1974a) also demonstrated that allogeneic skin grafts, leucocytes or lymph node cells placed into the uterine lumen sensitized the host into rejecting a subsequent skin graft. There is evidence that decidualized tissue in the uterus may confer a weak protective effect on the efferent arc of the immune response, since skin allografts placed in the decidualized uterine bed survive for longer (Beer & Billingham 1974b), but the decidua alone are not sufficient to prevent rejection of intra-uterine grafts in presensitized hosts. Thus the uterus does not seem to be protected from participation in immune reactions.

PLACENTAL BARRIER THEORY

Since the placenta represents the interface between mother and fetus, the question of whether HLA antigen is expressed on the outermost layer, i.e. the syncytiotrophoblast, is very important. Numerous research groups claim that class I and II antigenic expression is normal (Loke et al 1971, Lawler et al 1974, Doughty & Gelsthorpe 1976), whilst others have not been able to demonstrate any MHC expression (Faulk et al 1977, Sundqvist et al 1977). Inevitably there are some (Goodfellow et al 1976), who have taken a middle-of-the-road view by demonstrating low levels of antigens on the placental surface. The overall evidence seems to suggest that HLA antigen expression is probably absent or sparse on the human syncytiotrophoblast. Therefore, the conceptus is not analogous to an allograft in the context of MHC expression across this barrier. There is evidence that class II MHC antigen expression by antigen-presenting cells is inhibited by factors in human retroplacental serum. The mechanism is thought to be mediated by a sugar–sugar interaction between the carbohydrate moiety of the DR antigen and the serum inhibitory factor, causing masking of DR antigen presentation and thus immune non-reactivity (Nicholas et al 1986). Although HLA expression is absent, the trophoblast does express other allo-antigenic systems. There are at least 50 proteins on the trophoblast surface, which makes the answer to the question as to which of these is immunologically relevant very difficult (Faulk & Johnston 1977). Faulk et al (1978) have used serologically defined antigens raised in rabbits to identify trophoblast-specific minor histocompatibility antigens named TA_1 and TA_2 from trophoblast cell cultures, which are collectively called the TLX system (trophoblast lymphocyte cross-reacting antigens). TA_1 antigens are shared by trophoblasts and human cultured cell lines (HeLa and human amnion cells), whilst TA_2 antigens are shared by placental blood vessel endothelium and peripheral monocytes. It is suggested that the gene(s) responsible for the production of TLX antigens is (are) situated on chromosome 1.

The hypothesis is that during normal human pregnancy the maternal immune system recognizes the TA_2 antigen by producing anti-TA_2 antibodies, and thus there is non-recognition of TA_1. If TA_2 is not recognized, this may lead to recognition of TA_1 and subsequent termination of pregnancy, or it may lead to abnormal pregnancy. In vitro studies by Faulk have shown that TA_2 and anti-TA_2 antibodies are able to inhibit the MLR (mixed lymphocyte reaction) of maternal lymphocytes and allogeneic stimulator cells. In addition, these antibodies are both trophoblast- and species-specific (Faulk et al 1978). Faulk and McIntyre (1985) further suggest that sharing of TLX antigens between couples may lead to failed pregnancy, thus having similar functions to the transplantation antigens. Natural selection would favour HLA–TLX incompatible mating, thus perpetuating genetic diversity among the species.

SERUM BLOCKING FACTORS

Hellstrom et al (1969) described a shielding role for blocking antibodies in protecting antigenic tumour cells from sensitized lymphoid cells of the host. Similarly, anti-paternal antibodies may serve as blocking factors by binding to the placental trophoblast, thereby protecting the fetus from maternal cellular attack.

Chaouat et al (1979) have been able to elute these antibodies that could enhance the growth of tumour allografts of the paternal strain from the placenta (Fig. 1.2). These antibodies have been characterized as IgG, based on

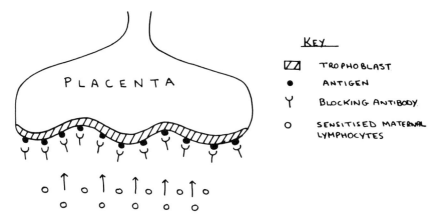

KEY

▨	TROPHOBLAST
●	ANTIGEN
Y	BLOCKING ANTIBODY
O	SENSITISED MATERNAL LYMPHOCYTES

Fig. 1.2 Possible mechanisms of trophoblast (fetal) survival

their electrophoretic mobility and their removal of inhibitory activity after passage of maternal sera over an anti-IgG affinity column (Rocklin et al 1976). Furthermore, absorption of these antibodies in maternal sera by paternal cells, and not pooled human platelets, suggests that they are directed mainly against class II MHC products of fetal tissues (Rocklin et al 1979). Women who recurrently abort have been shown to share HLA identity with their partners more commonly than would be expected (Rocklin et al 1976, Taylor & Faulk 1981). As a result of this tissue compatibility between mother and fetus, these women do not produce blocking antibodies (Stimson et al 1979). There is, however, evidence against this hypothesis, namely (1) anti-HLA-DR antibodies are not detectable in all normal pregnancies, and when they are found they occur late in pregnancy (Terasaki et al 1970), (2) it is difficult to reconcile how anti-HLA-DR antibodies can have such influence in early pregnancy when HLA-DR antigens are not expressed on placental tissues at that time (Faulk & Temple 1976), and (3) agammaglobulinaemic females have been reported to have normal pregnancies (Holland & Holland 1966).

MATERNAL IMMUNOCOMPETENCE

The in vivo evidence for depressed maternal cell-mediated immunity is by no means accepted (Table 1.2). It has been suggested that the incidence of certain bacterial and viral infections is increased during pregnancy. The balance of evidence suggests, however, that this is not the case. Siegel and Greenberg (1955) showed an increased incidence of poliomyelitis attributable

Table 1.2   In vivo evidence for depressed cell-mediated immunity in pregnancy

Depressed skin reactivity to tuberculin
Delayed skin graft rejection
Increased susceptibility to certain bacterial and viral infections including:
  herpes simplex
  rubella
  influenza
  poliomyelitis
  smallpox
Remission of rheumatoid arthritis

to parity and an associated increase in exposure, but decreased mortality. Similarly, the increased incidence of hepatitis in Bombay (D'Cruz et al 1968) was associated with severe anaemia and malnutrition in pregnant women. Purtilo (1975), investigating deaths from fungal infections in pregnancy, revealed that immunosuppression in these women was due to other clinical conditions and treatment, with the exception of coccidiomycosis. There does appear to be some increased risk in pregnancy of the dissemination of *Coccidioides immitis* (Purtilo 1975) and malaria (Van Zon & Eling 1980). Anergy to tuberculin skin testing has been reported in tuberculosis patients who subsequently became pregnant. Lichtenstein (1942) found evidence of anergy in 82 patients tested, as opposed to Finn et al (1972) who found no difference. His study did not, however, take into account the problems of difference in history of antigenic exposure (Jenkins & Scott 1972). Better studies were conducted by Montgomery et al (1968) and Comstock (1975), in which patients were followed longitudinally, thus acting as their own controls. The results of these two studies showed no indication of anergy to PPD (purified protein derivative) in pregnancy.

Pregnancy undoubtedly modifies the maternal immune system. However, systemic immunosuppression is an unlikely event since this would seriously jeopardize the mother's ability to resist life-threatening infections at a time when her defences should be least vulnerable. Consequently, non-specific local immunosuppression may be the cause of non-rejection, i.e. factor(s) acting at the feto-maternal interface.

PREGNANCY AND IL-2 METABOLISM

Work by Malkovsky and Medawar (1984) has shown that tolerance to antigens may arise because of either a lack of production or responsiveness to IL-2 by immune effector cells. In this context, Nicholas et al (1984) demonstrated decreased IL-2 production by factor(s) in human pregnancy serum when tested in the mixed lymphocyte reaction. Inhibitory activity was shown to correlate with increasing gestation and parity. Further studies have shown that these factors are produced at the fetomaternal interface, since IL-2 production was inhibited by all retroplacental blood sera, whilst only a few of the corresponding peripheral blood sera showed this effect (Nicholas & Panayi 1985).

IMMUNOSUPPRESSIVE AGENTS

Numerous protein and steroid hormones are elaborated during pregnancy, some of which are illustrated in Table 3. Some of these will be dealt with in further detail.

Table 1.3 Potential immunosuppressive agents in pregnancy

Proteins
　　Alphafetoprotein
　　Human chorionic gonadotrophin
　　Pregnancy-associated α2-glycoprotein
　　Early pregnancy factor
　　Human placental lactogen
　　Pregnancy-specific β1-glycoprotein

Steroids
　　Oestrogens
　　Progestogens
　　Cortisol

Antibodies
　　Blocking antibodies
　　Immune complexes

Human chorionic gonadotrophin (HCG)

HCG is produced by the syncytiotrophoblast and appears early in pregnancy, i.e. by about 8 days post-fertilization. It reaches a peak by 60 days after ovulation and is then followed by a fall by 80 days. The role of HCG is said to be luteotrophic, i.e. to maintain the corpus luteum which in turn produces other essential hormones necessary to maintain pregnancy; the corpus luteum then gives way to the placenta once it is formed. A number of groups have reported that HCG suppresses mitogen-induced blast transformation when added to adult male lymphocytes in vitro (Kaye & Jones 1971, Adcock et al 1973). These results were subsequently confirmed by others (Contractor & Davies 1973, Tomoda et al 1976). Similarly, mixed lymphocyte culture inhibition has been shown to occur when HCG was added in vitro to cultures (Jenkins et al 1972, Teasdale et al 1973).

However, all these studies have been carried out with commercially partially purified preparations. Caldwell et al (1975) observed immunosuppressive activity in mitogen-induced blast transformation using crude HCG preparations, but when HCG was purified it failed to show any immunosuppressive effects. Gunder et al (1975) obtained similar results. The in vitro phenomena exhibited by HCG have been suggested by Powell (1974) to be due to binding of HCG to phytohaemagglutinin (PHA). PHA has a natural propensity to combine with glycoproteins of which HCG has about a 31% carbohydrate moiety, and the glycoprotein nature of HCG may depress PHA stimulatory capacity on lymphocytes by neutralizing the mitogen rather than by competitive inhibition of surface receptor sites. The data then indicate that contaminating factors other than HCG are probably responsible for most of the immunosuppressive activity observed. Morse (1976) showed that these substances elute in the region of molecular weight 20–40 000, so that they are unlikely to be other steroid hormones such as oestrogen and progesterone unless they are bound to other heavier substances.

Sex steroids

There have been many conflicting reports on the effects of sex steroids, oestrogen and progestogens on immunological responses, both in adults and pregnancy (Siiteri et al 1977). Poskitt et al (1977) showed that high levels of progesterone were needed to affect the response of lymphocytes to PHA or pokeweed mitogen. Little effect was seen when pharmacological concentrations of progesterone were added to the cultures. Later, Mori et al (1977) demonstrated that progesterone at concentrations of 10^{-3}–10^{-4} per millilitre inhibited the uptake of tritiated thymidine by lymphocytes from non-pregnant women following PHA stimulation. Under these same conditions, oestrogens had no effect. Although the concentrations of progesterone are too high as compared with normal circulating levels in the peripheral blood, these levels are compatible with those found at the placental site. Clemens et al (1979) suggested that if the in vitro findings of progesterone are valid in vivo, then high concentrations of progesterone could produce a local immunosuppressive effect on maternal lymphocyte immunoreactivity, without any undue systemic effects.

Vitamin D

The relevance of 1,25-dihydroxyvitamin D_3 in mineral and skeletal metabolism is well known. Evidence demonstrating the presence of receptors for this hormone in tissues not generally regarded as being of importance in mineral metabolism has implied perhaps another biological role (Franceschi et al 1981). Rigby et al (1984) demonstrated the potent inhibitory effect of vitamin D_3 in PHA-induced lymphocyte proliferation. They showed that thymidine uptake was inhibited by 70% with concentrations of 10^{-7} mol/l vitamin D_3 (physiological levels) after 72 hours of culture. Moreover, this effect was shown to occur as a consequence of the inhibition of IL-2 production, which could be partially reversed by the re-addition of purified IL-2. Tsoukas et al (1984) confirmed these findings and concluded that the immunoregulatory effects of vitamin D_3 may be because: (1) vitamin D_3 may exert its effect directly on IL-2 by inhibiting its production or secretion or both; (2) vitamin D_3 may increase the 'consumption' of IL-2 by T cells with IL-2 receptors because of the changes in IL-2 receptor concentration; or (3) vitamin D_3 may promote the differentiation of suppressor lymphocytes, thus causing inhibition of IL-2 production. Vitamin D_3 is synthesized by successive hydroxylation of vitamin D in the liver and kidney. There is also good evidence to show that synthesis of the active metabolite, vitamin D_3, occurs in the placental region (Gray et al 1979, Weisman et al 1979). The relevance of this finding may be to indicate the local immunosuppression at the fetomaternal interface. There is also evidence that vitamin D_3 can induce the expression of class I and II HLA antigens on human macrophage cell lines, probably by inducing new RNA synthesis (Ball et al 1984).

Adrenal corticosteroids

Corticosteroids are produced mainly by the adrenal cortex, although the placenta also produces a small amount. Recent work has shown that both total and free plasma cortisol levels are increased during pregnancy (Nolten & Rueckert 1981), and that maternal tissues are exposed to levels of biologically active plasma-free cortisol which are approximately twice those found in the non-pregnant state. Initially, Kasakura (1971) postulated that cortisol was responsible for inhibiting the allogeneic MLR. Then, in 1973, Kasakura, analysing individual cases of plasma cortisol and inhibitory activity on the MLR, found no correlation to support his initial hypothesis. Tomoda et al (1976) showed a marked reduction in PHA transformation when steroids were added to the cultures. Hydrocortisone produced 45% suppression with levels of 400 $\mu g/ml$. Ramer and Yu (1978) were able to reduce Con-A stimulation of human lymphocytes by 70% using levels of methylprednisolone of 5×10^{-5} mmol/l. Interestingly, lymphocytes that had been pre-stimulated with PHA could not be suppressed subsequently, even with supra-optimal concentrations of corticosteroids (Ramer & Yu 1978). Glucocorticosteroids have anti-inflammatory and immunosuppressive effects, and the levels achieved during pregnancy may be responsible for remission of rheumatoid arthritis (RA) during pregnancy in a high proportion of cases (Persellin 1977). Unfortunately, not all patients who experience remission of disease activity in pregnancy have elevated cortisol levels, and some subjects having no change in RA activity actually have increased cortisol levels (Persellin 1977). Thus, it does not appear that increased cortisol levels in pregnancy are totally responsible for the remission of diseases like RA or fetal allograft tolerance.

Prostaglandins

Prostaglandins are derivatives of arachidonic acid and have immunological activity. They are produced by trophoblast cells, fetal adrenal glands (Mitchell et al 1982), lymphocytes and macrophages (Johnsen et al 1982). In adults, monocytes are the main source of prostaglandins. PGE_2 is the major species having immunosuppressive action. When added to cultures of T lymphocytes, it suppresses PHA and Con-A-induced proliferation (Goodwin et al 1978) and also suppresses lymphocyte cytotoxicity in the MLR (Darrow & Tomar 1980). PGE_2 is also synthesized by human fetal leucocytes at concentrations known to be immunosuppressive for adult human lymphocytes in vitro (Johnsen et al 1983a,b). Prostaglandins E_2 (PGE$_2$) and possibly PGF$_{2\alpha}$ mediate the decidual response (Peleg 1983, Kennedy 1985). PGF$_{2\alpha}$ stimulates natural killer cell activity, whilst PGE$_2$ is inhibitory (Szekeres-Bartho et al 1985a), and the balance between PGF$_{2\alpha}$ and PGE$_2$ has been shown to correlate with the ratio of oestrogen to progesterone, thus implying that prostaglandins may mediate some of the immunoregulatory effects of gestational hormones (Szekeres-Bartho et al 1985b). Furthermore, progesterone-treated lymphocytes release a 34 KDa soluble factor that inhibits PGF$_{2\alpha}$ production, thus allowing PGE$_2$ effects to become more prominent, i.e. they inhibit maternal T cell responses. The immunosuppressive effects of PGE$_2$ have been shown to be due to the inhibition of IL-2 production and the down-regulation of transferrin receptors (Chouaib et al 1985). Chouaib et al (1985) also showed that PGE$_2$ had no effect on IL-2 receptor expression. The degradation and turnover of PGE$_2$ is very rapid and thus suggests that prostaglandins act locally at the placenta, but have little or no effect in the maternal peripheral circulation.

Alphafetoprotein

Alphafetoprotein (AFP) is a major fetal protein initially produced by the yolk sac, then by the embryonal liver cells. The function of AFP is not known but it does have certain similarities to albumin, including a molecular weight of 64 000 (Nishi 1970), an amino acid composition similar to albumin, and the ability to bind oestrogens but not testosterone (Uriel et al 1972). AFP may have an immunosuppressive role (Murgita & Tomasi 1975, Murgita et al 1977); in particular it has been found to suppress in vitro mitogenic stimulation by Con-A and lipopolysaccharide (LPS), as well as inhibit the MLR (Yachnin & Lester 1976). The exact mechanism of immunosuppression by human AFP is not known, although Murgita et al (1977) have suggested that AFP induces the production of suppressor T cells, which alter T cell but not B cell function. Studies in mice indicate that murine AFP binds to the surface of murine T cells. For maximum effect AFP must be present at the start of interaction of lymphocytes with mitogen. Perhaps the long incubation time needed with AFP is to generate suppressor T cells which then control the level of responsiveness to T cell dependent antigens (Murgita et al 1977).

Recently, Nicholas and Panayi (1986) found no correlation between the serum concentrations of pregnancy-specific β1-glycoprotein, PAPP-A and pregnancy-associated α2-glycoprotein on retroplacental or peripheral blood sera and their abilities to inhibit the MLR. There was a negative correlation when serum AFP was analysed. Some possible explanations for discrepancies in the in vitro results may include the following: that AFP acquires its immunosuppressive effect during its isolation by physicochemical procedures which alter the sialic acid content of the protein (Lester et al 1977), or alternatively that AFP acts as a carrier protein, binding other cofactors or hormones such as prostaglandins, polyamines or free fatty acids, and thus conferring immunosuppressive activity on the molecule (Grosse & Belanger 1980).

Given that the in vitro results are ambiguous, it is even more difficult to accept an immunosuppressive role for AFP in fetomaternal interactions, since the human fetus with high AFP is not immunosuppressed and it can respond to antigenic stimulation early on in its development (Silverstein 1972). Patients with certain pathological conditions with raised serum AFP levels, i.e. hepatoma, tyrosinaemias and ataxia telangiectasia, are not immunosuppressed, and their lymphocytes show a normal response to PHA stimulation (Beldanger et al 1974). AFP may play a cardinal role in the immunological development of the neonate. HLA-DR expression on macrophages is said to be suppressed by AFP (Lu et al 1984), which would thus affect antigen presentation during this crucial period when acquisition of tolerance to self proteins is more advantageous, even at the risk of decreased immunosuppression. The role of AFP is still unresolved.

PAPP-A

Lin et al (1974) first isolated PAPP-A in 1974 as one of a group of pregnancy proteins present in the syncytiotrophoblast. It is also found in pregnancy plasma and endometrium, and the levels increase as pregnancy advances (50–4000 μg/ml). It peaks at delivery and has a short half-life of 55–73 hours. It is a glycoprotein with a molecular weight of 800 000, it has α_2 electrophoretic mobility (Bischof 1979), it binds heparin, and it will inhibit complement-mediated lysis, plasmin and urokinase activity.

The biological function of PAPP-A is still unanswered (Smart 1984). Since it is a placental product, one guess as to its role in vivo is to play a role in the immunological interactions between mother and fetus, thus preventing fetal allograft rejection. Both Bischof and Lin have independently demonstrated in vitro immunosuppressive activity of PAPP-A. Bischof showed that PAPP-A, either alone or in the presence of human serum (pregnancy or non-pregnancy), significantly inhibited PHA-induced lymphocyte transformation, and postulated that PAPP-A depressed cellular immunity by affecting the activity or production of lymphokines (Bischof et al 1982). McIntyre et al (1981), however, challenged these findings when they were unable to confirm Bischof's and Lin's findings. The evidence to date points to PAPP-A being a placental protein that inhibits complement fixation (Bischof 1981) and is bound to the fibrin overlying the chorionic villi (McIntyre et al 1981). PAPP-A may thus have a local immunosuppressive role by helping to maintain the defensive fibrin barrier between the trophoblast and maternal immunoreactive cells.

Pregnancy-associated $\alpha2$-glycoprotein ($\alpha2$-PAG)

$\alpha2$-PAG is a glycoprotein with a molecular weight ranging from 300 to 506 000. The reason for the variation in molecular weight may be explained either by molecular asymmetry (Stimson & Farquharson 1978) or by heterogeneity within the molecule (Towler & Horne 1977).

Levels of α2-PAG are usually greater in females than in males (Von Schoultz 1974), but more striking levels are noted in pregnancy. Maximum concentrations of α2-PAG occur around the twenty-fourth week of gestation (10–3000 μg/ml) (Wurz et al 1980) and thereafter plateau until 34–35 weeks, when levels start to fall (Straube et al 1980). About 10% of pregnant patients do not produce detectable amounts of α2-PAG (Von Schoultz 1974) although this bears no relation to fetal well-being (Beckman et al 1974). Post-delivery levels fall rapidly and by 6 weeks post-partum levels are equivalent to those of the pre-pregnant state (Stimson 1975).

However, several groups report elevated levels of α2-PAG until 3–6 months post partum (Stimson 1975, Lin et al 1976, Towler et al 1976). α2-PAG production is increased in vitro by oestrogens alone (Berne 1973), which agrees with the observation that women on the combined oestrogen–progesterone contraceptive pill have higher levels of the glycoprotein.

α2-PAG is said to have immunosuppressive activity in vitro as assessed by impairment of lymphocyte proliferation in response to plant mitogens (Von Schoultz et al 1973), antigens (Damber et al 1975) or allogeneic cells (Stimson 1976). Stimson (1980) artificially prepared a pregnancy 'super serum' containing high levels of pregnancy proteins to which immunosuppressive properties have been ascribed. These were HPL, SP1, AFP, α2-PAG and HCG. He then showed that, following sequential removal of the proteins individually by affinity chromatography, removal of α2-PAG reduced the suppressive effect of the serum on PHA and mixed lymphocyte responses.

α2-PAG expression on the surface of leucocytes is linked to that of HLA-DR antigens (Thomson et al 1979a). It has been postulated that α2-PAG may interfere with the expression of HLA-DR antigens on macrophages during gestation, and this could thus lead to maternal unresponsiveness towards the fetus. Thus, low α2-PAG levels in the plasma may result in inadequate suppression of cellular activation. In this context, several groups have found an association between low levels of α2-PAG in the first trimester of pregnancy and an increased risk of spontaneous abortion (Berne 1974, Thomson et al 1979b, Wurz et al 1980).

Pregnancy-specific β1-glycoprotein (SP1β)

Pregnancy-specific β1-glycoprotein (SP1β) is normally synthesized by the placenta and was first described in 1971 by Bohn. The serum concentration is high, relative to other pregnancy-specific proteins, ranging from 200 to 400 mg/l at term (Towler et al 1977a,b). It has aroused much attention because SP1 has been found in patients with trophoblast disease and other malignancies. The protein exists in two forms based on electrophoretic mobilities, and is thus referred to as SP1α and SP1β. The molecular weight of the alpha form is about 430 000 with a 29% carbohydrate content, whereas the beta form has a low molecular weight of 90–100 000 with the same carbohydrate content. Horne et al (1976) investigated the immunosuppressive activities of SP1 by demonstrating 75% inhibition of PHA-induced blast transformation at a concentration of 250 mg/l. There was no effect on the Con-A response. In another study Cerni et al (1977) found a smaller decrease in PHA responsiveness which was not dose-related. Johannsen et al (1976), using the mixed lymphocyte reaction, demonstrated that the 50% inhibition point occurred at a SP1 concentration of 1000 mg/l, which is well outside the physiological range.

On balance therefore it appears that SP1 is not inhibitory and that the maternal serum does not contain enough of the protein to be immunosuppressive in vivo.

MATERNAL HUMORAL-IMMUNITY

Immunoglobulin levels do not alter very markedly during pregnancy. IgG levels have been shown to fall by about 20% in pregnancy, being lowest in the third trimester (Amino et al 1978). The levels of IgA, IgE and IgM were found to be constant during pregnancy. IgD levels increase significantly to term, from 30 mg/l in the first and second trimester and in non-pregnant women to 85 mg/l at term (Studd 1971, Gusdon & Prichard 1972).

The estimation of immunoglobulin levels in absolute terms is of doubtful significance. Whether these antibodies are reduced in the circulation by being absorbed and sequestered by the placenta, or whether they are truly altered by pregnancy, remains to be clarified.

Undoubtedly, some pregnant women do develop anti-paternal allo-antibodies (anti-HLA) during pregnancy (Youtananukorn et al 1974, Winchester et al 1975), but there is considerable speculation as to their significance. Voisin (1984) suggests that these are protective antibodies, thus blocking any harmful immune response against the fetus. The presence of these antibodies poses a dilemma because if they are HLA antibodies, against what are they directed? The placental syncytiotrophoblast does not express MHC antigens. Herzenberg et al (1979), using a fluorescence-activated cell sorter and antibodies directed against paternal antigens absent in the mother which were used to detect the transplacental passage of fetal lymphocytes into the maternal circulation, found that fetal cells do not regularly cross into the maternal circulation during normal pregnancy. Furthermore, the mere fact that these antibodies are not found in all pregnancies makes it difficult to put forward any argument for their protective immune function.

CELL-MEDIATED IMMUNITY DURING PREGNANCY

In vitro evidence

The in vitro evidence for altered maternal cell-mediated immunity (CMI) is shown in Table 1.4. There is considerable disagreement between research

Table 1.4   In vitro evidence for diminished T lymphocyte responses

Reduced blast transformation following stimulation with plant mitogens and purified protein
 derivative
Depressed mixed lymphocyte responses
Altered T : B cell ratio
Increased T suppressor cell production

groups with the data obtained from in vitro tests of CMI. The reasons for
this are probably due to a combination of differences in types of media used,
cell culture techniques, reagents used and the subtle differences in methodology between laboratories. Furthermore, the results on in vitro tests need
not necessarily be a true reflection of events occurring in vivo. With this
in mind, I will elaborate on some of the in vivo findings in pregnancy and
try to explain the probable in vitro relevance.

Mixed lymphocyte reaction (MLR)

The MLR is an antigen-driven system used as an in vitro correlate of CMI.
It relies on the inherent ability of lymphocytes from two genetically different
individuals to be stimulated by each other when co-cultured. It is used either
as a two-way MLR when there is no need to discriminate between reactive
lymphocytes, or in a one-way MLR where the maternal cells are responders
and fetal cells are irradiated, thus acting as stimulators. The more genetically
diverse the lymphocytes are from each other when co-cultured, the greater
is the degree of cellular proliferation. In the same way the fetus and its mother
should, by virtue of their intimate anatomical relationship, initiate an in vivo
MLR, assuming that the integrity of their immune system is functional.
Using a unidirectional MLR system, many groups have demonstrated a
depressed response between maternal/paternal or maternal/fetal lymphocytes
when compared with unrelated individuals (Lewis et al 1966, Ceppellini et
al 1971, Kasakura 1971, Jenkins & Hancock 1972, Bonnard & Lemos 1972).
In addition to maternal lymphocytes being poor responders, they are also
poor stimulators to related cord blood lymphocytes (Ceppellini et al 1971).
This reciprocal hyporeactivity may be a reflection of maternal tolerance that
occurs as a result of the bi-directional passage of cells/antigens across the
placenta. Jenkins and Hancock (1972) showed that depression of the MLR
was more marked with increasing parity. Gatti et al (1973) implied that serum
factors were responsible for MLR inhibition by showing a depressed response
of maternal lymphocytes to husband, child and unrelated donor lymphocytes
in the presence of maternal serum. Curzen et al (1972) found that maternal
sera could non-specifically inhibit the MLR between unrelated pairs. Inhibition was more consistently found in late pregnancy sera than in early pregnancy sera. The ability to inhibit the MLR can be explained by the presence

of HLA-DR antibodies in pregnancy sera probably acting by masking the HLA-DR antigens on the antigen-presenting cells (Abrechtsen et al 1977). The overall evidence suggests that the intrinsic reactivity of maternal/fetal lymphocytes is essentially normal but that the observations of inhibition of the MLR occur as a result of non-specific immunosuppressive factor(s) present in the serum of either mother and/or fetus.

Lymphocyte populations in pregnancy

If CMI is altered in vivo, then there may be a change in lymphocyte populations in the systemic circulation during pregnancy. Although the total number of lymphocytes in the peripheral blood is not significantly altered (Strelkauskas et al 1975, Dodson et al 1977), a number of studies have looked for differences in T : B cell ratios. Several groups found no difference in the numbers of T and B cells between pregnant and non-pregnant individuals (Birkeland & Kristoffersen 1977, Dodson et al 1977, Birkeland et al 1979). Strelkauskas et al (1975) reported an inversion of the percentage of T and B cells during early pregnancy, such that the B cells rose to 70% and the T cells dropped to 25%, whilst the total lymphocyte count remained unchanged. Maximal changes occurred at about the tenth week and returned to normal ratios by the twenty-second week of gestation. Using a fluorescence-activated cell sorter, the same authors (1978) were able to confirm their initial findings of B and T cell inversion, with T cells decreasing to about 30% and B cells rising to 45–60%. These findings suggest that there is an absolute reduction in T cells with a corresponding increase in B cells, since the total number of lymphocytes remains constant. The depression in T lymphocytes could be due to suppressor cell reduction, and the B cell rise could assist fetal allograft acceptance by producing blocking antibodies.

The development of monoclonal antibodies has made it possible to characterize subpopulations of T lymphocytes in maternal blood and also to define differences in functional activities between T cell subsets. The monoclonal OKT3 recognizes >90% of adult peripheral T lymphocytes; OKT4 recognizes helper cells and comprises 50–60% of adult peripheral T cells; OKT8 recognizes the suppressor/cytotoxic T cells (Reinherz & Schlossman 1980). The levels of OKT3+ lymphocytes in the peripheral blood taken at term are similar to those in non-pregnant adults (69.0 and 71.5% respectively). There appears to be a slightly higher population of OKT4+ (helper) lymphocytes (48.5% and 41% respectively) and no difference in OKT8+ lymphocytes (31.0 and 29.5% respectively) (Jacoby & Oldstone 1983).

However, Coulam et al (1983), looking at T lymphocyte subsets in the peripheral blood of 31 pregnant women at various stages in pregnancy, found no change in percentages when compared with women on the combined oral contraceptive pill or women menstruating spontaneously. There is also evidence of heterogeneity even within T4/T8 lymphocyte subsets, such that there are both helper and suppressor cell inducer activities within each subpopulation (Reinherz et al 1982). Further experiments are needed to define their functional role in fetomaternal immune interactions.

FUTURE APPLICATIONS

Since the fetus resembles in many respects a malignant tumour which for a limited period of time evades rejection in an immunocompetent host, our understanding of the mechanisms involved in the maintenance of this symbiotic relationship should provide useful insights into the problems confronting tumour immunologists and the physiological methods that might be used to overcome the problems of organ transplantation. On a more clinical level, some immunological dysfunction may be instrumental in the aetiopathogenesis of certain clinical conditions, which include male and female infertility, recurrent spontaneous abortion, pre-eclampsia, abruptio placentae, trophoblastic disease and intra-uterine growth retardation. Also, isolation of these immunoactive serum factor(s) could result in their chemical biosynthesis and use as therapeutic agents in the treatment of rheumatoid arthritis, a condition known to improve in the vast majority of cases in pregnancy. The development of monoclonal antibodies and their application has increased dramatically over the last 5 years. This technique also provides an opportunity to look at cell surface structures and receptor sites that control the production of lymphokines. DNA probes will also enable the genetic basis of abnormal lymphokines, abnormalities in receptor sites and the control of lymphokine production to be investigated in a variety of diseases. All the pieces of the jigsaw must be found if we are to embark on therapeutic measures for some of the conditions mentioned above. Premature enthusiasm in treatment may actually do more harm than the good initially intended. For example, the deliberate immunization with paternal leucocytes of women who recurrently abort in an attempt to stimulate a blocking antibody response may actually act as a means of transmission of pathogenic viruses, i.e. the transmission of the Human Immunodeficiency Virus (HIV-III). Finally, a better understanding of reproductive immunology would assist us in using immunological manipulations in order to produce safe, effective and reversible methods of male and female contraception.

REFERENCES

Abrechtsen D, Solheim B G, Thorsey E 1977 Antiserum inhibition of the mixed lymphocyte culture (MLC) interaction. Inhibitory effect of antibodies reactive with HLA-D associated determinants. Cellular Immunology 28: 258–273
Adcock E W, Teasdale T, August C S et al 1973 Human chorionic gonadotrophin: its possible role in maternal lymphocyte suppression. Science 181: 845–847
Amino N, Tanizawa O, Miyai K et al 1978 Changes of serum immunoglobulins IgG, IgM and IgE during pregnancy. Obstetrics and Gynecology 52: 415–420

Ball E D, Guyre P B, Glynn J M, Rigby W F C, Fanger M W 1984 Modulation of Class I HLA antigens on HL-60 promyelocytic leukemic cells by serum-free medium: re-induction by gamma IFN and 1,25-dihydroxyvitamin D3 (calcitriol). Journal of Immunology 132: 2424–2428

Beckman G, Von Schoultz Z B, Stigbrand T 1974 The 'pregnancy zone' protein and fetal welfare. Acta Obstetricia et Gynecologica Scandinavica 53: 59–61

Beer A E, Billingham R E 1974a Host responses to intra-uterine tissue, cellular and fetal allografts. Journal of Reproduction and Fertility 21: 59–88

Beer A E, Billingham R E 1974b The embryo as a transplant. Scientific American 230: 36–46

Beldanger L, Warthe W I, Daguillard F, Larochelle J, Dufeur D 1974 Etude in vitro de l'esset de l'afp sur la reponse lymphocytaire. In: Masseyeff R (ed) L'Alpha-foetoproteine, pp 423–430. INSERM, Paris

Berne B H 1973 Alpha-2 pregnoglobulin—a pregnancy-associated macroglobulin elevated by oestrogen and oral contraceptive administration. IRCS Medical Science 1: 26 (abstract)

Berne B H 1974 Alpha-2 pregnoglobulin levels, a test of placental function in early pregnancy. Federation Proceedings 33: 290 (abstract)

Billingham R E 1964 Transplantation immunity and the maternal–fetal relation. New England Journal of Medicine 270: 667–672

Birkeland S A, Kristoffersen K 1977 Cellular immunity in pregnancy: blast transformation and rosette formation of maternal T and B lymphocytes. A cross-sectional analysis. Clinical and Experimental Immunology 30: 408–412

Birkeland S. A, Teisner B, Schilling W, Kemp E, Pedersen G T, Svehag S E 1979 Effect of pregnancy zone protein on leucocyte migration inhibition, lymphocyte transformation and rosette formation by lymphocytes. Acta Pathologica et Microbiologica Scandinavica (C) 87: 235–240

Bischof P 1979 Observations on the isolation of PAPP-A. In: Klopper A, Chard T (eds) Placental proteins, Springer-Verlag, New York, pp 105–118

Bischof P 1981 Pregnancy-associated plasma protein-A: an inhibitor of the complement system. Placenta 2: 29–34

Bischof P, Lauber K, De Wurstemberger B, Girrard J P 1982 Inhibition of lymphocyte transformation by pregnancy-associated plasma proteins. Journal of Clinical and Laboratory Immunology 7: 61–65

Bizhan U I, Schelykalina L A, Stoyanov N G 1978 Interferonogenesis in healthy non-pregnant women and in the physiologiical course of pregnancy. Akusherstvo I Ginekologiia (Moskva) 2: 17–20

Bohn H 1971 Detection and characterization of pregnancy proteins in the human placenta and their quantitative immunochemical determination in sera from pregnant women. Archives of Gynecology 210: 440–457

Bonnard G D, Lemos L 1972 The cellular immunity of mother versus child at delivery: sensitisation in unidirectional mixed lymphocyte culture and subsequent [13]Cr-release cytotoxicity test. Transplantation Proceedings 4: 177–180

Caldwell J L, Stites D P, Fudenberg H H 1975 Human chorionic gonadotrophin: effects of crude and purified preparations on lymphocyte responses to phytohaemagglutinin and allogeneic stimulation. Journal of Immunology 155: 1249–1253

Ceppellini R, Bonnard G D, Coppo F et al 1971 Mixed lymphocyte cultures and HLA antigens: 1. Reactivity of young fetuses, newborns and mothers at delivery. Transplantation Proceedings 3: 58–63

Cerni C, Tatra G, Bohn H 1977 Immunosuppression by human placental lactogen (HPL) and the pregnancy-specific beta 1-glycoprotein (SP-1). Inhibition of mitogen-induced lymphocyte transformation. Archives of Gynecology 223: 1–7

Chaouat G, Voisin G A, Escalier D, Robert P 1979 Facilitation reaction (enhancing antibodies and suppressor cells) and rejection reaction (sensitized cells) from the mother to the paternal antigens of the conceptus. Clinical and Experimental Immunology 35: 13–24

Chouaib S, Welte K, Mertelsmann R, Dupont B 1985 Prostaglandin E2 acts at two distinct pathways of T cell activation. Inhibition of interleukin-2 production and down-regulation of transferrin receptor expression. Journal of Immunology 135: 1172–1179

Clemens L E, Siiteri P K Stites D P 1979 Mechanism of immunosuppression of progesterone on maternal lymphocyte activation during pregnancy. Journal of Immunology 122: 1978–1985

Comstock G W 1975 Tuberculin sensitivity in pregnancy. American Review of Respiratory Disease 112: 413–416

Contractor S F, Davies H 1973 Effect of human chorionic gonadotrophin on phytohaemagglutinin induced lymphocyte transformation. Nature (New Biology) 243: 284–286

Coulam C B, Silverfield J C, Kazmar R E, Fathman C G 1983 T-lymphocyte subsets during pregnancy and the menstrual cycle. American Journal of Reproductive Immunology and Microbiology 4: 88–90

Curzen P, Jones E, Gaugas J 1972 Immunological responses in pregnancy. British Medical Journal 4: 49 (letter)

Damber M G, Von Schoultz B, Stigbrand T, Tarnvik A 1975 Inhibition of the mixed lymphocyte reaction by the pregnancy zone protein. FEBS Letters 58: 29–32

Darrow T L, Tomar R H 1980 Prostaglandin-mediated regulation of the mixed lymphocyte culture and generation of cytotoxic cells. Cellular Immunology 56: 172–183

D'Cruz I A, Balani S G, Lyer I S 1968 Infectious hepatitis and pregnancy. Obstetrics and Gynecology 31: 449–455

Djeu J Y, Heinbaugh J A, Holden H T, Herberman R B 1979 Augmentation of mouse natural killer cell activity by interferon and interferon inducers. Journal of Immunology 122: 175–181

Dodson M G, Kerman R H, Lange C F, Stefani S S, O'Leary J A 1977 T and B cells in pregnancy. Obstetrics and Gynecology 49: 299–302

Doughty R W, Gelsthorpe K 1976 Some parameters of lymphocyte antibody activity through pregnancy and further eluates of placental material. Tissue Antigens 8: 43–48

Faulk W P, Johnston P M 1977 Immunological studies of human placentae: identification and distribution of proteins in mature chorionic villi. Clinical and Experimental Immunology 27: 365–375

Faulk W P, McIntyre J A 1985 Immunology of placental antigens. In: Bischof P, Klopper A (eds) Proteins of the placenta. 5th International Congress on Placental Proteins, Karger, Basel, pp 26–53

Faulk W P, Temple A 1976 Distribution of beta-2 microglobulin and HLA in chorionic villi of human placentae. Nature 262: 799–802

Faulk W P, Sanderson A, Temple A 1977 Distribution of MHC antigens in human placentae. Transplantation Proceedings 9: 1379–1384

Faulk W P, Temple A, Lovins R E, Smith N 1978 Antigens of human trophoblasts: a working hypothesis for their role in normal and abnormal pregnancies. Proceedings of the National Academy of Sciences USA 75: 1947–1951

Finn R, St Hill C A, Govan A J, Ralfs I G, Gurney F J, Denye V 1972 Immunological responses in pregnancy and survival of fetal homografts. British Medical Journal 3: 150–152

Franceschi R T, Simpson R U, Deluca H F 1981 Binding proteins for vitamin D metabolites: serum carriers and intracellular receptors. Archives in Biochemistry and Biophysics 20: 1–13

Gatti R A, Yunis E J, Good R A 1973 Characterisation of a serum inhibitor of MLC reactions. Clinical and Experimental Immunology 13: 427–437

Goodfellow P N, Barnstaple C J, Bodmar W F, Snary D, Crumpton M J 1976 Expression of HLA system antigens on placenta. Transplantation 22: 595–603

Goodwin J S, Messner R P, Reak G T 1978 Prostaglandin suppression of mitogen-stimulated lymphocytes in vitro. Changes with mitogen dose and pre-incubation. Journal of Clinical Investigations 62: 753–760

Gray T K, Lester G E, Lorenc R S 1979 Evidence for extra-renal 1, alpha-hydroxylation of 25, hydroxyvitamin D_3 in pregnancy. Science 204: 1311–1313

Grose J, Belanger L, 1980 Binding of prostaglandins to α-fetoprotein. In: Peeters H (ed) Protides of the biological fluids. Proceedings of the 27th Colloquium, Pergamon Press, Oxford, pp 57–61

Gunder D, Merz W E, Hilgenfeldt V, Brossmer R 1975 Inability of highly purified preparations of HCG to inhibit PHA-induced stimulation of lymphocytes. FEBS Letters 53: 309–312

Gusdon J P, Prichard D 1972 Immunoglobulin D in pregnancy. American Journal of Obstetrics and Gynecology 112: 867 (letter)

Hellstrom K E, Hellstrom I, Brawn J 1969 Abrogation of cellular immunity to antigenically foreign mouse embryonic cells by a serum factor. Nature 224: 914–915

Herzenberg L A, Bianchi D W, Schroder J, Cann H M, Ivreson G M 1979 Fetal cells in the blood of pregnant women: detection and enrichment by fluorescence-activated cell sorting. Proceedings of the National Academy of Sciences USA 76: 1453–1455

Holland N H, Holland P 1966 Immunological maturation in an infant of an agammaglobulinaemic mother. Lancet ii: 1152–1155

Horne C H, Towler C M, Pugh-Humphreys R G, Thomson A W, Bohn H 1976 Pregnancy specific betaglycoprotein. A product of the syncytiotrophoblast. Experientia 32: 1197–1199

Jacoby D R, Oldstone M B A 1983 Delineation of suppressor and helper activity within the OKT4-defined T lymphocyte subset in human newborns. Journal of Immunology 131: 1765–1770

Jacoby D R, Olding L B, Oldstone M B A 1984 Immunologic regulation of fetal–maternal balance. Advances in Immunology 35: 157–208

Jenkins D M, Hancock K W 1972 Maternal unresponsiveness to paternal histocompatability antigens in human pregnancy. Transplantation 13: 618–619

Jenkins D M, Scott J S 1972 Immunological responses in pregnancy. British Medical Journal 3: 528–529

Jenkins D M, Acres M G, Peters J, Riley J 1972 Human chorionic gonadotrophin and the fetal allograft. American Journal of Obstetrics and Gynecology 114: 13–15

Johannsen R, Haupt H, Bohn H, Heide K, Seiler F R, Schwick H G 1976 Inhibition of the mixed leukocyte culture (MLC) by proteins: mechanism and specificity of the reaction (proceedings). Zeitschrift fur Immunitatsforschung Immunobiology 152: 280–285

Johnsen S A, Olding L B, Wersberg N G, Willhelmsson L 1982 Strong suppression by mononuclear leucocytes: mediation by prostaglandins. Clinical Immunology and Immunopathology 23: 606–615

Johnsen S A, Olding L B, Green K 1983a Conversion of arachidonic acid in human maternal and neonatal mononuclear leukocytes. Immunological Letters 6: 213–218

Johnsen S A, Olofsson A, Green K, Olding L B 1983b Strong suppression by mononuclear leukocytes from cord blood of human newborns on maternal leukocytes associated with differences in sensitivity to prostaglandin E2. American Journal of Reproductive Immunology and Microbiology 4: 45–49

Johnson H M, Blalock J E, Baron S 1977a Separation of mitogen-induced suppressor and helper cell activities during inhibition of interferon production by cyclic AMP. Cellular Immunology 33: 170–179

Johnson H M, Stanton G J, Barons S 1977b Relative ability of mitogens to stimulate production of interferon by lymphoid cells and to induce suppression of the in vitro immune response. Proceedings of the Society of Experimental Biology and Medicine 154: 138–141

Kasakura S 1971 A factor in maternal plasma during pregnancy that suppresses the reactivity of mixed leukocyte cultures. Journal of Immunology 107: 1296–1301

Kaye M D, Jones W R 1971 Effect of human chorionic gonodotrophin on in vitro lymphocyte transformation. American Journal of Obstetrics and Gynecology 109: 1029–1031

Kennedy T G 1985 Evidence for the role of prostaglandins throughout the decidual reaction in the rat. Biology of Reproduction 33: 140–146

Korsmeyer S J, Greene W C, Cossman J et al 1983 Rearrangement and expression of immunoglobulin genes and expression of Tac antigen in hairy cell leukaemia. Proceedings of the National Academy of Sciences USA 80: 4522–4526

Lawler S D, Klouda P T, Bagshawe K D 1974 Immunogenicity of molar pregnancies in the HL-A system. American Journal of Obstetrics and Gynecology 120: 857–861

Lewis J, Whang J, Nagel B, Oppenheim J J, Perry S 1966 Lymphocyte transformation in mixed lymphocyte cultures in women with normal pregnancy or tumors of placental origin. A preliminary report. American Journal of Obstetrics and Gynecology 96: 287–290

Lichtenstein M R 1942 Tuberculin reaction in tuberculosis during pregnancy. American Review of Tuberculosis 46: 89–92

Lin T M, Halbert S P, Kiefer D, Spellacy W N, Gall S 1974 Characterization of four human pregnancy-associated plasma proteins. American Journal of Obstetrics and Gynecology 118: 223–236

Lin T M, Halbert S P, Spellacy W N, Gall S 1976 Human pregnancy-associated plasma proteins during the postpartum period. American Journal of Obstetrics and Gynecology 124: 382–387

Loke Y W, Joysey V C, Borland R 1971 HL-A antigens on human trophoblast cells. Nature 232: 403–405

Lu C Y, Changelian P S, Unanue 1984 Alpha-fetoprotein inhibits macrophage expression of Ia antigens. Journal of Immunology 132: 1722–1727

Malkovsky M, Medawar P D 1984 Is immunological tolerance (non-responsiveness) a consequence of interleukin-2 deficit during the recognition of antigen? Immunology Today 5: 340–343

McIntyre J A, Hsi L B, Faulk W P, Klopper A, Thomson R 1981 Immunological studies of the human placenta: functional and morphological analysis of pregnancy-associated plasma protein-A (PAPP-A). Immunology 44: 577–583

Medawar P D 1953 Some immunological and endocrinological problems raised by the evolution of viviparity in vertebrates. In: Danielli J F, Brown R (eds) Symposia of the Society for Experimental Biology, vol VII, Oxford University Press, Oxford, pp 320–338

Meuer S C, Hussey R E, Cantrell D A et al 1984 Triggering of the T3-TI antigen–receptor complex results in clonal T-cell proliferation through an interleukin-2 dependent autocrine pathway. Proceedings of the National Academy of Sciences USA 81: 1509–1513

Mitchell D M, Carr B B, Mason J I, Simpson E R 1982 Prostaglandin biosynthesis in the human fetal adrenal gland regulation by glucocorticosteroids. Proceedings of the National Academy of Sciences USA 79: 7547–7551

Montgomery W P, Young R C, Achen M P, Harden H A 1968 The tuberculin test in pregnancy. American Journal of Obstetrics and Gynecology 100: 829–831

Mori T, Kabayashi H, Nishimura T, Mori T 1977 Possible role of progesterone in immunoregulation during pregnancy. In: Boettcher B (ed) Immunological influence on human fertility, Academic Press, Sydney, pp 175–180

Morse J H 1976 The effect of human chorionic gonadotrophin and placental lactogen on lymphocyte transformation in vitro. Scandinavian Journal of Immunology 5: 779–787

Murgita R A, Tomasi T B 1975 Suppression of the immune response by alpha fetoprotein. 1. The effect of mouse alpha fetoprotein on the primary and secondary antibody response. Journal of Experimental Medicine 141: 269–286

Murgita R A, Goidl E A, Kontiainen S, Wigzell H 1977 Alpha fetoprotein induces suppressor T cells in vitro. Nature 267: 257–259

Nicholas N S, Panayi G S 1985 Inhibition of interleukin-2 production by retroplacental sera: a possible mechanism for human fetal allograft survival. American Journal of Reproductive Immunology and Microbiology 9: 6–11

Nicholas N S, Panayi G S 1986 Immunosuppressive properties of pregnancy serum on the mixed lymphocyte reaction: correlation with serum levels of AFP, α_2PAG, PAPP-A and SP$_1$. British Journal of Obstetrics and Gynaecology 93: 1251–1255

Nicholas N S, Panayi G S, Nouri A M E 1984 Human pregnancy serum inhibits interleukin-2 production. Clinical and Experimental Immunology 58: 587–593

Nicholas N S, Panayi G S, Murphy J, Pitzalis C 1986 Human retroplacental sera inhibit the expression of Class II major histocompatibility antigens. Journal of Reproductive Immunology 9: 95–102

Nishi S 1970 Isolation and characterization of a human fetal alpha-globulin from the sera of fetuses and a hepatoma patient. Cancer Research 30: 2507–2513

Nolten W E, Rueckert P A 1981 Elevated free cortisol index in pregnancy: possible regulatory mechanism. American Journal of Obstetrics and Gynecology 139: 492–498

Olding L B 1979 Interactions between maternal and fetal/neonatal lymphocytes. Current Topics in Pathology 66: 83–104

Olding L B, Murgita R A, Wigzell H 1977 Mitogen-stimulated lymphoid cells from human newborns suppress the proliferation of maternal lymphocytes across a cell-impermeable membrane. Journal of Immunology 119: 1109–1114

Park W W 1971 In: Choriocarcinomona: a study of its pathology, Heinemann, London

Peleg S 1983 The modulation of decidual cell proliferation and differentiation by progesterone and prostaglandins. Journal of Steroid Biochemistry 19: 283–289

Persellin R H 1977 The effect of pregnancy on rheumatoid arthritis. Bulletin on the Rheumatic Diseases 27: 922–927

Poskitt P F K, Kurt E A, Paul B B, Selvaraj R J, Sharra A J, Mitchell G W 1977 Response to mitogen during pregnancy and postpartum period. Obstetrics and Gynaecology 50: 319–323

Powell A E 1974 Maternal lymphocytes. Suppression by human chorionic gonadotrophin. Science 184: 913–914 (letter)

Purtilo D T 1975 Opportunistic mycotic infections in pregnant women. American Journal of Obstetrics and Gynecology 122: 607–610

Ramer S J, Yu D T 1978 Effect of corticosteroids on committed lymphocytes. Clinical and Experimental Immunology 32: 545–553

Reinherz E L, Schlossman S F 1980 Current concepts in immunology. Regulation of the immune response—inducer and suppressor T lymphocyte subsets in human beings. New England Journal of Medicine 303: 370–373

Reinherz E L, Morimoto C, Fitzgerald K A, Hussey R E, Daley J F, Schlossman S F 1982 Heterogeneity of human T4+ inducer T cells defined by a monoclonal antibody that delineates two functional subpopulations. Journal of Immunology 128: 463–468

Rigby W F C, Stacy T, Fanger M W 1984 Inhibition of T lymphocyte mitogenesis by 1,25-dihydroxyvitamin D3 (Calcitriol). Journal of Clinical Investigation 74: 1451–1455

Rocklin R E, Kitzmiller J L, Carpenter C B, Garovoy M R, David J R 1976 Absence of an immunologic blocking factor from the serum of women with chronic abortion. New England Journal of Medicine 295: 1209–1213

Rocklin R E, Kitzmiller J L, Kaye M D 1979 Immunobiology of the maternal–fetal relationship. Annual Reviews in Medicine 30: 375–404

Santoli D, Trinchieri G, Koprowski H 1978 Cell-mediated cytotoxicity against virus-infected target cells in humans. II. Interferon induction and activation of natural killer cells. Journal of Immunology 121: 532–538

Schlesinger M 1962 Uterus of rodents as site for manifestation of transplantation immunity against transplantable tumors. Journal of the National Cancer Institute 28: 927–945

Seigler H F, Metzgar R S 1970 Embryonic development of human transplantation antigens. Transplantation 9: 478–486

Siegel M, Greenberg M 1955 Incidence of poliomyelitis in pregnancy. Its relation to maternal age, parity and gestational period. New England Journal of Medicine 253: 841–847

Siiteri P K, Febres F, Clemens L E, Chang R J, Gondos B, Stites D 1977 Progesterone and maintenance of pregnancy: is progesterone nature's immunosuppressant? Annals of the New York Academy of Sciences 286: 384–397

Silverstein A M 1972 Immunological maturation of the fetus: modulation of the pathogenesis of congenital infectious disease. In: Ontogeny of acquired immunity. Ciba Foundation Symposium, Associated Scientific Publications, Amsterdam, pp 17–25

Smart Y C 1984 Pregnancy-associated plasma protein-A (PAPP-A) an immunosuppressor in pregnancy? Fertility and Sterility 41: 508–510

Smith K A 1980 T-cell growth factor. Immunological Reviews 51: 337-357

Stagno S, Reynolds D, Tsiantos A et al 1975 Cervical cytomegalovirus excretion in pregnant and non pregnant women: suppression in early gestation. Journal of Infectious Diseases 131: 522–527

Stimson W H 1975 Variations in the serum concentration of a human pregnancy-associated-macroglobulin during pregnancy and after delivery. Journal of Reproductive Fertility 43: 579–582

Stimson W H 1976 Studies on the immunosuppressive properties of a pregnancy-associated-macroglobulin. Clinical and Experimental Immunology 25: 199–206

Stimson W H 1980 Are pregnancy-associated serum proteins responsible for the inhibition of lymphocyte transformation by pregnancy serum? Clinical and Experimental Immunology 40: 157–160

Stimson W H, Farquharson D M 1978 The molecular weight of pregnancy-associated alpha-2-glycoprotein and its subunits. International Journal of Biochemistry 9: 839–843

Stimson W H, Strachan A F, Shepherd A 1979 Studies in the maternal immune response to placental antigens: absence of a blocking factor from the blood of abortion-prone women. British Journal of Obstetrics and Gynaecology 86: 41–45

Straube W, Glockner E, Hofmann R, Klausch B, Semmler K 1980 Immunochemical investigations on the problems of the pregnancy zone protein. XII. Serum concentrations of pregnancy-associated alpha-2-glycoprotein in diabetic pregnancy. Archives of Gynecology 229: 271–278

Strelkauskas A J, Wilson B S, Dray S, Dodson M 1975 Inversion of levels of human T and B cells in early pregnancy. Nature 258: 331–332

Strelkauskas A J, Davies I J, Dray S 1978 Longitudinal studies showing alterations on the levels and functional responses of T and B lymphocytes in human pregnancy. Clinical and Experimental Immunology 32: 531–539

Studd J W W 1971 Immunoglobulins in normal pregnancy, pre-eclampsia and pregnancy complicated by the nephrotic syndrome. Journal of Obstetrics and Gynaecology of the British Commonwealth 78: 786–790

Sundqvist K G, Bergshom S, Hakansson S 1977 Surface antigens of human trophoblasts. Developmental and Comparative Immunology 1: 241–254

Szekeres-Bartho J, Falkay G, Torok A, Pasca A S 1985a The mechanism of the inhibitory effects of progesterone on lymphocyte cytotoxicity. II. Relationship between cytotoxicity and the cyclo-oxygenase pathway of arachadonic acid metabolism. American Journal of Reproductive Immunology and Microbiology 9: 19–22

Szekeres-Bartho J, Kilar F, Falkay G, Csernus V, Torok A, Pasca A S 1985b The mechanism of the inhibitory effects of progesterone on lymphocyte cytotoxicity. I. Progesterone-treated lymphocytes release a substance inhibiting cytotoxicity and prostaglandin synthesis. American Journal of Reproductive Immunology and Microbiology 9: 15–18

Taylor C, Faulk W P 1981 Prevention of recurrent abortion with leucocyte transfusions. Lancet ii: 68–69

Teasdale F, Adcock E W III, August C S, Cox S, Battaglia F C, Naught O 1973 Human chorionic gonadotrophin inhibitory effect on MLCs. Gynecologic Investigations 4: 263–269

Terasaki P I, Mickey M R, Yamazaki J N, Vredenore D 1970 Maternal–fetal incompatibility. 1. Incidence of HL-A antibodies and possible association with congenital anomalies. Transplantation 9: 538–543

Thomson A W, Hunter C B, Cruickshank N, Horn C H 1979a Study of pregnancy-associated alpha 2-glycoprotein in relation to populations of human blood leucocytes. International Archives of Allergy and Applied Immunology 58: 251–259

Thomson A W, Powrie J K, Horne C H 1979b Plasma pregnancy-associated alpha 2-glycoprotein concentrations in complications of pregnancy and foetal abnormality. Journal of Reproductive Immunology 1: 229–235

Tomoda Y, Fuma S, Miwa T, Saiki N, Ishizuka N 1976 Cell-mediated immunity in pregnant women. Gynecologic Investigations 7: 280–292

Towler C M, Horne C H 1977 Immunochemical investigations on the problem of the PZP. II. Serum concentrations of PAG in diabetic pregnancies. Archives of Gynecology 1229: 271–278

Towler C M, Jandial V, Horne C H W, Bohn H 1976 A serial study of pregnancy proteins in primigravidae. British Journal of Obstetrics and Gynaecology 83: 368–374

Towler C M, Horne C H, Jandial V, Campbell D M, MacGillivray I 1977a Plasma levels of pregnancy-specific beta 1-glycoprotein in complicated pregnancies. British Journal of Obstetrics and Gynaecology 84: 258–263

Towler C M, Horne C H, Jandial V, Chesworth J M 1977b A simple and sensitive radioimmunoassay for pregnancy-specific beta-glycoprotein. Journal of Obstetrics and Gynaecology 84: 580–584

Tsoukas C D, Provvedini D M, Manolagas S C 1984 1,25-dihydroxyvitamin D_3: a novel immunoregulatory hormone. Science 224: 1438–1440

Unander A M, Olding L B 1981 Ontogeny and postnatal persistence of a strong suppressor activity in man. Journal of Immunology 127: 1182–1186

Uriel J, De Nechaud B, Dupries M 1972 Estrogen-binding properties of rat, mouse and man fetospecific serum proteins. Demonstration by immuno-autoradiographic methods. Biochemical and Biophysical Research Communications 46: 1175–1180

Van Zon A J C, Eling W M C 1980 Depressed malarial immunity in pregnant mice. Infection and Immunity 28: 630–632

Voisin G A 1984 Enhancing antibodies and suppressor cells in pregnancy: role of the placentation. In: Isojima S, Billington W D (eds) Reproductive immunology, Elsevier, Amsterdam, pp 121–131

Von Schoultz B 1974 A quantitative study of the pregnancy zone protein in the sera of pregnant and puerperal women. American Journal of Obstetrics and Gynecology 119: 792–797

Von Schoultz B, Stigbrand T, Tarnvik A 1973 Inhibition of PHA-induced lymphocyte stimulation by the pregnancy zone protein. FEBS Letters 38: 23–26

Watson J, Moschizuki D 1980 Interleukin-2: a class of T-cell growth factors. Immunological Reviews 51: 257–278

Weisman Y, Harell A, Edelstein S, David M, Spirer Z, Golander A 1979 1-alpha, 25-dihydroxyvitamin D_3 and 24,25-dihydroxyvitamin D_3 in vitro synthesis by human decidua and placenta. Nature 281: 317–319

Winchester R J, Fu S M, Wernet P, Kunkel H G, Dupont B, Jersild C 1975 Recognition by pregnancy serum of non-HLA alloantigens selectively expressed on B lymphocytes. Journal of Experimental Medicine 141: 924–929

Wurz H, Geiger W, Kunzig H J, Courtral J, Linben G, Bohn H 1980 Determination of PAG (SP3) by RIA in maternal plasma during normal and pathological pregnancies. In: Klopper A, Genazzani A, Crosigani P G (eds) The human placenta: proteins and hormones, Accademic Press, London, pp 411–417

Yachnin S, Lester E 1976 Inhibition of human alphafetoprotein (HAFP): comparison of fetal and hepatoma HAFP and kinetic studies for in vitro immunosuppression. Clinical and Experimental Immunology 26: 484–490

Youtananukorn V, Matangkasombut P, Osathanondh V 1974 Onset of human maternal cell-mediated immune reaction to placental antigens during the first pregnancy. Clinical and Experimental Immunology 16: 593–598

The maternal blood supply to the placenta

INTRODUCTION

Throughout pregnancy and labour fetal well-being is dependent on the adequate supply of maternal blood to the placenta. Physiological adaptations of uterine spiral arteries are an essential requirement to facilitate the increase in blood flow to the placenta as pregnancy advances. The blood supply to the non-pregnant endometrium is only a few millilitres per minute, whereas the same vessels must deliver 600–800 ml of blood per minute to the placenta in late pregnancy. A reduced blood flow through the placenta and the myometrium has been shown in pregnancies complicated by maternal hypertension and fetal growth retardation (Browne & Veall 1953, Käär et al 1980). Using a continuous Doppler ultrasound system, abnormal maternal uterine artery wave forms have also been reported in pregnancies complicated by intra-uterine growth retardation (Trudinger et al 1985).

Morphological changes in the spiral arteries of the placental bed have been studied extensively since the end of the last century. Most of the early studies were inconclusive as the reports were based on material obtained from the delivered fetal placenta, and less often from hysterectomies and autopsy material. The introduction of the placental bed biopsy at caesarean section greatly increased our knowledge of uteroplacental vascular changes. This technique has now become widely used by several groups studying the physiological changes of normal pregnancy and uteroplacental vascular pathology in pregnancy complicated by hypertension and fetal growth retardation (Brosens & Robertson 1972, Brosens et al 1967, 1977, Sheppard & Bonnar 1974, 1976a, 1981, Gerretsen et al 1981).

Friedlander (1870) was the first to draw attention to the presence of large multinucleate cells in the walls of spiral arteries in late pregnancy. His view—that these cells were of fetal origin—was not shared by all subsequent investigators until the introduction of electron microscopy studies just over 12 years ago confirmed the trophoblastic origin of the multinucleate cells in the walls of modified uteroplacental arteries (De Wolf et al 1973, Sheppard & Bonnar 1974). The electron microscope has since been of major value in the study of uteroplacental vascular pathology associated with hypertensive pregnancy

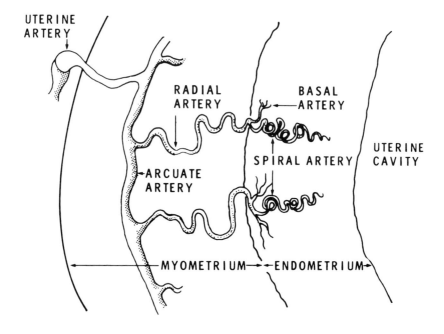

Fig. 2.1   Diagram of the arterial supply to the uterine endometrium

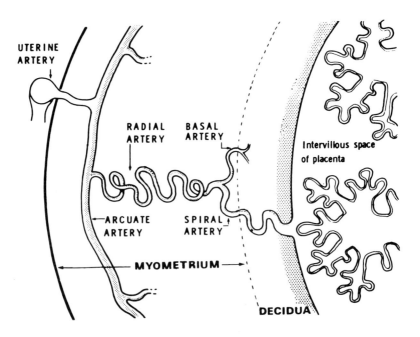

Fig. 2.2   Diagram of the arterial supply to the placenta in normal pregnancy

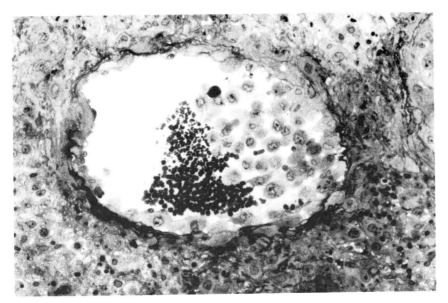

Fig. 2.3 Decidual spiral artery at 12 weeks of pregnancy. Much trophoblast may be seen within the lumen, forming a new intima and invading the media below the endothelium (× 225)

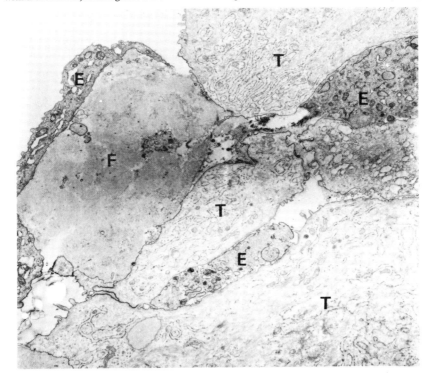

Fig. 2.4 Electron micrograph of the intima of a decidual spiral artery at 12 weeks of pregnancy. Invasion of trophoblast (T) is associated with the degeneration of endothelium (E) and the accumulation of fibrinoid material (F) and trophoblast within the media (× 5000)

and intra-uterine fetal growth retardation (De Wolf et al 1975, Sheppard & Bonnar 1976a, 1981).

DEVELOPMENT OF THE UTEROPLACENTAL BLOOD SUPPLY IN NORMAL PREGNANCY

In the non-pregnant uterus, the spiral arteries are the terminations of the radial arteries (Fig. 2.1) The spiral, or coiled, arteries are muscular arteries measuring 2–300μm in diameter and containing a prominent internal elastic lamina which becomes more tenuous as the vessels penetrate the endometrium. Smaller, basal or straight arteries are also branches of the radial arteries which terminate in the basal endometrium. Unlike the spiral arteries which open into the intervillous space (Fig. 2.2), the basal arteries undergo only minor changes during pregnancy.

In early pregnancy, trophoblast proliferating from the cytotrophoblastic shell of the implanting blastocyst penetrates the basal decidua and may be seen within the lumen of decidual spiral arteries (Fig. 2.3) This endovascular trophoblast invades the vessel wall (Fig. 2.4), replacing much of the intimal lining of the endothelium. The disruption of the vessel media results in the loss of musculo-elastic tissue and the appearance of trophoblast surrounded by fibrinoid material, which by electron microscopy has been shown to contain fibrin (Sheppard & Bonnar 1974).

Trophoblast invasion of the uteroplacental vasculature appears to occur in two stages—the decidual segments are structurally modified during the first trimester, and later, in the second trimester, a second wave of endovascular trophoblast begins to convert the myometrial segments of these vessels (Pijnenborg et al 1980, 1981, 1983). As in the decidua, trophoblast replacement of much of the endothelium is associated with a loss of elastic tissue and smooth muscle from the media of the myometrial segments of the placental bed spiral arteries, and may even involve the terminal segments of the radial arteries. These fully developed physiological changes, seen in the myometrium in late pregnancy (Figs 2.5 and 2.6), allow the progressive enlargement of the vessels to accommodate the increased uteroplacental blood flow.

The loss of the musculo-elastic tissue renders the vessels incapable of responding to vasomotor influences. The overall effect of the endovascular trophoblast invasion is to convert the uteroplacental spiral arteries into tortuous, distended, funnel-shaped vessels emptying into the placenta. The physiological dilatation induced by these morphological changes to the uteroplacental vasculature is also associated with a reduction in vascular resistance (Moll et al 1975), creating a low-pressure high flow system into the placenta. In the physiology of the third stage of labour, the vascular changes facilitate the placental separation, which involves the tearing of the terminal part of the uteroplacental vessels and their closure by the contraction of the myometrium. The placental site that bleeds in both placenta praevia and 'accidental' haemorrhage arises from these vessels.

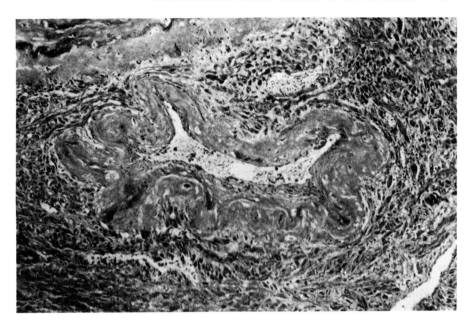

Fig. 2.5   Spiral artery showing physiological changes within the placental bed myometrium at term in normal pregnancy. The vessel wall is distended, containing intramural trophoblast cells surrounded by fibrinoid material ($\times$ 150)

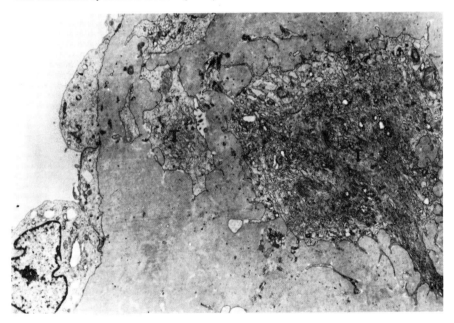

Fig. 2.6   Electron micrograph of part of the wall of the spiral artery in Figure 2.5 showing part of a trophoblast cell (T) and fibrinoid material of the media ($\times$ 4000)

UTEROPLACENTAL ARTERIES IN HYPERTENSIVE PREGNANCY AND INTRA-UTERINE FETAL GROWTH RETARDATION

For many years studies have reported on the pathology of spiral arteries in association with pregnancy complicated by hypertension, irrespective of the fetal outcome of the pregnancy (Dixon & Robertson 1958, Marais 1962, Brosens 1964, Robertson et al 1967). More recently, however, attention has been directed towards uterine pathology in pregnancy complicated by intra-uterine fetal growth retardation, not only in pre-eclampsia but also in the normotensive patient (Sheppard & Bonnar 1976a, 1981, Brosens et al 1977, Gerretsen et al 1981). Although several factors are known to be associated with the aetiology of intra-uterine fetal growth retardation, no morphological explanation for this pregnancy complication had previously been forth-coming—and such a concept is still not agreed by all.

The relationship between uteroplacental vascular pathology, hypertension in pregnancy and intra-uterine fetal growth retardation remains a subject of controversy. The two main areas of contention have been: (1) the extent of physiological adaptations of the uteroplacental spiral arteries in pre-eclampsia and intra-uterine fetal growth retardation, and (2) the specificity of the placental bed vascular lesion, 'acute atherosis', to pre-eclampsia. Attempts to elucidate these complex relationships have been further complicated by lack of uniformity of clinical definitions in pre-eclampsia (Chesley 1985) and to a lesser extent in fetal growth retardation.

HYPERTENSIVE PREGNANCY

The vascular lesion termed 'acute atherosis' is ascribed to Zeek & Assali (1950) who confirmed the presence of the lesions which Hertig (1945) had found in the spiral arteries of patients with 'hypertensive albuminuric toxae-mia of pregnancy'. The lesions were characterised by fibrinoid necrosis with accumulation of lipid-containing cells in the intima and media of the vessel walls. It was later suggested that the lesion only occurred in pre-eclampsia (Brosens et al 1967) and that the physiological adaptations of placental bed spiral arteries were limited, without exception, to the decidual segments of the vessels (Brosens & Robertson 1972). Although hypertension of pregnancy has been considered as a compensatory mechanism to ensure an adequate blood supply to the placenta when the vascular physiological changes have failed to occur (Gerretsen et al 1981), it is unlikely that the inadequate response of the myometrial spiral arteries or the occurrence of arteriopathy is the causal factor of pre-eclampsia. Indeed, we have found in pre-eclampsia, where the birth weight of the infant is appropriate for gestational age, that uteroplacental spiral arteries may show the physiological changes in myometrial segments, coupled with vascular lesions (Fig. 2.7).

Where the pre-eclampsia is superimposed on essential hypertension, the restrictions of the physiological changes are similar to those observed in spiral

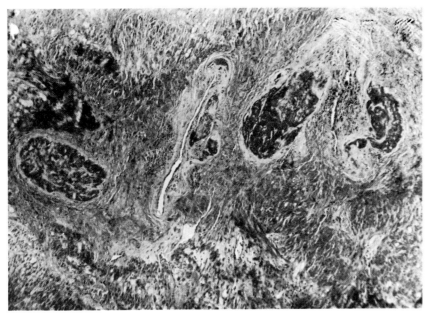

Fig. 2.7 Myometrial spiral artery in a pregnancy complicated by pre-eclampsia where the birthweight of the infant was appropriate for gestational age. The vessel (centre segment) shows the morphological adaptations of pregnancy whereas the adjacent segments of the same artery are occluded with fibrin and lipid-containing cells ($\times$ 150)

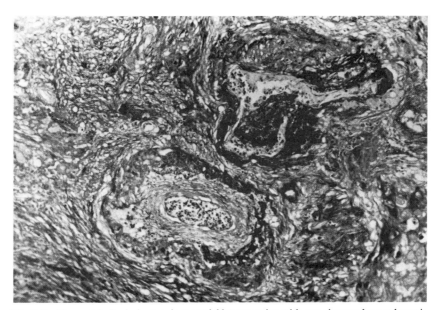

Fig. 2.8 Myometrical spiral artery in essential hypertension with superimposed pre-eclampsia. The lesion exhibits intimal smooth muscle hyperplasia with an accumulation of fibrin and lipid-laden cells in the media. There is no evidence of the physiological changes of pregnancy ($\times$ 150)

arteries of the myometrium in pre-eclampsia alone. Fibrin deposition and lipid-laden cells are the main features within the media below intimal smooth muscle hyperplasia in lesions of the myometrial spiral arteries (Fig. 2.8) In patients with essential hypertension who do not develop pre-eclampsia, the myometrial spiral arteries often undergo the physiological changes of pregnancy. However, myo-intimal smooth muscle hyperplasia has been reported in myometrial placental bed spiral arteries which have not undergone physiological changes of pregnancy, and which still retain a prominent internal elastic lamina in essential hypertension where the pregnancy has resulted in the delivery of a growth-retarded infant (Sheppard & Bonnar 1981).

INTRA-UTERINE FETAL GROWTH RETARDATION

In 1976 we described the uteroplacental vasculature in 15 well-documented pregnancies with severe intra-uterine fetal growth retardation of mixed aetiology. Extensive placental infarction, occlusive uteroplacental vascular lesions and an absence of physiological changes in myometrial spiral arteries were common findings, not only in hypertensive but also in normotensive pregnancies complicated by intra-uterine fetal growth retardation (Sheppard & Bonnar 1976a). In a retrospective study, Brosens et al (1977), although confirming our findings of restricted physiological changes, only found vascular lesions in intra-uterine fetal growth retardation where the pregnancy was complicated by pre-eclampsia. However, De Wolf et al (1980) from the same group were able to find lesions characterised by less well developed physiological morphological changes, by extensive intimal thickening, by fibrinoid degeneration of the media and by acute atherosis in patients with fetal growth retardation in pregnancies with no or only a moderate and transient rise in blood pressure.

We subsequently confirmed our original findings in a larger detailed study using both light and electron microscopy (Sheppard & Bonnar 1981). We found a failure of the physiological adaptations to extend into the myometrial segments of spiral arteries of the placental bed (Fig. 2.9), and the vascular lesions exhibited fibrin deposition and the accumulation of lipid-laden cells in pregnancy complicated by intra-uterine fetal growth retardation, whether maternal hypertension was present or not. These lesions are found in the uteroplacental spiral arteries of the basal decidua and to a lesser extent in the spiral arteries of the placental bed myometrium (Fig. 2.10). As the lesions we observed in spiral arteries in normotensive pregnancy complicated by intra-uterine fetal growth retardation were morphologically similar to those seen in pre-eclampsia, even when examined by electron microscopy (Fig. 2.11), we concluded that 'acute atherosis' was not pathognomonic for pre-eclampsia. However, it is still possible that the lesion in intra-uterine growth retardation is analogous to, but not identical with, acute atherosis. It is now clear from our own studies and those of others that a failure of complete trophoblast invasion often occurs in intra-uterine fetal growth retardation

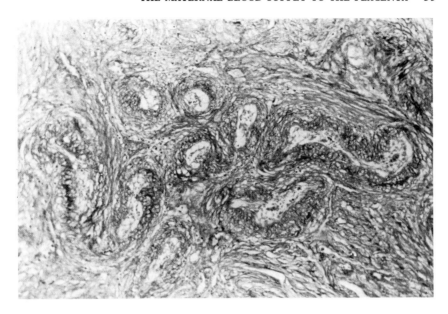

Fig. 2.9 Myometrial spiral artery showing a complete absence of the physiological adaptations of pregnancy in a normotensive pregnancy complicated by severe intra-uterine fetal growth retardation (× 150)

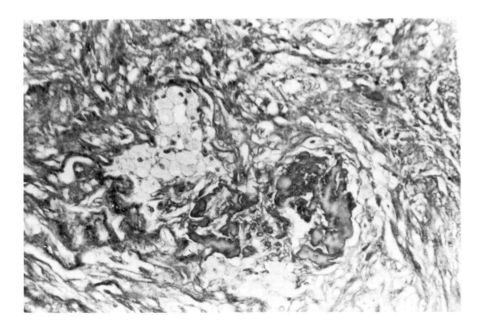

Fig. 2.10 Myometrial spiral artery. Severe intra-uterine fetal growth retardation where the pregnancy remained normotensive. The vessel is occluded with fibrin and large lipid-containing cells (× 225)

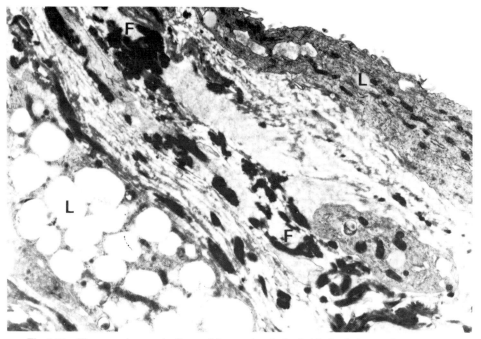

Fig. 2.11 Electron micrograph of part of the vessel wall of a decidual spiral artery in normotenisve intra-uterine fetal growth retardation. Lipid (L) is seen within the endothelium and within underlying cells of the vessel wall surrounded by fibrinous material containing electron-dense fibrin (F) (× 9000)

and hypertension. However, little information is available on the function of endovascular trophoblasts which do invade uteroplacental spiral arteries in such pregnancies.

Trophoblast cells lining decidual spiral arteries are known to have a reduced capacity for fibrinolysis, even in normal pregnancy (Sheppard & Bonnar 1976b), and placentae from pregnancies complicated by fetal growth retardation but without hypertension have an increased ability to inhibit urokinase-induced fibrinolysis when compared with normal placentae (Elder & Myatt 1976). The precise location of the inhibitors in the placenta has, however, not been identified. Trophoblast cells from pregnancies complicated by intra-uterine fetal growth retardation also have a greatly reduced ability to produce prostacyclin compared with those from normal pregnancies (Jogee et al 1983). Prostacyclin is a potent vasodilator and platelet anti-aggregator; a localised decidual decrease in production by the intravascular trophoblast could result in the increased platelet aggregation and fibrin deposition seen in the uteroplacental vasculature in intra-uterine fetal growth retardation. An increase of platelet deposition, which has been described in early normal pregnancy (Sheppard & Bonnar 1974), would account for the shortened life span of platelets in pregnancy complicated by intra-uterine growth retardation (Wallenburg & van Kessell 1979).

Although decreased prostacyclin production and increased fibrin deposition may be aetiological factors in the thrombotic occlusion of the uteroplacental circulation which impairs fetal growth, other vascular factors, such as a reduction in the size and number of spiral arteries, may also be involved in pregnancies complicated by intra-uterine fetal growth retardation. In normal pregnancy, between 120 and 150 spiral arteries supply the placenta at term (Brosens & Dixon 1966). It is quite possible that in intra-uterine fetal growth retardation the vessels observed in the myometrium without physiological changes represent spiral arteries which were never 'opened up' to the intervillous space of the placenta in early pregnancy. This would result in not only smaller, narrower vessels restricted to decidual adaptations, but also a reduced number of vessels supplying the placenta in intra-uterine fetal growth retardation. In fetal growth retardation, as in pre-eclampsia, much of the vasculopathy in the maternal supply line to the placenta seen in late pregnancy is most likely to be due to a failure of adequate placentation during the first and early second trimesters. The reason for failure of trophoblast invasion to effect complete physiological adaptations of the placental bed spiral arteries in some pregnancies still remains unclear.

Although recent studies have improved our basic knowledge of uterine vascular morphology during pregnancy, further studies, perhaps incorporating local uterine haemostatic changes, are required to ascertain the significance of uterine arteriopathy in pre-eclampsia and intra-uterine fetal growth retardation. A greater understanding of the complex relationship between uteroplacental vascular changes in complications of pregnancy is required if advances are to be made in any therapeutic control to improve the maternal blood flow to the placenta, thus preventing impairment of fetal growth.

REFERENCES

Brosens I 1964 A study of the spiral arteries of the decidua basalis in normotensive and hypertensive pregnancies. Journal of Obstetrics and Gynaecology of the British Commonwealth 71: 222–229
Brosens I, Dixon H G 1966 The anatomy of the maternal side of the placenta. Journal of Obstetrics and Gynaecology of the British Commonwealth 73: 357–363
Brosens I, Robertson W B 1972 The role of the spiral arteries in the pathogenesis of pre-eclampsia. In: Wynn R M (ed) Obstetrics and gynecology annual, vol. 1, Appleton-Century-Croft, New York, pp 177–191
Brosens I, Robertson W B, Dixon H G 1967 The physiological response of the vessels of the placental bed to normal pregnancy. Journal of Pathology and Bacteriology 93: 569–579
Brosens I, Dixon H G, Robertson W B 1977 Fetal growth retardation and the arteries of the placental bed. British Journal of Obstetrics and Gynaecology 84: 656–663
Browne J C M, Veall N 1953 The maternal placental blood flow in normotensive and hypertensive women. Journal of Obstetrics and Gynaecology of the British Empire 60: 141–147
Chesley L C 1985 Diagnosis of pre-eclampsia. Obstetrics and Gynecology 65: 423–425
De Wolf F, De Wolf P C, Brosens I 1973 Ultrastructure of the spiral arteries in the human placental bed at the end of the normal pregnancy. American Journal of Obstetrics and Gynecology 117: 833–848
De Wolf F, Robertson W B, Brosens I 1975 The ultrastructure of acute atherosis in hypertensive pregnancy. American Journal of Obstetrics and Gynecology 123: 164–174

De Wolf F, Brosens I, Renaer M 1980 Fetal growth retardation and the maternal arterial supply of the human placenta in the absence of sustained hypertension. British Journal of Obstetrics and Gynaecology 87: 678–685

Dixon H G, Robertson W B 1958 A study of the vessels of the placental bed in normotensive and hypertensive women. Journal of Obstetrics and Gynaecology of the British Empire 65: 803–809

Elder M G, Myatt L 1976 Coagulation and fibrinolysis in pregnancies complicated by fetal growth retardation. British Journal of Obstetrics and Gynaecology 83: 355–360

Friedlander C 1870 Physiologisch-anatomische untersuchungen uber den uterus, Leipzig University Press, Leipzig, p 32

Gerretsen G, Hinsjes H J, Elema J D 1981 Morphological changes of the spiral arteries in the placental bed in relation to pre-eclampsia and fetal growth retardation. British Journal of Obstetrics and Gynaecology 88: 876–881

Hertig A T 1945 Vascular pathology in the hypertensive albuminuric toxemias of pregnancy. Clinics 4: 602–613

Jogee M, Myatt L, Elder M G 1983 Decreased prostacyclin production by placental cells in culture from pregnancies complicated by fetal growth retardation. British Journal of Obstetrics and Gynaecology 90: 247–250

Käär K, Jouppila P, Kuikka J, Luotola H, Toivanen J, Rekonen A 1980 Intervillous blood flow in normal and complicated late pregnancy measured by intravenous ^{133}Xe method. Acta Obstetricia et Gynecologica Scandinavica 59: 7–10

Marais W D 1962 Human decidual spiral arterial studies. IV. Human atherosis of a few weeks duration. Histopathogenesis. Journal of Obstetrics and Gynaecology of the British Commonwealth 69: 234–240

Moll W, Kinzel W, Hoberger J 1975 Haemodynamic implications of haemochemical placentations. European Journal of Obstetrics, Gynecology, and Reproductive Biology 5: 67–74

Pijnenborg R, Dixon H G, Robertson W B, Brosens I 1980 Trophoblast invasion of human decidua from 8 to 18 weeks of pregnancy. Placenta 1: 3–19

Pijnenborg R, Bland J M, Robertson W B, Dixon G, Brosens I 1981 The pattern of interstitial trophoblastic invasion of the myometrium in early human pregnancy. Placenta 2: 303–316

Pijnenborg R, Bland J M, Robertson W B, Brosens I 1983 Uteroplacental arterial changes related to interstitial trophoblast migration in early human pregnancy. Placenta 4: 397–414

Robertson W B, Brosens I, Dixon H G 1967 The pathological response of the vessels of the placental bed to hypertensive pregnancy. Journal of Pathology and Bacteriology 93: 581–592

Sheppard B L, Bonnar J 1974 The ultrastructure of the arterial supply of the human placenta in early and late pregnancy. Journal of Obstetrics and Gynaecology of the British Commonwealth 81: 497–511

Sheppard B L, Bonnar J 1976a The ultrastructure of the arterial supply of the human placenta in pregnancy complicated by intrauterine growth retardation. British Journal of Obstetrics and Gynaecology 83: 948–959

Sheppard B L, Bonnar J 1976b Fibrinolysis in decidual spiral arteries in late pregnancy. Thrombosis and Haemostasis 39: 751–758

Sheppard B L, Bonnar J 1981 An ultrastructural study of the uteroplacental spiral arteries in hypertensive and normotensive pregnancy and fetal growth retardation. British Journal of Obstetrics and Gynaecology 88: 695–705

Trudinger B J, Giles W B, Cook C M 1985 Uteroplacental blood flow velocity-time waveforms in normal and complicated pregnancy. British Journal of Obstetrics and Gynaecology 92: 39–45

Wallenburg H C S, Van Kessell P H 1979 Platelet life span in pregnancies resulting in small-for-gestational age infants. American Journal of Obstetrics and Gynecology 134: 739–742

Zeek P M, Assali N S 1950 Vascular changes in the decidua associated with eclamptogenic toxemia of pregnancy. American Journal of Clinical Pathology 20: 1099–1109

3   *David J. H. Brock*

Gene probe analysis

INTRODUCTION

The history of medical genetics can be divided into three phases. The first
followed the rediscovery of Mendel's laws around the turn of the century,
and was concerned with analysis of the inheritance patterns of genetic disorders and with their division into autosomal and X-linked dominant and
recessive traits. The second phase started in the late 1940s, when it was
discovered that mutant genes could be followed through the proteins they
controlled. The classic example is sickle cell anaemia, a recessively inherited
disease which can be tracked by measurement of an abnormal haemoglobin
molecule in red blood cells. The third phase, sometimes called 'the new
genetics', stems from technologies developed in the late 1970s which allow
direct analysis of genes themselves. Although each phase has added to the
power of the preceding one, the potential of gene analysis for the diagnosis
of genetic disorders is almost without limit.

For the obstetrician, the major impact of the new genetics has been in
expanding the range of prenatal diagnosis and in changing its timing. Traditional methods of diagnosis of genetic disorders use second-trimester amniocentesis, culture of amniotic fluid cells and measurement of enzyme activities
after several weeks of cell growth. Prenatal diagnosis is not possible if the
expressed protein abnormality in the genetic disorder is unknown (e.g. cystic
fibrosis, muscular dystrophy). It is also impossible if the known protein abnormality is not expressed in cultured amniotic fluid cells (e.g. as in phenylketonuria). The power of gene probe analysis lies in the fact that it concentrates
on the genetic material itself rather than on the protein products. Thus,
diagnosis is possible on some disorders where the protein pathology is completely obscure, and on others where amniotic fluid cells are unsuitable for
enzymatic analysis. Furthermore, since adequate samples of DNA may be
extracted from a few milligrams of chorionic villus, the new genetics is beginning to shift the timing of prenatal diagnosis from the second to the first
trimester.

TECHNOLOGY OF GENE PROBE ANALYSIS

Restriction enzymes

Several new techniques have contributed to the success of gene probe analysis. One of these was the discovery of restriction endonucleases—bacterial enzymes which cleave double-stranded DNA in a highly specific and reproducible manner. For example, the restriction enzyme *Taq* I cuts DNA at the four-base recognition site TCGA, and only at that site, while *Hind* III cuts selectively at the six-base site AAGCTT. Well over 100 restriction enzymes are now commercially available, each one recognizing particular sites in DNA for cleavage. Extraction of DNA from a chorionic villus sample and digestion with a restriction enzyme will produce a set of specific fragments for subsequent manipulation and analysis. Since the genomic DNA of each person is unique (except for monozygous twins), it is possible in principle to find a restriction enzyme which will produce an individual-specific set of cleavage products. In practice this is tedious and unnecessary. Since genetic disorders are inherited, it is usually sufficient to employ a restriction enzyme (or set of restriction enzymes) which allows the transmission of the mutant gene from the parents to the fetus to be followed.

Southern blots

The central procedure in gene analysis is the Southern blot, named after its inventor, E. M. Southern (1975). A schematic representation of this technique is shown in Figure 3.1. Genomic double-stranded DNA can be extracted by standard methods from any nucleated cell. Favoured sources are white blood cells, cultured skin fibroblasts or amniotic fluid cells, and chorionic villus samples. The DNA is digested to completion with an appropriate restriction enzyme to give a mixture of fragments ranging in length from about 0.5 to 20 kilobases (kb). The mixture is fractionated by agarose gel electrophoresis so that the smaller fragments move furthest while the larger fragments stay near the origin. The DNA is denatured or rendered single-stranded by soaking in alkali, and is then transferred by blotting onto a nitrocellulose or nylon membrane. Both types of membrane bind single-stranded DNA, so that the 'blot' becomes a perfect single-stranded replica of the original double-stranded electrophoresis gel.

Single-stranded DNA will hybridize or anneal to any other DNA which contains complementary sequences (referred to as a DNA probe). The strength of hybridization depends on the degree of complementarity and the stringency of the washing solution. If the DNA probe is radioactively tagged, the fragment of DNA to which it anneals on the Southern blot can be visualized by autoradiography. The position on the blot (distance from the origin) gives an indication of the size of the DNA fragments detected. Sizes are measured in kilobases, 1 kb representing a sequence of 1000 nucleotide bases.

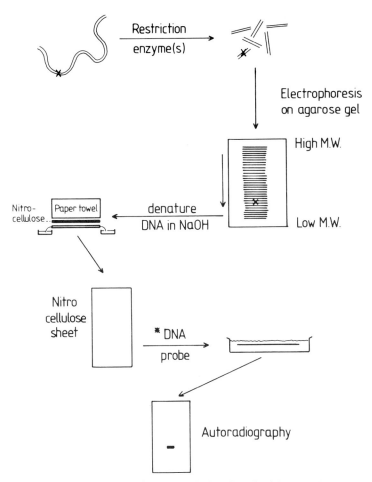

Fig. 3.1 Schematic representation of Southern blotting. Details of the procedures are given in the text. The cross represents a stretch of DNA in the original extract to which the radioactively labelled probe will hybridize

DNA probes

Identification of a DNA fragment on a Southern blot depends on hybridization—the ability of a radioactively labelled single-stranded DNA molecule (the probe) to recognize an immobilized strand on the blot which has complementary sequences. Probes can be obtained in a number of ways: they may be pieces of genomic DNA which have been amplified by cloning and thus greatly enriched for a particular sequence (genomic probes); they may be synthesized by preparing a DNA copy of a messenger-RNA sequence using enzymes known as reverse transcriptases (complementary DNA or cDNA probes); or they may be synthesized chemically by linking together a short stretch of nucleotides of an exactly specified sequence. Although most DNA fragments on a Southern blot are quite large (500–20 000 base pairs or

0.5–20 kb), a stretch of 17–20 bases usually has enough specificity to recognize a unique sequence in the fragment. These short stretches, or oligonucleotides, can now be made rapidly and specifically in machines called 'DNA synthesizers'. All probes, whatever their origin, must be tagged in some way (usually by radioactive labelling with ^{32}P) to be useful.

The jargon

Molecular biology is full of baffling and often incomprehensible jargon. The key pieces of terminology necessary for understanding gene probe analysis are:

1. *Extraction*—isolation of DNA from an appropriate tissue;
2. *Digestion*—specific cleavage of DNA by restriction enzymes;
3. *Blotting*—separation of DNA fragments by molecular weight size and transfer to a membrane;
4. *Probing*—identification of a DNA fragment by hybridization with a radioactively tagged probe. The probe can be genomic DNA, cDNA or an oligonucleotide.

An excellent account of the practical aspects of gene probe analysis is given in Davies (1986).

DIRECT ANALYSIS OF GENETIC DISEASES

Use of gene probes

Most genetic disorders are the consequence of quite subtle modifications of the gene in question, often a single base change in a sequence of 1000 or more nucleotides. For example, sickle cell anaemia is caused by a point mutation in the β-globin gene, and the consequent haemoglobin S (Hb S) differs from the normal haemoglobin A (Hb A) by one amino acid in the complete stretch of 146 amino acids. If a β-globin gene probe were used to try and detect the Hb S gene, it would not be able to distinguish it from the Hb A gene and would simply score the Hb S gene on a Southern blot as 'present'.

There are two ways in which gene probes can be used in prenatal diagnosis. The first is when there is a major change in the mutant gene, with either a complete deletion, a partial deletion or a substantial rearrangement. Thus, in most cases of α-thalassaemia, all four α-globin genes in the affected homozygote are deleted, and the use of an α-globin gene probe will demonstrate this loss on a Southern blot (Liming et al 1986). However, gene deletions are comparatively rare, and even when they do occur (e.g. in muscular dystrophy, haemophilias A and B, and β-thalassaemia) they are an infrequent occurrence in the spectrum of mutations making up the particular genetic disorder. Probably as few as 2% of cases of haemophilia A are the result of gene deletions (Gitschier et al 1985b), the remainder being made up of less dramatic mutations. Similar proportions are found in hypercholesterolaemia (Humphries et al 1985).

The second way in which gene probes can be used depends on the fact that a mutation (even a point mutation) may alter a restriction endonuclease recognition site within the gene. This can be illustrated by the example of sickle cell anaemia. The point mutation, leading to the substitution of glutamic acid by valine at position 6 in the β-globin chain, is an adenine (A) to thymine (T) change (Fig. 3.2). This has the effect of abolishing the recognition site

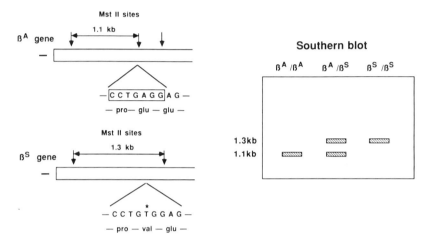

Fig. 3.2 Use of a β-globin gene probe to detect the β^S mutation which abolishes a recognition site for the restriction enzyme *Mst* II. The relevant portions of the nucleotide and amino acid sequences where the mutation has occurred are shown at the left. The Southern blot patterns for the three different genotypes are shown on the right

CCTGAGG for the restriction enzyme *Mst* II, and replacing it with CCTGTGG which *Mst* II does not cleave. Digestion of the DNA from an individual homozygous for Hb S with *Mst* II, and probing of the resulting Southern blot with a β-globin probe, produces a larger fragment than that seen in an individual homozygous for Hb A (Wilson et al 1982). Note that the heterozygous parents (β^A/β^S) have both large (1.3 kb) and normal (1.1 kb) fragments, so that the actual transmission of the mutant sickle cell gene can be followed (Fig. 3.2).

Use of oligonucleotide probes

When the exact nature of a point mutation leading to a genetic disease is known, it is possible to synthesize an oligonucleotide probe which will recognize the altered sequence. Conversely, it is possible to make an oligonucleotide which will recognize a similar sequence in the normal gene, but not in the mutant gene. In fact, oligonucleotide probes are conventionally used in pairs, one member having specificity for the normal gene and one having specificity for the mutant gene. Although oligonucleotides are usually only 17–20 base pairs in length, they can be designed to have the specificity to hybridize to DNA fragments of up to 100 times this size and to distinguish a point mutation in a sequence of several thousand base pairs.

Oligonucleotides have now been designed and used for several genetic disorders, including haemophilia B (Winship & Brownlee 1986), α_1-antitrypsin deficiency (Kidd et al 1983), phenylketonuria (Dilella et al 1986) and β-chain haemoglobinopathies (Conner et al 1983). An example can be given for one form of β-thalassaemia where a defined mutation occurs at quite high frequencies in some Mediterranean populations (Fig. 3.3). A 19-base-pair oligonucleotide (known as a 19-mer) is synthesized which is complementary to the

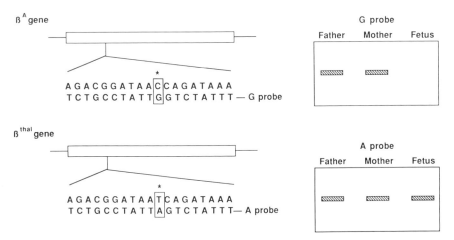

Fig. 3.3   Use of the 19-mer oligonucleotide probes to detect the mutation responsible for one form of β-thalassaemia. The G probe is complementary to the normal sequence and the A probe to the mutant sequence. As shown on the Southern blots at the right, both probes detect genes in the heterozygous parents, but the G probe shows the absence of the normal gene in the homozygous affected fetus

sequence surrounding the mutant site in the β-globin gene (A probe), while at the same time another 19-mer is made complementary to the same sequence in the normal β-globin gene (G probe). After digestion of genomic DNA from individuals at risk, and Southern blotting of the resulting fragments, the two radioactively tagged 19-mer probes are separately hybridized to the separated DNA. As shown in Figure 3.3, the G probe only recognizes the normal gene, while the A probe recognizes the mutant gene. Since the disorder is a recessive trait, the parents will be obligate heterozygotes and will be scored by both A and G probes—a useful control experiment (Weatherall 1985).

INDIRECT ANALYSIS OF GENETIC DISEASES

Principles of linkage analysis

In general, different genes tend to segregate independently of one another during transmission from one generation to the next, a fact first noted by Mendel and incorporated into his law of independent assortment. The exception occurs when genes are situated near to one another on a chromosome and when they can sometimes be transmitted together as a linked unit. This behaviour is a function of the physical distance between two genes; the closer they are together the more likely they are to stay as a unit during meiosis, while the further apart they are the more likely they are to cross over or show recombination during the scrambling process of meiosis. However, even when genes are contiguous on a chromosome, there is always a finite chance of crossing over, and it is never entirely safe to assume that linked genes will stay together in parent-to-child transmission. The frequency of crossing over, or recombination, can be measured empirically for any pair of genes by making observations on large numbers of meioses. The recombination fraction, which measures this tendency, ranges from 0.5 (independent assortment) to less than 0.01 (tight linkage).

For practical purposes linkage analysis can be used when the recombination fraction is 0.05 or less. At 0.05, linked genes will be transmitted as a unit in 95% of meioses, while in 5% of cases there will be recombination. Thus, in using linkage analysis there will be a built-in error rate in using one gene to give information on the behaviour of another.

Restriction fragment length polymorphisms

Although linkage analysis has been used for many years in the diagnosis of genetic diseases, its power has been greatly enhanced in recent years by the new techniques of molecular biology. Two factors have contributed to these advances. The first is the availability of large numbers of DNA fragments, sometimes representing actual genes and sometimes being 'anonymous' fragments, which can be used as markers of disease genes. The function of anonymous fragments does not need to be known; indeed many may not have the property of coding for specific proteins. Their linkage to a disease gene is their important attribute, and they are usually simply given a code number.

The second factor is one which could not have been predicted 10 years ago. Throughout the human genome there is a great deal of variation in individual base pairs making up the DNA, much of it occurring in regions which do not encode specific messenger-RNA or carry regulatory sequences. This variation appears to have no discernible effect on the phenotype and is referred to as neutral mutation or polymorphism. Many of these neutral mutations alter existing restriction enzyme recognition sites, either by abolishing them or by introducing new ones. Thus, digestion of genomic DNA from two different individuals with a battery of restriction enzymes will always produce a set of DNA fragments which are individual-specific. However, recognition of the variation in fragments depends on having an appropriate probe.

When a suitable probe is available it can be used to follow mutation in a restriction site on a Southern blot. If mutation has abolished the site the resulting fragment will be larger and will travel less far in the agarose gel electrophoresis, which precedes blotting (Fig. 3.4). Conversely, if a new recognition site has been introduced, a smaller fragment will run further on the

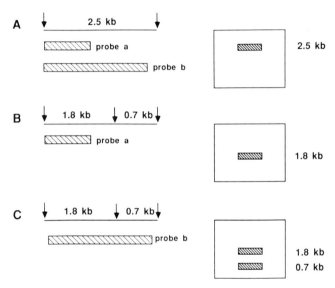

Fig. 3.4 RFLPs generated by variation in a restriction enzyme recognition site. In A the 2.5 kb fragment is detected by both probes. In B and C a new restriction site divides the 2.5 kb fragment into 1.8 kb and 0.7 kb fragments. In B the smaller probe (probe a) recognizes only the 1.8 kb fragment, while in C the larger probe (probe b) detects both 1.8 kb and 0.7 kb fragments

gel and will be identified towards the anodic end. Since the variation identified by restriction enzymes is in the size or length of the fragments, they are known as restriction fragment length polymorphisms or RFLPs. We must note that since humans are diploid organisms, individuals can be either homozygous or heterozygous for a particular RFLP (the exception is when a probe recognizes an RFLP on the X chromosome in a male). We must also note that the actual fragments recognized depend not only on the presence or absence of specific cleavage sites, but also on the size of the probe used in detection (Fig. 3.4). A probe need only be complementary to part of a DNA fragment for hybridization to occur.

Establishing phase relationships

When an RFLP is found to be linked to a particular disease gene, it can be used to track the gene through several generations of a family. However, it is not usually known in advance which of the two (or more) polymorphic variants segregates with the disease gene and which segregates with the normal gene. Thus, in any form of linkage analysis (or indirect gene analysis), establishing the phase relationship of gene and marker is of critical importance.

The rules for establishing phase relationships can sometimes be difficult for the non-specialist to interpret, and are best outlined with examples from autosomal dominant, autosomal recessive and X-linked recessive modes of inheritance. In each case critical information must be obtained from an index-affected case, and it is usually very difficult to be certain about the relationship between disease gene and marker if index individuals are not available for genotyping.

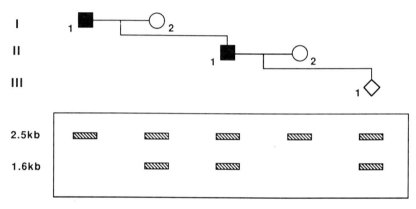

Fig. 3.5   An example of prenatal diagnosis in an autosomal dominantly inherited disorder. Heavy shading in the pedigree indicates an affected individual. Southern blot patterns for each individual in the pedigree are shown directly below in the box. In this case the at-risk fetus (III-1) is deemed unaffected. See text for details

The example shown in Figure 3.5 illustrates a prenatal exclusion of the autosomal dominant condition, myotonic dystrophy, on a chorionic villus sample, using an RFLP linked to the disease and detected by an apolipoprotein CII gene probe (Lunt et al 1986). Two fragments are detected by the probe, one measuring 2.5 kb and the other measuring 1.6 kb. The affected father (II-1) is heterozygous for the RFLP and must have inherited the myotonic gene on his 2.5 kb fragment, since his own affected father (I-1) is homozygous for this fragment. Thus, it is established that in this pedigree the myotonic gene is 'in phase' with a 2.5 kb DNA fragment. The pregnant wife (II-2) is homozygous for the 2.5 kb fragment and must transmit a normal gene also in phase with this fragment to her unborn child (III-1). By the rules of Mendelian genetics the fetus must therefore inherit the 1.6 kb fragment from its affected father, and this is not the fragment in phase with the myotonic gene. Thus, the fetus has not inherited the myotonic gene and, barring recombination, can be pronounced normal. Note that if the fetus had been homozygous for the 2.5 kb fragment it would probably have been affected.

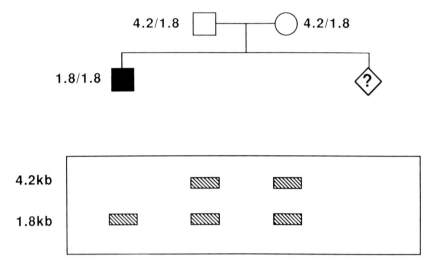

Fig. 3.6   Prenatal diagnosis of a condition inherited as an autosomal recessive. The index-affected child in the pedigree is shaded. If the fetus at risk has a single band at 1.8 kb, it will be affected. See text for details

Figure 3.6 illustrates the prenatal diagnosis of cystic fibrosis (CF), inherited as an autosomal recessive condition. Here a random DNA probe, called pJ3.11, recognizes an RFLP tightly linked to the CF gene (Wainwright et al 1985). Genomic DNA, extracted from blood of the parents and index-affected child and digested with the restriction enzyme *Msp* I, can produce two fragments of lengths measuring 4.2 or 1.8 kb. If both parents are heterozygous for the fragments (4.2/1.8), while the index-affected child is homozygous (1.8/1.8), it can be inferred that the CF gene is in phase with the 1.8 kb fragment in both paternal and maternal branches of the family. Genotyping of a chorionic villus sample produces an unambiguous result; 1.8/1.8 signals an affected fetus, 4.2/1.8 a heterozygous normal fetus and 4.2/4.2 a homozygous normal fetus.

An example of the use of RFLP analysis in the prenatal diagnosis of the X-linked recessive condition, haemophilia A, is shown in Figure 3.7 (Gitschier et al 1985a). The patient seeking advice (II-2) has an affected brother, and therefore has a 50% chance of carrying the haemophilia gene. A factor VIII gene probe detects a common polymorphism, with restriction enzyme *Bcl* I giving fragment lengths of 1.2 and 0.9 kb. The consultand is heterozygous for this polymorphism, while her affected brother (II-1) is hemizygous for the 0.9 kb fragment. Since the fetus at risk (III-1) has not inherited this chromosome, he can be assumed to be a normal male. (In X-linked recessive

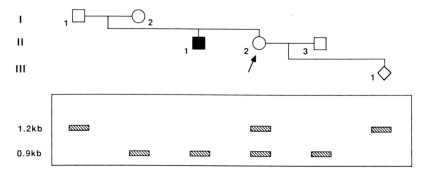

Fig. 3.7 Prenatal diagnosis of an X-linked recessive condition. The brother (II-1) of the proband (arrowed) is affected. The fetus at risk (III-1) is deemed to be an unaffected male. See text for details

inheritance, males are hemizygous, while females can be heterozygous or homozygous.)

Informativeness

It often happens that RFLPs do not give adequate information on the phase relationships in a family. For example, Figure 3.8 is a variation of the CF

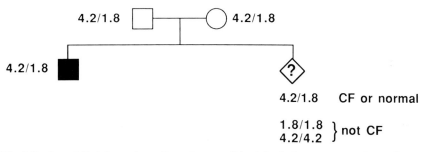

Fig. 3.8 A partially informative pedigree for a condition inherited as an autosomal recessive. The index-affected child has the same genotype as each of its parents. The diagnosis on the fetus at risk will be either 'not CF' or 'not known'

pedigree of Figure 3.6, but in this case the index-affected child has the same band pattern as its parents. This means that it is not known whether it is the 4.2 kb fragment in the father which is in phase with the CF gene, or whether it is the 4.2 kb fragment in the mother. However, since the affected child must inherit a CF gene from each parent, some predictions can be made on a chorionic villus sample. Homozygous band patterns (1.8/1.8 or 4.2/4.2) show that the fetus does not have the disease. A heterozygous band pattern (4.2/1.8) is uninformative, and the fetus has a 50% chance of being affected and an equal chance of being normal. Such situations are referred to as being 'partially informative'.

Table 3.1 Genetic disorders where a first-trimester prenatal diagnosis has been carried out by the use of DNA-based methodology (December 1986)

Genetic disorder	Mode of inheritance*	References
α-Thalassaemia	AR	Old et al 1986
		Liming et al 1986
β-Thalassaemia	AR	Old et al 1982, 1986
Sickle cell anaemia	AR	Old et al 1982, 1986
Cystic fibrosis	AR	Farrall et al 1986
Phenylketonuria	AR	Lidsky et al 1985
α_1-Antitrypsin deficiency	AR	Kidd et al 1984
		Hejtmancik et al 1986
Haemophilia A	XR	Tonnesen et al 1984b
		Gitschier et al 1985a
Haemophilia B	XR	Tonnesen et al 1984a
Duchenne muscular dystrophy	XR	Bakker et al 1985
Ornithine transcarbamylase deficiency	XR	Old et al 1985
		Pembrey et al 1985
Choroideraemia	XR	Robertson et al 1986
Polycystic kidney disease	AD	Reeders et al 1986
Myotonic dystrophy	AD	Lunt et al 1986

* AR autosomal recessive, XR X-linked recessive, AD autosomal dominant

Informativeness can be increased by using a probe which recognizes an RFLP with multiple alleles, so that the chance of any individual having a unique pattern is high. Alternatively, several different probes can be used, provided that each recognizes an RFLP tightly linked to the gene in question. For example, there are now eight different probes available which detect DNA polymorphisms linked to the CF gene. If all eight probes are used, virtually every family in which this gene is segregating becomes fully informative.

Error rates

The use of gene probes in diagnosis is not without error. Direct probing for a gene deletion or a variant restriction enzyme site within the gene is theoretically error-free, as is the use of oligonucleotides for the detection of defined mutations. However, most forms of gene probe analysis currently depend on the analysis of RFLPs co-segregating with a disease. Here the recombination rate between the marker and the gene is a finite source of error and must not be overlooked in counselling.

In the example shown in Figure 3.5 it was stated that the fetus 'can be pronounced normal'. However, it is known that recombination between the myotonic gene and the apolipoprotein CII locus occurs in about 4% of meioses (Lunt et al 1986). Thus, correct counselling would point out that, in the pedigree in Figure 3.5, the odds of an affected fetus have been reduced from 50% to 4%, and that there is still a residual risk of the child developing myotonic dystrophy in later life. These inherent error rates can be reduced by finding RFLPs with tighter linkage to the gene in question, but they can never be entirely eliminated.

ACHIEVEMENTS

The principles and methodology of gene probe analysis have been outlined in the preceding sections. Much of the technology is evolving, and its application to actual first-trimester prenatal diagnoses is still limited. Considerable experience in the use of DNA probes on the major haemoglobinopathies—α-thalassaemia, β-thalassaemia and sickle cell anaemia (Old et al 1986, Liming et al 1986)—has accumulated. In other disorders (Table 3.1) the examples of successful diagnoses are still sparse. But there is little doubt that the 'new genetics' will play an increasingly important role in the first-trimester diagnosis of Mendelian disorders in the coming years.

REFERENCES

Bakker E, Hofker M H, Goor N et al 1985 Prenatal diagnosis and carrier detection of Duchenne muscular dystrophy with closely linked RFLPs. Lancet i: 655–658
Conner B J, Reyes A A, Morin C et al 1983 Detection of sickle cell β^S-globin allele by hybridisation with synthetic oligonucleotides. Proceedings of the National Academy of Sciences 80: 278–282
Davies K E 1986 Human genetic diseases: a practical approach, IRL Press, Oxford
Dilella A G, Marvit J, Lidsky A S et al 1986 Tight linkage between a splicing mutation and a specific DNA haplotype in phenylketonuria. Nature 322: 799–803
Farrall M, Law H Y, Rodeck D H et al 1986 First-trimester prenatal diagnosis of cystic fibrosis with linked DNA probes. Lancet i: 1402–1405
Gitschier J, Lawn R M, Rotblat F et al 1985a Antenatal diagnosis and carrier detection of haemophilia A using Factor VIII gene probe. Lancet i: 1093–1094
Gitschier J, Wood W I, Tuddenham E G D et al 1985b Detection and sequence of mutations in the Factor VIII gene of haemophiliacs. Nature 315: 427–430
Hejtmancik J F, Sifers R N, Ward P A et al 1986 Prenatal diagnosis of α_1-antitrypsin deficiency by direct analysis of the mutation site in the gene. Lancet ii: 767–770
Humphries S E, Kessling A M, Horsthemke B et al 1985 A common DNA polymorphism of the low-density lipoprotein (LDL) receptor gene and its use in diagnosis. Lancet i: 1003–1005
Kidd V J, Wallace R B, Itakura K et al 1983 α_1-Antitrypsin deficiency detection by direct analysis of the mutation in the gene. Nature 304: 230–234
Kidd V J, Golbus M S, Wallace R B et al 1984 Prenatal diagnosis of α-1-antitrypsin deficiency by direct analysis of the mutation site in the gene. New England Journal of Medicine 310: 639–642
Lidsky A S, Guttler F, Woo S L C 1985 Prenatal diagnosis of classic phenylketonuria by DNA analysis. Lancet i: 549–551
Liming W, Junwu Z, Guanyun W et al 1986 First-trimester prenatal diagnosis of severe α-thalassaemia. Prenatal Diagnosis 6: 89–95
Lunt P W, Meredith A L, Harper P S 1986 First-trimester prediction in fetus at risk for myotonic dystrophy. Lancet ii: 350–351
Old J M, Ward R H T, Petrou M et al 1982 First-trimester diagnosis for haemoglobinopathies. Three cases. Lancet ii: 1413–1416
Old J M, Briand P L, Purvis-Smith et al 1985 Prenatal exclusion of ornithine transcarbamylase deficiency by direct gene analysis. Lancet i: 73–75
Old J M, Fitches A, Heath C et al 1986 First-trimester fetal diagnosis for haemoglobinopathies: report on 200 cases. Lancet ii: 763–767
Pembrey M E, Old J M, Leonard J V et al 1985 Prenatal diagnosis of ornithine carbamoyl transferase deficiency using a gene-specific probe. Journal of Medical Genetics 22: 462–465
Reeders S T, Zerres K, Gal A et al 1986 Prenatal diagnosis of autosomal dominant polycystic kidney disease with a DNA probe. Lancet ii: 6–8
Robertson M E, Hodgson S V, Fisher J A et al 1986 Prenatal exclusion in a family where choroideraemia is associated with a small Xq deletion. Journal of Medical Genetics 22: 472

Southern E M 1975 Detection of specific sequences among DNA fragments separated by gel electrophoresis. Journal of Molecular Biology 98: 503–517

Tonnesen T, Sondergaard F, Guttler F et al 1984a Exclusion of haemophilia B in male fetus by chorionic villus biopsy. Lancet ii: 932

Tonnesen T, Sondergaard B, Mikkelson M et al 1984b X-chromosome-specific probe DX13 for carrier detection and first trimester prenatal diagnosis in haemophilia A. Lancet ii: 1269–1270

Wainwright B J, Scambler P J, Schmidtke J et al 1985 Localisation of cystic fibrosis locus to human chromosome 7cen-q22. Nature 318: 384–385

Weatherall D J 1985 The new genetics and clinical practice, 2nd edn, Oxford University Press, London

Wilson J T, Milner P F, Summer M E et al 1982 Use of restriction endonucleases for mapping the allele for β^S-globin. Proceedings of the National Academy of Sciences 79: 3628–3631

Winship P R, Brownlee G G 1986 Diagnosis of haemophilia B carriers using intragenic oligonucleotide probes. Lancet ii: 218–219

High-risk pregnancies

INTRODUCTION

A 'high-risk pregnancy' is defined as a pregnancy in which there is a risk of a serious adverse outcome in the mother and/or the baby that is greater than the incidence of that outcome in the general population.

All pregnancies receive conventional antenatal care which, in quantity and quality, is based on the resources and personnel available. When a factor is identified in an individual mother that is associated with an increased risk of a specific adverse outcome (and the pregnancy is thus labelled 'high risk'), additional antenatal care is given which either prevents, anticipates, treats or minimises the effect of that adverse outcome. Once again, the nature and amount of this additional antenatal care is determined by the resources available.

The following approach will be used for this chapter:

1. What are the more important risk factors in pregnancy?
2. What are the specific risks associated with those factors
   (a) for the mother?
   (b) for the baby?
3. What additional antenatal care, over and above that provided routinely, would be appropriate for pregnancies where such specific high-risk factors are identified?

SOCIOMEDICAL RISK FACTORS

Age

The maternal mortality rate (MMR) and the perinatal mortality rate (PNMR) are lowest for mothers in their twenties. Both maternal and perinatal mortality rates rise progressively with maternal age, mothers aged over 40 years having a MMR nearly ten times and a PNMR over three times that of mothers in their mid-twenties (OPCS 1984, DHSS 1986). Specific complications of pregnancy that are commoner in the older woman include hypertension,

Table 4.1 Maternal age and risk of fetal chromosomal abnormality (Data from Harper 1984)

Maternal age (years)	All chromosomal abnormalities (rate per 1000 amniocenteses)	Down's syndrome	
		Rate per 1000 births	Risk
All ages		1.5	1:650
35	8.7	2.2	1:450
36	10.1	2.5	1:400
37	12.2	4.0	1:250
38	14.8	5.0	1:200
39	18.4	6.5	1:150
40	23.0	10.0	1:100
44	96.0	25.0	1:40

placental abruption and intra-uterine growth retardation. Thus, with a woman in her late thirties, vigilance should be maintained for these complications.

Fetal chromosomal abnormalities are also commoner in the older woman. The mother at booking should be counselled as to the risks (Table 4.1) (Harper 1984). For the woman aged 32–37, the wisdom of offering prenatal diagnosis can be judged on the basis of estimating a combined risk based on her age and the value of her serum alpha-fetoprotein estimation (Murday & Slack 1985). A combined risk greater than one in 200 might be considered to be a suitable cut-off point for offering prenatal diagnosis. Prenatal diagnosis should be offered to all women aged over 38 years. Prenatal diagnosis in the form of chorion villus sampling (CVS) (at 8–12 weeks) or amniocentesis (at 16 weeks) is not without risks, including abortion, intra-uterine death, amniotic fluid leak, infection, haematoma and rhesus isoimmunisation (Rodeck 1984).

Teenagers also have higher maternal and perinatal mortality rates. In older teenagers, however, who are receiving adequate antenatal care, pregnancy does not appear as hazardous as was previously thought; nevertheless, they present late in pregnancy and are poor clinic attenders. For younger teenagers, pregnancy is more serious. They are at greater risk of hypertension and pre-term labour, though from a practical point of view all that can be done is to maintain a greater degree of vigilance for these complications in such mothers. Probably of most value during pregnancy and the puerperium, if appropriate, is social worker involvement to help with domestic and schooling problems, sympathetic midwifery support to help these mothers to learn more about mothering, and satisfactory contraceptive counselling (Bury 1985).

Ethnic group

All non-whites should be screened for evidence of haemoglobinopathy. If carrier status is confirmed, then the partner should also be tested. If similarly he is positive, then the couple should be counselled regarding possible prenatal diagnosis either by CVS, amniocentesis or fetal blood sampling (Rodeck 1984).

The mother with sickle cell disease is at special risk. Maternal complications commoner in such pregnancies include infection, sickling crises, pre-eclampsia and, more rarely, renal compromise and jaundice. The fetus is at risk of growth retardation and acute hypoxia, especially during a crisis and in labour. During pregnancy the mother's haemoglobin (Hb) should be regularly measured and the percentage of Hb A estimated. Donations of fresh, carefully cross-matched blood (at least two units at a time) are transfused weekly until the Hb is over 11.0 g/dl and the HB A is over 70%. Though antibiotics are not given prophylactically during the antenatal period, vigilance must be maintained for any evidence of infection. Bacteriuria should be excluded regularly. There should be a low threshold for the prescription of antibiotics. With any clinical indication of infection the mother should be admitted to hospital to ensure adequate hydration, warmth and oxygenation in addition to the antibiotics. Fetal growth and renal and liver function should be monitored regularly. Vigilance for hypertensive problems must be maintained. If a crisis is suspected than admission to hospital is mandatory. A cause should be sought (especially an infective one) and adequate hydration, oxygenation and antibiotic ensured. The principles regarding labour and delivery are to ensure adequate hydration and oxygenation and to perform continuous fetal heart rate monitoring. Labour, delivery and the first 2 weeks of the puerperium should be covered with prophylactic antibiotics (Morrison 1982, Letsky 1984).

Oriental women should be screened for hepatitis B surface antigen (HB Ag). If this is found to be positive, then their e-antigen status should be determined so that their infectivity (both to attendants and to the baby) can be determined more precisely. Special precautions should be taken when handling blood samples from such patients and during labour. Most units have well-documented protocols for such procedures. The paediatricians should be informed since the baby may have to be given HB immunoglobulin and/or HB vaccine (Sever et al 1979).

Smoking

Cigarette smoking during pregnancy is associated with a higher incidence of spontaneous abortion, a lower birth weight (shown in both pre-term delivery and growth retardation) and perinatal mortality. The risk varies with the number of cigarettes smoked daily and the presence of other risk factors (Bottoms 1982).

Attempts to stop the mother smoking are likely to be unsuccessful in the majority of cases (Lumley 1987). Nevertheless, the woman should be encouraged to stop or reduce her smoking and the risks explained. This is especially important where there are additional risk factors such as intra-uterine growth retardation, hypertension or diabetes.

Alcohol

Alcohol consumption during the first trimester of pregnancy is associated with an increased incidence of spontaneous abortion and congenital abnormality. Later on in pregnancy, drinking 100 g of alcohol per week has a significant effect on fetal growth (10 g of alcohol is equivalent to one glass of wine, one short or half a pint of beer or lager). Women who drink to excess (over 80 g of alcohol per day) in their pregnancy are at risk of producing the fetal alcohol syndrome (the syndrome includes moderate mental retardation, microcephaly, poor co-ordination and tone, behavioural abnormalities, growth retardation and certain facial abnormalities) (Zuspan 1982, Wright 1983).

All mothers should be encouraged to avoid alcohol ingestion during pregnancy. Those with chronic alcoholism present a number of problems. The first is in diagnosis, the woman perhaps not admitting to her addiction. An elevated mean corpuscular cell volume or gamma-glutamyl transferase might be helpful in this respect. Once such a mother is identified then appropriate experienced help and psychological support should be offered.

Drug abuse

Anaemia, premature rupture of the membranes, sexually transmitted diseases, urinary infection and fetal and neonatal dependence are all problems in mothers addicted to drugs.

Experienced psychiatric input is essential for such pregnancies. Dietary review is advisable since such patients frequently have a poor diet. Iron and folate supplements should be given. Regular laboratory investigations undertaken throughout the pregnancy include tests for haemoglobin, liver and renal function, HB Ag, urine culture and sexually transmitted diseases (such as syphilis, trichomoniasis, chlamydiosis, herpes simplex, gonorrhoea, hepatitis B and AIDS).

If fetal compromise is suspected, then assessment of fetal health can be difficult. Urinary and serum oestriol values are often low without necessarily reflecting poor fetoplacental function. Non-stress cardiotocography can also be unhelpful since an addicted fetus can often be inactive. Biophysical profile testing (plus stress testing if abnormal) perhaps is the best method of assessing the fetus.

Whilst a detoxification programme may be instituted in pregnancy, coupled perhaps with methadone substitution, total abstinence from drugs should be avoided since fetal withdrawal may be fatal.

The newborn will need supervision and treatment if withdrawal symptoms occur (Zuspan 1982).

MEDICAL RISK FACTORS

Mothers presenting in pregnancy with pre-existing medical or surgical problems known to carry an increased risk in the pregnancy are probably best managed with an established protocol which is reviewed from time to time in the light of experience and new developments (Queenan & Hobbins 1982).

Hypertension

Much debate centres around the definition of 'hypertension'. The main points to make are as follows. Blood pressure should be measured with a relaxed mother in the semi-recumbent position with a cuff which is large enough for the arm and with the base of the sphigmomanometer level with the patient's heart. Phases I and IV of the Korotkoff sounds identify the systolic and diastolic pressures respectively. A single reading is insufficient to characterise the patient's blood pressure accurately. A blood pressure of 140/90 mmHg is the conventional dividing line for obstetric hypertension. In the first half of pregnancy this is appropriate, though in the second half a higher cut-off point is advisable.

Broadly speaking, hypertension can be either caused by the pregnancy itself (pre-eclampsia) or by a long-standing problem pre-dating the pregnancy (chronic hypertension).

Pre-eclampsia is a systemic condition peculiar to the second half of pregnancy, is of unknown aetiology, and runs a progressive course until the pregnancy is completed. Hypertension is an early sign of pre-eclampsia, and vasoconstriction and reduced circulating blood volume are the pathophysiological correlates. Renal involvement with fluid retention and uricaemia is common; proteinuria occurs at a later phase in the illness and renal failure is a terminal event. Other complications of the condition include involvement of the central nervous system (cerebral oedema, convulsions, cerebral haemorrhage), liver (jaundice, hepatic rupture), coagulation system (disseminated intravascular coagulation, DIC), lungs (pulmonary oedema) and placenta (fetal growth retardation, fetal death, placental abruption).

The principles of management of the patient with pre-eclampsia are to monitor the maternal and fetal conditions, recognise early features of the more serious complications, and deliver (and hence cure) the patient either before they develop or before they jeopardise the mother or baby. In practice, the patient with early/mild disease (b.p. <160/100 mmHg, no proteinuria and no other complications) could be managed as an outpatient. In addition to monitoring the blood pressure and testing for proteinuria, fetal growth and health, renal function, clotting, liver function and the presence of symptoms should be recorded in such patients. Severe hypertension (170/110 mmHg or more) should be treated with agents such as methyldopa, beta-blockers or labetalol. Uncontrollable hypertension is an ominous feature. There is no place for the use of long-term anticonvulsants or sedatives. The only indication for diuretics is pulmonary oedema. Intravenous phenytoin or diazepam should be used for imminent or actual eclampsia.

The absolute indications in pre-eclampsia for delivery are eclampsia, renal failure (rising urea), DIC, liver involvement, acute fetal compromise and uncontrollable hypertension. The relative indications for delivery are gestation of 37 weeks or more with chronic fetal compromise and/or proteinuria.

Mothers with chronic hypertension (essential hypertension, renal disease and other rare conditions) are at greater risk of developing pre-eclampsia, and the first priority is to monitor for this condition. If anti-hypertensive therapy has been started before conception, this should be continued. There is no evidence of teratogenic effects associated with the commonly used agents. The indications for starting treatment in pregnancy are more debatable. When the maternal health is at risk (with b.p. values of 170/110 mmHG or more), then antihypertensive therapy is mandatory. At levels lower than this, the maternal health is unlikely to be at risk and, furthermore, there is no evidence that starting treatment will reduce the likelihood of pre-eclampsia developing (Redman 1984).

Chronic renal disease

Normal pregnancy is rare when plasma creatinine and urea levels exceed 275 μmol/l and 10 mmol/l respectively. These values probably represent more than 50% loss of function.

The effect of the renal disease on pregnancy is subject to some debate. The glomerular filtration rate in women with chronic renal disease, though lower than normal, nevertheless still increases during pregnancy and tends to fall towards term. Increased proteinuria is common (occurring in 50% of pregnancies) and when high (in excess of 3 g per 24 hours) carries a risk of the nephrotic syndrome. One in five women with chronic pyelonephritis have a 20% risk of recurrence of urinary infection. Pre-eclampsia is certainly commoner in patients with chronic renal disease, but it is not easy to diagnose since there may be pre-existing hypertension, proteinuria and hyperuricaemia. Perinatal mortality, pre-term delivery and fetal growth retardation are commoner.

The effect of the pregnancy on the renal disease is also a controversial area. It would appear that pregnancy has no permanent effect on renal parenchymal disease provided that renal function is only moderately compromised and that there is no hypertension. Hypertension, including pre-eclampsia, would appear to increase the risk of further renal damage.

There is little published information on long-term dialysis in pregnancy. The reports that exist would seem to indicate a high incidence (possibly 80%) of fetal loss (either as spontaneous abortion or perinatal death).

Management of such patients should be under the joint supervision of a renal physician and obstetrician. The principles of management include careful monitoring of blood pressure and treatment when elevated, assessment of renal function and fluid balance, quantifying proteinuria (when present) and serum albumin levels, detection of superimposed pre-eclampsia (can be difficult) and monitoring fetal growth and health. For most, this approach can be as an outpatient. Uncontrollable hypertension, deteriorating renal function, severe proteinuria, especially when associated with hypoalbuminaemia (<30 g/l), pre-eclampsia and fetal compromise are factors which will influence both the decision to admit a patient and also the timing of the delivery.

The prognosis for the pregnant patient with a renal transplant is very good, both for the mother and the baby. Immunosuppression with low-dose prednisolone and azathioprine does not appear to be associated with any significant teratogenic risk. Similarly, at the end of pregnancy the normal doses of these two drugs do not appear to carry any great risks to the fetus. High doses of azathioprine sufficient to produce marrow suppression in the mother may have a similar effect in the fetus and, subsequently, in the newborn infant. There is no evidence of increased graft rejection greater than that to be expected during a 40-week period. In contrast, cyclosporin A immunosuppression may be associated with a higher risk of decline of renal function. Caesarean section is commoner in these women, but this is not predominantly due to the transplant preventing vaginal delivery (Davison 1984).

Diabetes

The risks to the diabetic mother who is pregnant include pre-term labour and delivery (sometimes iatrogenic), pre-eclampsia (especially in those patients with vascular disease), vaginal bleeding, traumatic delivery and/or caesarean section and poor diabetic control (though keto-acidosis is rare).

The risks to the baby include increased perinatal mortality rate, congenital malformations (especially musculoskeletal and cardiac), macrosomia, hydramnios, fetal death, respiratory distress, metabolic problems (hypoglycaemia, hypocalcaemia, hypomagnesaemia), jaundice and the risk of diabetes in later life.

Pre-pregnancy/pre-conception counselling is now recognised as an important aspect of management of the pregnancy associated with diabetes. The main aim is to stress the importance of euglycaemia in the first trimester in reducing congenital abnormalities. It also provides the opportunity of reviewing the diabetes in general, including the diet, and discussing contraception. Good pre-conception diabetic control is established with 24-hour capillary glucose profiles (samples pre- and post-prandial, at bedtime and, if possible, during the night).

During pregnancy, management should be the joint responsibility of a diabetologist and obstetrician. Outpatient care should be the aim. The diet (high-fibre carbohydrate comprising approximately 35–40% of calories) should be reviewed; some women may be managed on diet alone. Fundoscopy should be performed every 3 months. Oral hypoglycaemic agents are best avoided. Blood glucose control is assessed by 24-hour capillary glucose profiles. These are usually performed by the patient (1–3 times weekly). The aim should be to keep pre-prandial values at less than 5.0 mmol/l and post-prandial values at less than 7.0 mmol/l. Most diabetics will require insulin to maintain these strict values. The choice of insulin and method of administration vary. Most centres use a twice daily mixture of quick and intermediate insulins (human preferably). The glycosylated haemoglobin provides a retrospective assessment of the preceding 12 weeks control. Renal function is assessed at booking and vigilance is maintained for hypertension. Fetal normality is confirmed with a detailed ultrasonic scan at 18–20 weeks. Fetal growth is monitored during the latter half of pregnancy and fetal health over the last trimester (see p. 69).

Delivery is undertaken at term in well-controlled, uncomplicated pregnancies. In the latent phase of labour the normal diet and insulin dosage are continued. In the active phase of labour it is advisable to keep the patient 'nil by mouth' and to control the blood glucose with a double-infusion regimen (5% dextrose and potassium chloride in one and a quick-acting insulin in normal saline in the other). The same strict criteria for euglycaemia apply in labour as before (see above). This double-infusion technique is suitable for caesarean section and following delivery until the mother is eating and drinking again. After delivery, the patient's insulin requirements drop dramatically to approximately one-third of their pre-delivery levels.

Screening for diabetes in pregnancy raises a number of dilemmas. The first is whether the whole population should be screened or only those at special risk (e.g. those with glycosuria, a family history of diabetes, a previous unexplained stillbirth or large baby, hydramnios). The fact that perhaps as many as 50% of patients with impaired glucose tolerance in pregnancy will be missed with a selective programme supports a whole population approach. The next dilemma is which screening test to use. Many have been described and evaluated but the simplest is a random blood glucose test, with the upper limits for normality set by the normal range for the local population. Those mothers with an elevated random blood glucose level should then receive a formal 75 g glucose tolerance test for definitive diagnosis. It is probably wise to screen for impaired glucose tolerance on more than one occasion during the pregnancy (approximately 5% are identified by screening in the first half of pregnancy, 75% by screening at the start of the last trimester), but that still leaves 25% that are only recognised during the last trimester (Gillmer 1983, Speidel 1983).

Cardiac disease

Cardiovascular disease is now found in only 1% of all pregnancies, with congenital heart disease as frequent as rheumatic heart disease. Nevertheless, heart disease remains the leading non-obstetric cause of maternal death (DHSS, 1986).

Certain forms of cardiovascular disease place the pregnant woman at considerable risk of major handicap and death, and in such cases pregnancy is ill advised. For example, the maternal mortality rate in association with pulmonary hypertension (irrespective of the cause), Marfan's syndrome and peripartum cardiomyopathy (with its high recurrence rate) ranges from 30 to 50%. Among patients with rheumatic heart disease, those with severe mitral stenosis are at greatest risk. The tighter the stenosis, the greater the risk. When found in association with atrial fibrillation, the mortality rate from mitral stenosis in pregnancy is approximately 15%. After the first trimester, labour and delivery represent the time of the highest risk of complications and death to the mother.

Risks to the fetus include spontaneous abortion, low birth weight (pre-term delivery and growth retardation) and death. These risks are related to the degree of maternal cyanosis. Finally, if one parent has congenital heart disease, the incidence of congenital heart disease in the offspring increases six-fold overall.

Diagnosis can be difficult in pregnancy. However, certain clinical features make the possibility of cardiovascular abnormality more likely. These include symptoms such as severe dyspnoea, syncope with exertion, haemoptysis, paroxysmal nocturnal dyspnoea and chest pain on exertion. The following signs are also highly suspicious: cyanosis, clubbing, a diastolic murmur, a cardiac arrhythmia, a harsh systolic murmur and cardiomegaly. Cardiological opinion, together with an electrocardiograph (ECG), echocardiography and even a chest X-ray, is mandatory when cardiovascular abnormality is suspected.

Close liaison between obstetricians and cardiologists is mandatory. The principles regarding management are as follows. Firm support, consistent information and reassurance are important. Termination of pregnancy in the first trimester should be considered if the maternal risks are great (see above). Physical activity should be limited, though whether this necessitates hospital admission depends on the individual circumstances. Iron and folate supplements are advisable. Prompt recognition and treatment of anaemia and infection are essential. Medical treatment (e.g. with digoxin, diuretics and beta-blockers) should be implemented as appropriate. Ultraonsic monitoring of fetal growth should be undertaken. Cardiovascular surgery should be reserved for those with severe disability which does not respond to conservative measures. Such surgery apparently carries no greater risk to the mother but is associated with an increased fetal loss (especially with open heart surgery and cardiopulmonary bypass).

During labour, women at risk of infective endocarditis should receive antibiotic prophylaxis for 48 hours after delivery. Such patients, in addition to the normal intrapartum observations, should have close monitoring of their clinical condition, fluid balance, ECG, fetal heart rate and, if indicated, maternal Pao_2. Caval compression should be avoided. Extra oxygen is administered via a face mask. Cardiac drugs (digoxin, diuretics, aminophylline, lignocaine, beta-blockers) should be readily available. Analgesia must be adequate. An epidural is not contraindicated except in cases where there is outflow obstruction. A short second stage avoiding undue maternal effort is advisable, and no ergot-containing preparations should be used for the third stage.

After delivery, breast feeding is to be encouraged. Contraception and even sterilisation should be discussed (Ueland 1982, de Swiet 1984a).

Auto-immune thrombocytopenic purpura (AITP)

Maternal problems in pregnancy complicated by AITP can include petechiae and bleeding from various sites, especially episiotomies and abdominal and wound incisions. This is unlikely to be serious if the platelet count is greater than 35×10^9 per litre.

Fetal and neonatal thrombocytopenia can occur because of the transplacental passage of immunoglobulin (IgG), accounting for increased perinatal morbidity and mortality, especially from intracranial haemorrhage. The baby is likely to be thrombocytopenic in 70% of cases where the maternal platelet count is less than 100×10^9 per litre. But even when the mother's count is over 100×10^9 per litre there is a 20% risk of thrombocytopenia in the infant. The risk to the baby is greater if the mother has had a splenectomy.

During pregnancy the priority should be to maintain the maternal platelet count in excess of 30×10^9 per litre by the administration of steroids. Very severely thrombocytopenic patients may require intravenous immunoglobulin.

The timing and method of delivery are important, yet difficult, decisions. Some advocate that if the maternal platelet count is above 100×10^9 per litre then vaginal delivery should be safe, and that fetal scalp sampling early in the labour showing a fetal platelet count over 50×10^9 per litre is an indication to allow the labour to continue towards a vaginal delivery. Maternal and fetal values of less than these figures are indications for caesarean section under maternal platelet cover.

The introduction of intravenous immunoglobulin has made such decisions easier. If such infusions are started 10–14 days before the expected delivery, vaginal delivery will be safe, the baby will have an adequate platelet count and even if a caesarean section is necessary subsequently, then this will be safe (Cruikshank 1982, Hegde 1985).

Epilepsy

Epilepsy is found in 0.5% of pregnancies. Nearly half of these patients will require an increase in anticonvulsant dosage to control a rise in seizure frequency occurring during pregnancy. The main risks are of uncontrolled status epilepticus producing hypoxia to the fetus and trauma to the mother. Another risk to the mother taking phenytoin is folate deficiency.

There are risks to the fetus from anticonvulsant drugs. Phenytoin produces the classic hydantoin syndrome in a few cases (growth retardation, mild mental retardation, cranial and facial abnormalities and hypoplasia of the distal phalanges with small nails). Cleft lip and palate have been reported to be commoner in babies of mothers taking phenytoin during pregnancy. Sodium valproate has been demonstrated to be associated with a higher incidence of neural tube defects. Carbamazepine has not been linked with any fetal abnormalities. It should be stressed that the incidence of congenital abnormalities associated with the use of anticonvulsant drugs during the first trimester is not greater than double the normal population rate (in other words less than 6%). Phenytoin and phenobarbitone (the latter no longer commonly used in epilepsy) carry an increased risk of neonatal bleeding due to deficiency in clotting factors II, VII, IX and X.

Ideally, epileptic patients should be seen before pregnancy so that anticonvulsant medication can be reviewed (aiming for the lowest dose of the least number of agents that controls fits) and the potential complications in pregnancy discussed.

During pregnancy, the effectiveness of seizure control should be monitored both clinically (enquiring not only for fit frequency but also for the presence of auras) and in the laboratory with various anticonvulsant levels. The aim is to keep the patient fit-free on the lowest dose of anticonvulsant. Vigilance should be maintained for features of anticonvulsant toxicity (such as ataxia, nystagmus and vertigo). Women taking phenytoin should receive extra folic acid (5 mg daily).

The newborn infant should be given vitamin K and carefully examined to exclude abnormality.

After delivery, anticonvulsant therapy in the mother should be reviewed (Kochenour 1982, Hopkins 1987).

Myasthenia gravis

In some mothers with myasthenia there is little change in their condition during the pregnancy. A few improve and some deteriorate in the second trimester. However, the most likely time for deterioration is in the immediate postnatal period. Whilst spontaneous vaginal delivery is possible, there is a higher incidence of instrumental deliveries in such patients. Muscle relaxants should be avoided if general anaesthesia is necessary since they are poorly tolerated by such women.

About 1 in 10 babies born to myasthenic mothers will have transient neonatal myasthenia requiring short-term anti-cholinesterase treatment (Hopkins 1984).

Thyroid disease

Hyperthyroidism in pregnancy, though uncommon, is an important condition to recognise because untreated it is associated with risks to the mother of pre-eclampsia and occasionally thyroid 'storm' or crisis at delivery. The risks to the baby are of growth retardation, pre-term birth, cardiac failure and death. Clinical diagnosis is difficult because of the similarity between some clinical features and those normally associated with pregnancy. Persistent tachycardia and lack of weight gain are common signs; eye signs are less frequently seen. Laboratory diagnosis is made by the demonstration of an elevated free thyroxine index.

Anti-thyroid drugs, especially carbimazole, are the treatment of choice in the management of hyperthyroidism in pregnancy. The aim of therapy is to keep the patient clinically and biochemically euthyroid on the minimum medication. Subtotal thyroidectomy should only be considered in the extremely rare case where the mother is 'resistant' to oral agents.

In approximately 2% of patients with hyperthyroidism, the cause is thyroid-stimulating IgG. The babies of such women are at risk of developing intra-uterine thyrotoxicosis (fetal tachycardia followed eventually by cardiac failure and death) due to the transplacental transmission of the antibodies. Therefore, fetal heart rate monitoring should be undertaken monthly during the last trimester to exclude this complication. An alternative approach is to characterise the nature of any thyroid-stimulating antibody (usually via a supraregional chemical pathology service) and to reserve the fetal heart rate monitoring for those patients with IgG. Should fetal tachycardia develop and delivery be deemed inappropriate because of prematurity, maternal treatment with propranolol can control the fetal condition until a gestational age is reached when elective delivery is considered to be safer.

In theory, infants born to mothers treated with hypothyroid agents could be transiently hypothyroid with goitre formation. However, this risk is minimised if the mother is given the minimum dosage that keeps her euthyroid.

Untreated hypothyroid women rarely become pregnant since ovulation is uncommon. Hypothyroid women treated with thyroxine can become pregnant and usually go through pregnancy with few complications. Some treated patients may require a slight increase in L-thyroxine dosage during the pregnancy (though very seldom in excess of 0.2 mg per 24 hours). The indications for such an increase would be the development of clinical features of hypothyrodism, confirmed by a low free thyroxine index and an elevated serum stimulating hormone concentration.

Infants of hypothyroid mothers appear to have no increased risk of congenital hypothyroidism (Mestman 1982, Ramsay 1984).

Prolactinoma

When a patient has been successfully treated for a prolactinoma, bromocriptine treatment is usually stopped once a pregnancy is diagnosed. There is no evidence of risk to the fetus of women given bromocriptine during pregnancy, but the drug does cross the placenta and can reduce fetal prolactin levels, though this seems to be of no clinical consequence. Routine assessment of visual fields is not indicated since tumour expansion, when it occurs, does so rapidly. Serial measurements of prolactin are not helpful. If pituitary expansion does occur, it results in headache and impaired vision. It can be confirmed with a CT scan of the head and bromocriptine treatment can be recommenced immediately (Tan & Jacobs 1986).

Systemic lupus erythematosus (SLE)

The effects of SLE on pregnancy include an increased risk of spontaneous abortion, low birth weight (pre-term delivery and growth retardation), super-imposed pre-eclampsia and congenital heart block, haematological complications and skin lesions in the newborn.

The patient should have monthly measurements of complement 3 and 4 levels. Sharp falls in these can herald an exacerbation of the condition, and prompt intervention in the form of starting or increasing steroid therapy may be necessary. Regular assessment of blood pressure and renal function is important, the frequency depending on the degree of renal involvement. Ultrasonic monitoring of fetal growth is essential. Fetal heart rate testing should be carried out in the last trimester to exclude congenital heart block.

More intensive assessment of maternal and fetal health would be necessary if exacerbation of SLE, pre-eclampsia or retardation of fetal growth were recognised. Similarly, the timing of delivery would be determined by the maternal and/or fetal condition. Continuous fetal heart rate monitoring in labour is mandatory.

The mother with SLE should be closely watched in the immediate puerperium, a time when exacerbation of the condition is common (Pitkin 1982, de Swiet 1984b).

Infections

There are many maternal infections which are associated with an increased risk to the fetus. Space does not permit a detailed discussion of these and the reader is referred to more exhaustive texts (Sever et al 1979).

AIDS, caused by human lymphotrophic virus type III (HTLV-III), is an infection which has only been reported in a few pregnancies to date. These early reports suggest that AIDS in pregnancy is associated with a high infection rate in the baby and that when the infant is infected the mortality is high. It should be stressed, however, that the data relating to the perinatal period are limited at present, and before rigid guidelines are established more information is needed. This applies equally to breast-feeding advice. The present practice in most units is to manage such pregnancies as for patients who are HB Ag positive, especially around labour and delivery.

Prescribed drugs

The risks (especially to the fetus) of drugs prescribed in pregnancy have been well documented (British National Formulary 1987, Rubin 1987). Table 4.2 summarises guidelines for prescribing specific drugs during pregnancy and lactation. It is not possible in this chapter to discuss comprehensively the risks associated with specific drugs and the indications for their use.

Table 4.2   Summary of guidelines for prescribing drugs during pregnancy and lactation

1. Most drugs cross the placenta and are excreted in breast milk.

2. Drugs should only be prescribed for the mother when the indications are clear and specific and the expected benefit to the mother is greater than the risk to the fetus.

3. All drugs should be avoided during the first trimester if possible.

4. Drugs used should be those with a well-documented pedigree in pregnancy rather than newer preparations.

5. The smallest effective therapeutic dose should be used for the smallest possible time.

6. Drugs contraindicated in pregnancy are as follows:
   Iodides and radio-active iodine
   Methotrexate for psoriasis
   Mono-amine oxidase inhibitors
   Oral hypoglycaemic agents
   Live viral vaccines (rubella, smallpox, measles, polio and yellow fever)
   Oral progestagens
   Ketonazole
   Reserpine
   Tetracyclines
   Phenindione

7. Drugs best avoided during pregnancy are as follows:

First trimester	*All pregnancy*	*Lactation*
Antacids	Amiodarone	Amiodarone
Iron supplements	Clofibrate	Chloramphenicol
Metronidazole	Diazoxide	Laxatives
Salicylates	Diuretics	Iodide cough mixtures
	Enalapril	
	Ergotamine	
	Hypnotics	
	Iodide cough mixtures	
	Probenecid	
	Propranolol	
	Prostaglandin synthetase inhibitors	

18. Drugs to be used under specialist supervision and with unequivocal indications are as follows:
    Anticonvulsants
    Anti-thyroid drugs
    Aminoglycoside antibiotics
    Cytotoxic drugs
    Hypotensive agents
    Lithium carbonate
    Systemic corticosteroids
    Warfarin sodium

(Data from the British National Formulary 1987, Rubin 1987)

OBSTETRIC RISK FACTORS

Previous stillbirth or neonatal death

When a mother has had a previous perinatal death it is important to accurately establish the cause. Only once this has been determined can the appropriate management for the current pregnancy be decided. For example, the patient who has lost a baby previously due to cytomegalovirus infection is at a very low risk of recurrence and does not merit intensive fetal surveillance during the pregnancy for obstetric reasons. In contrast, the woman whose previous perinatal death was due to severe proteinuric pre-eclampsia should have close monitoring of fetal and maternal health during the pregnancy, since she has at least a 10% risk of recurrence of the condition.

Previous congenital abnormality

Where there is a history of a previous child being born with a congenital abnormality either to the mother herself or in the family, the first course of action must be to obtain details of the abnormality. Then the likelihood of recurrence can be established and the mother counselled accordingly, especially with regard to prenatal diagnosis (Harper 1984).

Multiple pregnancy

All pregnancy complications occur more frequently in mothers with a multiple pregnancy (especially anaemia, placenta praevia, placental abruption, pre-term labour and post-partum haemorrhage). This fact should be reflected in their antenatal care. Thus, these patients should receive iron and folate supplements and ultrasonic evaluation of fetal growth and well-being, especially in the latter half of their pregnancy. Whilst pre-term delivery complicates as many as one-third of such pregnancies (10% deliver before 28 weeks), there is no evidence that prophylactic tocolytic agents prevent it or that regular assessment of the cervix (either clinically or by ultrasound) anticipates this complication. It is normal practice to undertake elective delivery at 38–40 weeks.

Pre-term uterine activity

More women are admitted to hospital complaining of contractions than are those in pre-term labour. The first priority, therefore, when evaluating the mother with pre-term uterine activity is to establish whether there is any evidence that she is in pre-term labour and consequently at risk of pre-term delivery. The strength and frequency of uterine contractions are only part of the necessary clinical assessment. The woman with an unengaged presenting fetal part and a cervix which is uneffaced and closed is unlikely to be in labour.

Once a clinical diagnosis of pre-term labour has been made, the second priority is to establish a cause, if possible. Thus, maternal infection (especially urinary), premature rupture of the membranes, antepartum haemorrhage, multiple pregnancy, hydramnios, uterine abnormalities, cervical incompetence, fetal abnormality or death should all be considered.

Only after these two priorities have been addressed can reasonable management plans be established. For example, if the cervix is 4 or more centimetres dilated, it is unlikely that any attempts to arrest the pre-term labour (from whatever cause) will be successful. The cause will directly influence the decision to use tocolytic agents; their use is ill-advised/contraindicated with antepartum haemorrhage, premature rupture of the membranes and fetal abnormality or death, and with sepsis as the cause the concomitant use of antibiotics is mandatory.

Finally, gestation is important. Pre-term labour at 34 weeks or more should not be suppressed as the outlook for a normal fetus beyond this gestation is excellent. The mother with pre-term labour at 28–32 weeks could be considered for steroid therapy to stimulate surfactant production, but the number of cases where a 48-hour course can be completed is limited (Pett et al 1983).

Premature rupture of the membranes (PROM)

This is defined as rupture of the membranes before the onset of regular uterine contractions. It occurs in only 10% of all pregnancies but in over 33% of pre-term deliveries.

The two main risks or consequences of PROM are (1) labour and delivery and (2) infection of the mother (pelvic sepsis) and/or baby (chorio-amnionitis). Gestational age is fundamentally important as both the incidence and effects of labour and sepsis following PROM vary with gestation. In general, if PROM occurs before 34 weeks, the risks of pre-term delivery far outweigh the risks of infection, whereas infection is more common and comprises the predominant risk after 33 weeks (Mead 1983).

Infection surveillance should be implemented when the duration of membrane rupture exceeds 24 hours. The diagnosis of intra-auterine infection is not easy. Gram stain and culture of the liquor are the best indicators of intra-uterine infection. The presence of group A or B streptococci or *Neisseria gonorrhoeae* in vaginal liquor is an indication to deliver. The discovery of other organisms is an indication to attempt amniocentesis for definitive diagnosis, though this will only be successful in 50% of cases.

If intra-uterine infection is confirmed, the patient is given antibiotics and delivered. The vaginal route is not contraindicated. Caesarean section is undertaken for the normal obstetric indications.

There is no evidence to support the use of prophylactic antibiotics in PROM. Labour occurring after PROM should not be suppressed.

With PROM before 34 weeks it is advisable to transfer the patient to a regional perinatal unit with facilities for neonatal intensive care. Indications for delivery include labour, the presence of phosphatidylglycerol in the liquor (tested daily if possible), fetal distress or intra-uterine infection. If these signs are absent, the management may vary with gestation. An aggressive approach (systemic steroids for 48 hours and then delivery) is more reasonable towards 33 weeks, and a conservative approach (no steroids and waiting) is advisable around 28 weeks.

With PROM after 33 weeks there are also two approaches. The aggressive approach involves inducing labour as soon as possible after PROM; there is no evidence that this approach results in less infection. The conservative approach involves waiting for 24 hours for spontaneous labour (85% success). Induction is only necessary in the 15% not in labour after that time. This method probably produces fewer caesarean sections. It is advisable at 34 and 35 weeks (James 1983).

Abnormal uterine size

In the following discussion it will be assumed that the 'dates' are correct and confirmed by ultrasonic scan in the first half of pregnancy. Thus the discussion relates to pathologically abnormal uterine size.

When a patient has a uterus that is 'small-for-dates', the cause must be ascertained. Maternal-related causes include excessive alcohol ingestion, pre-eclampsia, placental abruption and systemic lupus erythematosus. Clinical and laboratory investigations should be directed towards excluding these conditions. Whilst smoking, racial and genetic factors result in a small baby, severe growth retardation is not common.

A detailed ultrasonic scan of the fetus is performed to establish not only fetal size (by measurement of biparietal diameter, head circumference, abdominal circumference and head-to-abdomen ratio) but also ultrasonic fetal normality. Chromosomal abnormality or fetal viral infection are other important causes to consider and it may be that fetal blood sampling is necessary to exclude these (Sabbagha & Tamura 1983, Rodeck 1984).

Naturally, the management will depend on the cause. If the fetus is normal and the decision is that pregnancy should continue until a more mature gestation is achieved, then fetal health should be closely monitored with regular cardiotocography (CTG) or biophysical profiles (BPP) (Chamberlain & Manning 1983). The frequency of testing will depend on the severity of the retardation but should be at least twice weekly with CTGs and at least weekly with BPPs.

The patient with a uterus that is 'large-for-dates' should have a detailed ultrasonic scan to exclude multiple pregnancy, fetal abnormality (especially those producing intestinal obstruction) and hydramnios. Glucose tolerance should be tested.

Prolonged pregnancy

The continuing debate over the risks associated with and the management of prolonged pregnancy has been well reviewed by Steer (1986). Whilst most studies have shown an increase in perinatal mortality (PNM) at 42 weeks or more, this is only slight and certainly much less than the overall population PNM rate and the rate prior to 37 weeks. Despite such relatively small differences there have been large increases in induction rates for prolonged pregnancy over recent years, with reassuring falls in prolonged pregnancy PNM rates (though these are proportionately much smaller). Overall, the evidence

would not seem to support a causative association between the two observations. Furthermore, there is reason to suspect that the rise in the induction
rate might be producing an increase in the caesarean section rate.

Whilst many obstetricians will continue to feel that induction of labour
for prolonged pregnancy is a reasonable approach, there is good evidence
that techniques used in the evaluation of the fetus suspected of growth failure
(see above) are effective in the safe conservative management of 'postmaturity'.
Perhaps in otherwise uncomplicated but prolonged pregnancies the better
course of action is to implement such fetal surveillance, and in the absence
of signs of fetal compromise await the spontaneous onset of labour?

Rhesus antibodies

Rhesus disease still occurs, though much less commonly than 30 years ago
due to the advent of prophylaxis. The frequency, however, is such that severe
cases are probably best managed in a regional centre.

When rhesus antibodies are detected in a mother by routine antenatal serological surveillance, the rhesus genotype of her consort should be determined.
Antibody quantitation should carried out at least monthly. If the anti-D antibody concentration remains below $0.5 \mu g/ml$, term delivery without prior
amniocentesis is safe. Values above this merit amniocentesis, the timing of
this being determined by the absolute concentration, the rate of concentration
rise and the past obstetric history. Thus a level over $4.0 \mu g/ml$, a rapidly
rising concentration and a previously severely affected fetus warrant early
(20–22 weeks) amniocentesis. The severity of the fetal haemolytic process
is best assessed by estimating the amniotic fluid content (by measuring the
optical density difference at 450 nm) and relating the value to prediction zones
for the gestation (as described for example by Liley). Ultrasonic evaluation
for evidence of fetal or placental oedema, fetal ascites or pleural effusions
and polyhydramnios is essential.

The severity of the rhesus disease, as estimated from the amniocentesis
coupled with ultrasound examination, will determine the optimum management. This can vary from mild disease requiring no more than delivery at
37–38 weeks, to moderate disease requiring moderate pre-term delivery (e.g.
32–36 weeks), to more severe disease requiring some additional therapy. Such
additional therapy can itself vary.

Rescue by 48-hour steroid treatment followed by very early delivery (28–32
weeks) is considered by some to be the optimum approach, especially when
high-quality neonatal intensive care facilities exist. Amniotic fluid phospho-
lipid analysis for fetal surfactant production is a useful adjunct to decision-
making.

Intra-uterine transfusion (IUT) (either intraperitoneally or intravenously)
under ultrasound control remains a fetal life-saving procedure with severe
disease, especially before 28 weeks. Very stringent indications must be applied
for the use of this technique. IUT has recently been demonstrated to dramati-

cally improve the prognosis, even for fetuses with hydrops, with the hydrops actually resolving in many cases.

Some centres advocate intensive plasmapheresis started in early pregnancy. The advantage of this technique is that it can be started at a very early stage in pregnancy. It is, however, expensive and not without some risk to the mother. It has not been subjected to controlled clinical trial. Finally, it is possible to subject a patient, with a history of a previously affected pregnancy, to a programme of plasmapheresis on the basis of relatively high rhesus-antibody levels in early pregnancy, only to find that the fetus is rhesus-negative and unaffected (Whitfield 1983).

ALPHA-FETOPROTEIN (AFP)

The AFP screening programme is designed to identify those women at high risk of carrying a fetus with an open neural tube defect (NTD). Since there is an overlap between the distribution of values for mothers with normal fetuses and that for mothers with affected fetuses, there is no particular level which discriminates totally between normal and abnormal cases. A low 'cut-off' level, whilst including all affected pregnancies, would include a high proportion of normal pregnancies. Conversely, a high 'cut-off' level would exclude normal pregnancies but miss more affected pregnancies. Thus, each centre offering an AFP service chooses an arbitrary 'cut-off' level which is determined by its local experience. This is usually between 2.3 and 2.5 multiples of the normal median value. For example, operating a maternal AFP 'cut-off' level of 2.5 will detect 90% of cases of anencephaly and 80% of cases of open NTDs, but will include 3% of normal pregnancies. The subject is further complicated in that values for AFP in the maternal serum vary with gestation and also that values must be adjusted for maternal weight.

When an elevated maternal serum AFP is discovered at 16–18 weeks, a detailed ultrasonic scan must be performed to confirm gestational age and exclude multiple pregnancy (a benign cause of elevated AFP) and obvious fetal abnormality (especially anterior abdominal wall defects in addition to NTD). Whilst centres of excellence suggest that a detailed scan at 18–20 weeks may supplant the need for an AFP screening programme for most units, the two procedures are probably complementary. If there is no obvious abnormality on the scan and the second AFP is still raised, then an amniocentesis should be undertaken not only for liquor AFP concentration but also for the presence of acetyl-cholinesterase. The latter distinguishes open NTDs from other abnormalities associated with elevated AFP levels.

In the absence of a fetal abnormality, an elevated maternal serum AFP value is associated with a higher incidence of fetal growth retardation and pre-eclampsia later in the pregnancy. Thus in such a pregnancy, once a fetal abnormality has been excluded by the protocol described above, vigilance for the development of hypertension and ultrasonic monitoring of fetal growth should be undertaken.

The use of low AFP values in identifying mothers at increased risk for Down's syndrome has been discussed above (see p. 54). (UK collaborative study 1977, Evans & Stokes 1984).

FURTHER READING AND SELECTED REFERENCES

Bottoms S 1982 Smoking. In: Queenan J T, Hobbins J C (eds) Protocols for high risk pregnancies, Medical Economics Books, New Jersey, pp 14–16
British National Formulary No 13 1987 British Medical Association and Pharmaceutical Society of Great Britain, London
Bury J K 1985 Teenage pregnancy. British Journal of Obstetrics and Gynaecology 92: 1081–1085
Chamberlain P, Manning F 1983 Biophysical approach to fetal assessment. Medicine (International) 35: 1658–1660
Cruikshank D P 1982 Idiopathic thrombocytopenic purpura. In: Queenan J T, Hobbins J C (eds) Protocols for high risk pregnancies, Medical Economics Books, New Jersey, pp 89–92
Davison J 1984 Renal disease. In: de Swiet M (ed) Medical disorders in obstetric practice, Blackwell Scientific, Oxford, pp 192–259
de Swiet M 1984a Heart disease in pregnancy. In: de Swiet M (ed) Medical disorders in obstetric practice, Blackwell Scientific, Oxford, pp 116–148
de Swiet M 1984b Systemic lupus erythematosus and other connective tissue diseases. In: de Swiet M (ed) Medical disorders in obstetric practice, Blackwell Scientific, Oxford, pp 260–269
DHSS 1986 Report on confidential enquiries into maternal deaths in England and Wales 1979–1981. DHSS Report on Health and Social Subjects No 29, HMSO, London
Evans J, Stokes I M 1984 Outcome of pregnancies associated with raised serum and normal amniotic fluid AFP concentrations. British Medical Journal 288: 1494
Gillmer M D G 1983 Diabetes in pregnancy. Medicine (International) 35: 1639–1640
Harper P S 1984 Practical genetic counselling, John Wright, Bristol
Hegde U M 1985 Immune thromboyctopenia in pregnancy and the newborn (leader article). British Journal of Obstetrics and Gynaecology 92: 657–659
Hopkins A 1984 Neurological disorders. In: de Swiet M (ed) Medical disorders in obstetrics practice, Blackwell Scientific, Oxford, pp 456–482
Hopkins A 1987 Epilepsy and anticonvulsant drugs. In: Rubin P C (ed) Prescribing in pregnancy, British Medical Journal, London, pp 96–110
Hytten F E 1980 Weight gain in pregnancy. In: Hytten F E, Chamberlain G (eds) Clinical physiology in obstetrics, Blackwell Scientific, Oxford, pp 193–233
James D 1983 Premature rupture of the membranes. Medicine (International) 1(35): 1654–1655
Kochenour N K 1982 Epilepsy. In: Queenan J T, Hobbins J C (eds) Protocols for high risk pregnancies, Medical Economics Books, New Jersey, pp 135–139
Letsky E 1984 Blood volume, haematinics, anaemia. In: de Swiet M (ed) Medical disorders in obstetic practice, Blackwell Scientific, Oxford, pp 35–69
Lumley J 1987 Stopping smoking (leader article). British Journal of Obstetrics and Gynaecology 94: 289–292
Mead P B 1983 Premature rupture of the membranes. In: Chiswick M L (ed) Recent advances in perinatal medicine, 1. Churchill Livingstone, Edinburgh, pp 77–94
Mestman J H 1982 Hyperthyroidism and hypothyroidism. In: Queenan J T, Hobbins J C (eds) Protocols for high risk pregnancies, Medical Economics Books, New Jersey, pp 119–125
Morrison J C 1982 Sickle cell disease. In: Queenan J T, Hobbins J C (eds) Protocols for high risk pregnancies, Medical Economics Books, New Jersey, pp 85–88
Murday V, Slack J 1985 Screening for Down's syndrome in the North East Thames Region. British Medical Journal 291: 1315–1318
OPCS 1984 Perinatal, neonatal and infant mortality for England and Wales 1981, OPCS DH3 84/3, London
Pett S, Dunlop P, Elder M 1983 Pre-term labour. Medicine (International) 35: 1646–1649
Pitkin R M 1982 Systemic lupus erythematosus. In: Queenan J T, Hobbins J C (eds) Protocols for high risk pregnancies, Medical Economics Books, New Jersey, pp 93–95

Queenan J T, Hobbins J C (eds) 1982 Protocols for high-risk pregnancies, Medical Economics Books, Oradel, New Jersey

Ramsay I 1984 Thyroid disease. In: de Swiet M (ed) Medical disorders in obstetric practice, Blackwell Scientific, Oxford, pp 385–404

Redman C 1984 Hypertension in pregnancy. In: de Swiet M (ed) Medical disorders in obstetrics, Blackwell Scientific, Oxford, pp 149–191

Rodeck C H 1984 Obstetric techniques in prenatal diagnosis. In: Rodeck C H, Nicolaides, K H (eds) Prenatal diagnosis, RCOG, London, pp 15–28

Rubin P C (ed) 1987 Prescribing in pregnancy. British Medical Journal, London

Sabbagha R E, Tamura R K 1983 Intrauterine growth retardation. Medicine (International) 35: 1656–1657

Sever J L, Larsen J W, Grossman J H 1979 Handbook of perinatal infections, Little Brown, Boston

Speidel B D 1983 Infant of the diabetic mother. Medicine (International) 35: 1641–1642

Steer P J 1986 Postmaturity—much ado about nothing. British Journal of Obstetrics and Gynaecology 93: 105–108

Tan S L, Jacobs H S 1986 Management of prolactinomas—1986. British Journal of Obstetrics and Gynaecology 93: 1025–1029

Ueland K 1982 Cardiac disease. In: Queenan J T, Hobbins J C (eds) Protocols for high risk pregnancies, Medical Economics Books, New Jersey, pp 96–101

UK collaborative study on AFP in relation to NTD 1977 Maternal serum AFP measurement in antenatal screening for anencephaly and spina bifida in early pregnancy. Lancet i: 1323–1332

Whitfield C R 1983 Haemolytic disease of the newborn—a continuing problem. In: Chiswick M L (ed) Recent advances in perinatal medicine, 1. Churchill Livingstone, Edinburgh, pp 95–115

Wright J T 1983 Alcohol and drug abuse in pregnancy. Medicine (International) 35: 1630–1631

Zuspan F P 1982 Drug and alcohol addiction. In: Queenan J T, Hobbins J C (eds) Protocols for high risk pregnancies, Medical Economics Books, New Jersey, pp 3–9

Schoolgirl pregnancies

'I didn't really know what was wrong with me and I was feeling sort of funny. Then I got scared 'cos I could feel my stomach sort of moving about. I told my dad I didn't feel well and he took me to the doctor. First he said it was probably wind and "come back next week" but I thought I had something really serious, like maybe cancer or something, so I went back and then he checked me over and he said I was pregnant.' (Susie, 13)

Each year in England and Wales 10 000 schoolgirls make this same discovery.

The media would have us believe that there has been a 'tragic rise in schoolgirl pregnancies'! Is this truly the case? The actual number of pregnancies to schoolgirls has shown fluctuations from year to year but has not substantially altered since 1972. There are, however, proportionately more births in the younger age ranges. In 1973, under-14s accounted for 4% of schoolgirl pregnancies, rising to 6% in 1983 (OPCS 1983) (Table 5.1).

Table 5.1 Number of schoolgirl pregnancies* in England and Wales

	All schoolgirls	Under-16s	Under-14s
1973	10 650	9700	400
1974	10 100	9300	400
1975	10 050	9200	400
1976	9900	9100	400
1977	9800	9000	400
1978	10 000	9100	400
1979	10 000	9100	400
1980	9350	8500	400
1981	9400	8500	400
1982	10 400	9100	500
1983	10 500	9100	600

* These were estimated values (including under-16 conception figures plus figures for a proportion of 16-year-olds).

Nationally, the general fertility rate has fallen. Taking the three decades 1951–1981, numbers of births per 1000 women aged 15–44 years rose by 19% from 1951 to 1961, while births per 1000 girls aged 15–19 years rose alarmingly by 76%. During the next 10 years, rates slowed, showing a fall of 6.7% in the general fertility rate with a smaller rise of 38% in the 15–19-year age group; this trend continued in the period 1971–1981, with a fall of −26%

for all women and a fall of −45% in teenagers (OPCS 1981). The lowest birth rate among teenagers for 20 years occurred in 1981 (Bury 1984).

In considering fertility rates and statistical data on schoolgirls, it is important to differentiate data on under-16s from information on 'teenagers' (the 15–19-year age group). The presence of this younger group of high-risk girls needs to be emphasised since their figures are often masked by analysing data on teenagers as a whole (Stanley & Straton 1981).

The dramatic fall in teenage fertility has been attributed to better contraceptive services. However, while older teenagers (over 16 years) have, to an increasing extent, been protected from unwanted pregnancy by better availability and use of contraception, this has not been the case for the under-16-year age group.

The conception rate for under-16s peaked in the early 1970s, the peak fertility rate for 15- and 16-year-olds being for girls born in 1955. Rates then fell until 1979, but from then on abortion rates have increased and the birth rate has also shown an upward trend since 1982 (Hansard 1983) (Fig. 5.1).

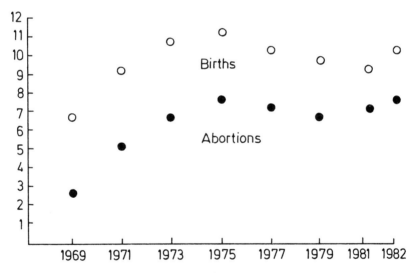

Fig. 5.1 Total pregnancies (○) and abortions (●) per thousand in 15-year-old girls in England and Wales (from Hansard 1983)

SOCIETY AND THE FAMILY

In Britain, schoolgirl pregnancy is part of a culture of poverty and deprivation. Pregnant schoolgirls live in areas of poor housing, overcrowding and unemployment (Fig. 5.2). A 6-year longitudinal study of pregnant schoolgirls in an inner city area, Camberwell (Birch 1986), revealed that 40% of such families are already known to social service agencies before their daughter's pregnancy, and that 20% of the girls had been in care. 13% of girls have been on the social services 'child abuse' register. The family background is often a violent one (in 29% of cases), with frequent brushes with the law.

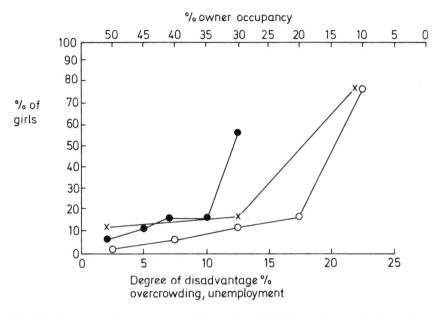

Fig. 5.2   Percentage of pregnant schoolgirls living in ACORN (a classification of residential neighbourhoods) districts with varying degrees of deprivation. ○ = male unemployment; ● = overcrowding; × = housing

The 'typical' pregnant schoolgirl is a member of a large single-parent family (McEwan et al 1974, Birch 1986). In South London, 70% of girls do not live with both of their natural parents, 16% have no mother and 65% have no father. Of those who have a father, one-third have a poor relationship with him and 12% of fathers suffer from mental illness, including severe alcoholism (Birch 1986).

The absence of a father is a critical feature. Fatherless teenage girls may become sexually involved in an attempt to find a kind of paternal caring which is absent in their homes (Zongker 1977, Gispert et al 1984). A poor relationship between pregnant girls and their fathers, who are often ineffectual or absent, may result in girls lacking affirmation of their femininity and thus initiating relationships with immature men who are drug abusers, alcoholics or in jail and with whom they cannot establish a stable relationship (Landy et al 1983).

Pregnant schoolgirls' families fall into three groups as regards the relation-

ship between the girl and her mother (Birch 1986): those where the relationship is a good one (25% of cases), those where the relationship is very poor
or the mother is absent (54% of cases), and a third group where there is
an 'over-close', suffocating relationship between mother and daughter (21%).
This relationship largely results in the exclusion of peers and the father and
in the mother assuming control and care of her daughter's baby. Characteristi-
cally, the mother is always present at interview and answers questions on
her daughter's behalf. 'She also contradicted her daughter's response to questions about the baby' (Parks & Jenkins 1983). The pattern of weak father/dom-
inant mother has been described as a family syndrome which can identify
an 'at risk' group (Landy et al 1983).

Despite their single-parent status, families are large with an average of
five children, a consequence of a repeating pattern of having a man coming
and going and fathering children without living permanently in the household.

Two-thirds of schoolgirl mothers in South London have a family history
of teenage pregnancy, and in 35% their mothers have had the same experience.
43% of girls have sisters who are also teenage mothers (Birch 1986) and,
interestingly, the same percentage of 'baby fathers' (teenage fathers) also
have brothers who are teenage parents (Hendricks & Montgomery 1983).

SEXUALITY AND SEX EDUCATION

As one might expect, in view of the difficult family circumstances, very few
pregnant girls have had any sex education at home. 87% of Camberwell
girls have learned nothing from their parents about the facts of life, and
a further 8% have picked up a very small amount of information from home.
This ignorance is further compounded by the fact that 64% of girls have
also had no sex education at school. Many become pregnant before the sex
education course begins, but most miss out because of truancy. In fact, 62%
of pregnant schoolgirls are persistent truants, of whom 20% have been out
of school for more than 1 year (Birch 1986), the result being that the most
common source of sex education is information picked up from friends, which
is often unreliable and inaccurate (Reichelt & Werley 1975, Ashken & Soddy
1980, Birch 1986) (Fig. 5.3, SD 2). These findings clearly refute the often-
quoted opinion that sex education in schools encourages promiscuity, while
supporting the premise that it is 'those young people most in ignorance who
tend to experiment early and to suffer the consequences of unwanted pregnancies and sexually transmitted diseases' (Christopher 1978).

Contrary to popular belief, pregnant schoolgirls are not a promiscuous
group. They tend to have long-standing relationships or to follow a pattern
of 'serial monogamy', having a series of fairly long relationships in which
they are 'faithful' to that one person (Farrell 1978, Ashken & Soddy 1980,
Bury 1984, Tobin 1985). Most pregnancies are unplanned (98% of cases)
but arise out of a regular sexual relationship (59%). For two-thirds of girls

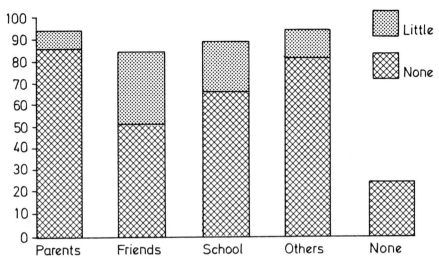

Fig. 5.3 Sex education sources

this is their first sexual relationship, and 5% conceive the first time they sleep with a boy. In South London, this first sexual encounter occurs at an average age of 13.5 years, 1 year later than the mean menarche of 12.5 years (Birch 1986).

Although most pregnant girls have stable relationships with boys and 77% have known their 'baby fathers' for more than 6 months, a subgroup of girls can be identified who have been sexually abused (11%), involved in an incestuous relationship (6%) or introduced to prostitution (9%). This subgroup of sexually exploited young girls has a very poor prognosis. A review of their circumstances 2 years after the birth of their babies revealed that half had become involved in prostitution and an equal number were drug abusers; moreover, their babies constituted 60% of the cases of child abuse occurring within the sample (Birch 1986).

REALISATIONS AND DECISIONS

Being largely ignorant of the facts of life, it is hardly surprising to find that girls do not immediately realise that they are pregnant. One-third of Camberwell girls did not realise the significance of missed periods or did not realise that they were late, and 90% were unsure of the date of their last period; those that did miss periods generally missed three before suspecting pregnancy. Younger girls took longer to realise that they were pregnant; only 33% of those aged 12–13 years eventually realised the significance of amenorrhoea, as opposed to 68% at 14 years and 78% at 15 years. 4% of girls were alerted to pregnancy by fetal movements and 1% by actual labour, and 20% were informed of their pregnancies by a sister or mother who realised that she was putting on weight or had not used sanitary towels for some time (Birch 1986).

Realisation of pregnancy can be a crisis point. Many girls cannot cope with this realisation and deny it to themselves, or they may try to hide their pregnancies, fearing discovery by their parents or teachers or to prevent their boyfriends from getting into trouble.

> 'I kept convincing myself I wasn't—I kept missing periods but I kept putting it off, saying nay, it's just ... I was saying to myself, I've had sex so it's most probably changing my body or something. Just giving myself any old excuse.' (Janet, 15, 'Schoolgirl Mum' 1985)

Faced with the monumental decision of what to do, who to tell and who to trust, the reaction of many girls is to do nothing and tell nobody. The 'average' pregnant schoolgirl takes no action until 15 weeks' gestation; her boyfriend is usually the first to be told, followed by her parents or family doctor. Most girls find it very difficult to tell their parents about their pregnancies. They avoid the problem by asking a sister to tell them or using ploys such as semi-deliberately leaving their antenatal appointment cards where their parents will find it. One-third of girls never tell their parents, but in half of these cases the parents notice themselves (Birch 1986).

Nationally 2 out of 3 pregnant schoolgirls decide to terminate their pregnancies; however, in areas of socioeconomic deprivation a higher proportion of girls go to term (Simkins 1984, Straton & Stanley 1983). In Camberwell, only 1 in 4 girls choose abortion (Birch 1986, Dean 1984).

Younger teenagers present late for abortion due to failure to realise that they are pregnant, concealment of pregnancy, and conflicts with parents. They thus have a higher rate of late, more dangerous abortions. 81% of Newcastle girls aged under 16 years presented for termination after 10 weeks' gestation as opposed to 75% of 17–19-year-old teenagers (Russell 1983). This later presentation produced a 4% increase in lacerated cervix, a 5% increase in retained products, a 4% increase in uterine infection and a higher mortality. In the United States, where schoolgirl pregnancies show the highest rate of a 'developed' country, mortality from legal abortions rose from 0.5 in 100 000 at 8 weeks' gestation to 1.4 at 10 weeks, 2.3 at 12 weeks and 6.7 at 15 weeks (National Center for Health Statistics 1976). However, 'the later a girl applies for an abortion—the more she needs it' (Ketting 1982, Savage 1985).

Three-quarters of girls who eventually keep their babies make this decision as soon as they realise that they are pregnant (Birch 1986). Others decide to terminate and later change their minds, often under family pressure, and 10% present too late for abortion. In 62% of cases the decision of girl, boyfriend and parents concur, but when disagreement occurs a great deal of stress and unhappiness results. 13% of Camberwell schoolgirls were forced either to abort their pregnancies or to keep their babies against their wills, often with the result that they became pregnant again or rejected their children. Adoption is not a popular option. In America, only 7% of girls chose adoption (Block et al 1981), while in Camberwell the 2% who did so were strongly pressured by their families who sent them to London to have their babies in secret (Birch 1986).

ANTENATAL CARE

In the 1950s and 1960s the social stigma attached to a teenage pregnancy discouraged young girls from attending hospital, resulting in poor antenatal care and thus higher obstetric risks (Marchetti & Menaker 1950, Morrison 1953, Hassan & Falls 1964, Mussio 1962).

The general standard of care has improved over the last 20 years, but many girls book late and attend hospital irregularly with the result that 'the antenatal care of pregnant teenagers is often grossly deficient' (Block et al 1981). One-fifth of teenagers under 20 years of age do not consult their general practitioners until they are more than 20 weeks pregnant (Simms & Smith 1983).

The situation for younger, school-age teenagers is even worse: over half (52%) of South London schoolgirls book for antenatal care after 20 weeks gestation (Birch 1986). Girls do not realise that they are pregnant and conceal their pregnancies. Some girls wait until they are 16 years old before coming to the clinic, 'risking their health and that of their future child because of the state of the law' (McEwan et al 1974). Problems of diagnosis also occur; there is a tendency for some professionals not to want to believe that a very young girl could be pregnant.

> 'My mum sent me to the doctor's when I was about four months, because I hadn't been on the periods. So the doctor said it was just puppy fat. So then she sent me back when I was seven and a half months and he said it was wind . . . (Kirsty, 14, 'Schoolgirl Mum')

'He said I definitely was not pregnant but my mother said I was because I was too fat so she made him write a letter for the hospital.' Julie was an emergency admission from the termination counselling clinic at 38 weeks' gestation with severe pre-eclampsia. Her baby died at 10 months of age—a 'cot death'.

If antenatal care is adequate, the risks of childbearing do not appear to be greater for the teenager than for older women, but the risks to the baby are increased, particularly for very young mothers (Straton & Stanley 1983). Multiparous mothers are more likely to have small-for-dates babies if they are younger and have little prenatal care, but in the case of primiparous mothers poor care exerts a more powerful influence than young age (Elster 1984).

Many studies have reported higher rates of anaemia in teenage patients than in older pregnant women and the rates of anaemia (defined as less than 10 g of haemoglobin per 100 ml) have been shown to be inversely proportional to the age of the sample group (Jovanovitch 1972, Elliott & Beazley 1980,

Osbourne & Howat 1981, Scholl et al 1984, Miller & Field 1984). The rates of anaemia in these studies were in the region of 14% (mainly in the 16-year and under age group).

The increased frequency of anaemia in teenagers is related to socioeconomic circumstances (Russell 1983, Miller & Field 1984). In Liverpool, young girls attending hospital in a deprived area of the city were more likely to be anaemic (18%) than in the more affluent areas (6%) (Elliott & Beazley 1980). The incidence of anaemia in pregnant Camberwell schoolgirls is high at 19% (Birch 1986).

Camberwell has a deprived population where 57% of pregnant schoolgirls have no employed parent and 33% have a grossly inadequate diet. If one excludes girls with an associated haemoglobinopathy—HbS or HbC—which are present in 10% of the overall sample, the rate of antenatal anaemia is still 16%. White anaemic girls are more likely to come from homes with no employed parent (100%), have a poor diet (86%) and book late for antenatal care (65%). The mean time of booking for anaemic girls is at 24 weeks' gestation as opposed to 20 weeks for all schoolgirls. Hence it would appear that those girls most in need of antenatal care are less likely to receive it.

Studies have varied in their findings regarding hypertension in pregnant teenagers. In Australia a higher incidence of pre-eclampsia was found in the under 16s (16.6%) than in older mothers aged 20–25 years (14.7%), although hypertension alone was shown not to be significant (O'Brien et al 1982). Other workers have found hypertension to be more common (Duenhoelter et al 1975). In Camberwell, the overall incidence of hypertension (defined as a diastolic measurement of 90+ mmHg) was found to be 18%, with an increased incidence in the upper range of schoolgirls (16 years and over) which was associated with an increase in smoking and drinking alcohol during pregnancy (Birch 1986) (Fig. 5.4).

THE BIRTH

'Obstetric complications are bedevilled with conflicting reports using different control groups' (Block et al 1981). 'With the exception of preeclempsia and a small bony pelvis the majority of complications are due to lack of prenatal care rather than maternal age' (McKenry et al 1979).

Maternal mortality rates can give a false picture if age groups are not considered separately. The maternal mortality for girls aged 16–19 years at 9.6 in 100 000 (OPCS 1981) is actually considerably better than the national mean of 13 in 100 000, whereas the mortality for mothers aged less than 16 years is very high at 49 in 100 000. These parameters can equal out if all teenage births are taken together, thus giving a false impression that there is little difference in maternal mortality rates for all teenagers and older mothers.

In Glasgow, obstetric risks were not significantly different in all teenagers (under 20 years) than in older women (20–24 years), but an 'at risk' group of younger teenagers who remained single was defined. They were more

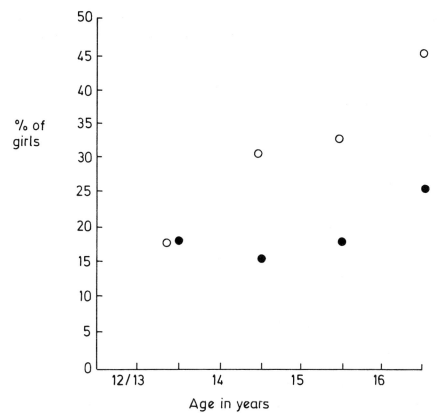

Fig. 5.4   Percentage of cases of high blood pressure (●) by age group (○ = smoking/alcohol)

likely to go into premature labour and had a higher perinatal mortality than those who married.

It might be expected that the teenager's pelvis may not be fully grown by the time she delivers her baby, thus giving high rates of cephalo-pelvic disproportion and caesarean section. Russell (1983) did not find a high caesarean section rate in Newcastle girls, while Glaswegian teenagers actually had a lower rate (9.2%) than women 20–24 years (14.7%) (Osbourne et al 1981), nor was the incidence of operative delivery increased in Liverpool in the under-16s (Elliott & Beazley 1980).

In the United States, Duenhoelter et al (1975) found that, while the rates of contracted pelvis were high, the caesarean section rate was not raised significantly. Dwyer (1974) found very low rates of all delivery complications and particularly a low caesarean rate—2.6% overall (6% current hospital average). He concluded that the female pelvis is not contracted because it is fully grown before a girl is physiologically old enough to reproduce.

Possibly there are not more operative deliveries because although the teenager's pelvis is smaller, the babies are of lower birthweights. In Camberwell,

77% of schoolgirls experienced a normal delivery, the caesarean section rate was 10% (Birch 1986). Some of the 'problem deliveries' presented difficulties not normally recorded in obstetric textbooks—such as Sabrina, who delivered at home by candle-light when the electricity was cut off; or Kim, who was so afraid that she tried to get up and go home when her baby's head appeared; or sexually abused Marie, whose waters broke prematurely in my car on our way from seeing a psychiatrist.

BIRTHWEIGHT AND PERINATAL MORTALITY

Figures from the National Birthday Trust and Royal College of Obstetricians and Gynaecologists survey (1970) showed perinatal mortality for babies of mothers under 20 years to be one of the highest.

Illegitimacy, independent of age, is a predictor of low birth weight and high perinatal mortality. The important factors which have been shown to be more important than age for teenage mothers are marital status at conception [Gill et al (Aberdeen) 1970, Osbourne & Howat (Glasgow) 1981, Ventura & Hendershot (USA) 1984], timing of antenatal care (Ventura & Hendershot 1984) and socioeconomic status (Phipps-Yonas 1980).

Whereas in general second babies have a lower risk of perinatal mortality, the highest mortality rates are among children of teenage mothers who have already borne a child (Lambert 1976). This higher perinatal mortality in multipara is unfortunate since 25% of girls are pregnant again within 12 months (Block et al 1981, Birch 1986).

The precise effect of nutrition on pregnancy outcome is not entirely clear, although studies would suggest that attention to adequate food intake and quality of diet can only be beneficial to the pregnant schoolgirl and her developing baby (Block et al 1981). Alton, in 1979, studied dietary habits in pregnant schoolgirls enrolled in an American school-based pregnancy programme and found that, even in this relatively well cared for group, 75% of girls had diets that were deficient in protein content.

In the Camberwell study, one-third of girls were regarded as having a poor diet. These girls had a diet that was grossly deficient in both quantity and quality. Two were clinically anaemic due to dietary causes and two were generally debilitated, very thin and weak because they had too little to eat. All families were on low incomes so that they were unable to spend much money on food, and two-thirds were surviving on supplementary benefit only. The younger girls had poorer diets than the older girls. This was associated with the birth of smaller babies (Birch 1986) (Fig. 5.5).

In Liverpool, 10% of under-16s gave birth to babies weighing less than 2500 g (Elliott & Beazley 1980) and this same figure was recorded in Camberwell primiparous schoolgirls (Birch 1986), where the number of small babies was inversely proportional to the girl's age and increased with repeat pregnancies (16%).

Dietary supplements have been provided for women considered to be 'nutri-

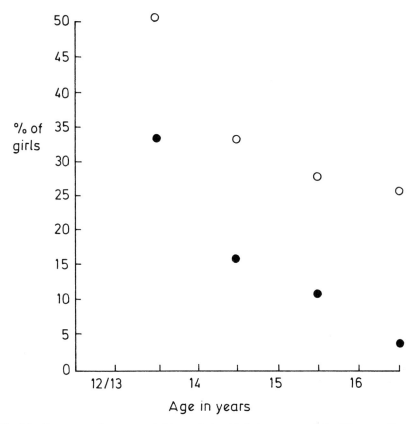

Fig. 5.5   Percentage of premature babies—relationship between age and diet (○ = poor diet; ● = premature delivery)

tionally at risk', with the result of an improved obstetric outcome [Blackwell et al (Taiwan) 1973, Lechtig et al (Guatemala) 1975, Scholl et al (USA) 1984]. Teenagers on relatively good diets have been shown to have similar pregnancy weight gains to older women, while still giving birth to smaller babies. Girls on poor diets have poor weight gains and even smaller babies [Frisancho et al (Peru) 1983].

'Health and social factors are more important to fetal outcome among primiparous mothers than adolescent status' (Zuckerman 1983). 'The prevalence of low birthweight is not due to their age but to sociodemographic features of women of this age who carry their pregnancies to term' (Horon et al 1985). Thus it would appear that factors other than maternal age per se influence the obstetric outcome and numbers of small babies borne by young mothers. The diet and social habits of young people are important. Young people start smoking because they perceive it to be an adult behaviour (Bewley 1984). These same teenagers are likely to be those experimenting in other 'adult behaviours' such as sexual activity, drinking alcohol or using drugs.

It has been estimated that smoking less than 20 cigarettes per day during pregnancy results in a 150–200 mg reduction in birth weight and a 20% increase in neonatal death rate (Martin 1982), while heavy smoking more than doubles the chances of a girl losing her baby at or near birth (Surgeon General 1980).

Few estimates have been made of the drinking and smoking habits of pregnant schoolgirls. In Camberwell, 33% smoked and 30% had more than the occasional drink. These figures are likely to be underestimates due to the common problem of under-reporting and denial of alcoholism. Alcohol abuse and drug-taking are well known to affect fetal growth (Ghishan & Greene 1983, Meadows et al 1981). Less well known are the effects of solvent abuse or 'glue sniffing' which is becoming more prevalent among young people. It is to some extent a substitute for alcohol in the young since it is cheaper and often more readily available to under-age, under-privileged teenagers.

WHY DO SCHOOLGIRLS BECOME PREGANT?

Why do so many girls become pregnant at an early age? A multitude of factors are involved which are equally applicable to the often-forgotten teenage 'baby father'. Social and family problems deprive boys and girls of love and self-worth. These emotionally immature young people are brought together by their loneliness and, by virtue of their lack of knowledge and motivation to control their reproductive ability, have unprotected sex, resulting in school-age pregnancy.

The majority of schoolgirls become pregnant as the 'inadvertent consequence of a normal erotic relationship in itself desired and rewarding, abnormal only in that the usual social taboos had not been effective . . .' (Anderson et al 1960). Social taboos may be broken down by social deprivation; absent or working mothers unable to talk to their daughters and set examples of behaviour; overcrowding causing lack of privacy; boredom and frustration encouraging early sexual experimentation; and the model of peers and siblings who may also be sexually active.

Some pregnant girls seem to have an unconscious desire to get pregnant, are trapped in a culture of poverty (McKenry et al 1979) and use pregnancy as a supposed avenue of escape from an unhappy life and to resolve their own sense of dependency and deprivation (Phipps-Yonas 1980). Others are seen to be re-enacting unhappy circumstances rather than escaping from them. 'They need to do so largely to understand and excuse their mothers' behaviour towards themselves' (Gough 1966).

Pregnant schoolgirls have difficulty in developing and sustaining interpersonal relationships (Cohen 1983); both peer and family relationships are poor (Elster 1983, Landy et al 1983). These young people are lonely, feel unloved and may become involved in a sexual relationship to cope with their loneliness. A sexual relationship is merely part of the spectrum of possible relationships, and some girls may inadvertently become pregnant while exploring the possibilities of such a relationship and attempting to define their own boundaries.

An experience of failure, for instance in poor school performance and in failing to be lovable, is common in young pregnant girls (Elster 1983, Ulvedal & Feeg 1983), resulting in a feeling that 'the only thing I can do right is have a baby' (Rosenstock 1980).

Physical maturity may be coupled with psychological immaturity. Lacking the adolescent change from concrete to abstract reasoning (Blum & Resnick 1982), a young girl has no clear sense of a personal future (Babikian & Goldman 1971); she is thus unable to plan ahead. Such a girl is unable to visualise how having a baby might change her life. She is unable to appreciate the consequences of her actions in that having sex might result in a baby and is therefore unable to take steps to protect herself by using contraception.

Older teenagers (16–19 years) have been using contraception more effectively (Bury 1984), but this has not been the case for sexually active, under-16s who continue to have a very low rate of contraceptive use (Zelnik et al 1979, Miller 1984, Schinke 1984).

Contraceptive use among the British under-16s is difficult to quantify. The extensive studies of Schofield in the 1960s and by Farrell and Dunnell in the 1970s relate mainly to older teenagers (15–19 years). There is a vast difference in contraceptive use between under- and over-16s, both in motivation to use, knowledge of and availability of contraception. Contraceptive use prior to pregnancy in an American sample was only 9% for girls aged 12–15 years and 25% for older teenagers (Miller 1984).

Knowledge of contraception among pregnant teenagers in Camberwell in 1974 was poor and frequently inappropriate. 17% of under-17s used spermicides or withdrawal only and 49% had never used anything (McEwan et al 1974). Only 7% of a younger sample of pregnant Camberwell schoolgirls had ever used any contraception prior to their first pregnancy (Birch 1986). Girls gave varied reasons for non-use of contraception, the most common being that they did not think that they could get pregnant and they had not expected to have sex.

> 'I never thought I could get pregnant, I thought I was too young. I mean you hear about girls at school getting pregnant and you think, "She's having sex", you don't think you are, you don't think it'll happen to you, do you?' (Annette, 15)

Young girls do not want to use contraceptives because this implies that they are planning to have sex, which indicates promiscuity. If they use contraceptives they are acknowledging that they are sexually active, something which they are denying to themselves.

> 'If my mum knew I was on the pill she would think I was sleeping around.' (Janet, 15)

> 'Let's face it—good girls don't—so they don't need the pill; bad girls go out and do it anyway!' (Dianne, 16)

The low rate of contraceptive use results in it being a rarity for young people seeking contraceptive advice not to have been involved in unprotected sex. Half of pregnancies occur in the first 6 months after a girl starts to have intercourse, and 20% occur in the first month (Zabin et al 1979). We must therefore reach teenagers before they begin sexual activity in order to be effective with family planning programmes. The median delay for contraceptive clinic attendance is 12 months, but the median delay for pregnancy is 6 months (Zabin et al 1979).

After giving birth to unplanned babies, and in many cases unwanted babies, schoolgirl mothers still demonstrate low levels of contraceptive use and high failure rates. In Camberwell, one-third never used any contraception during a 2-year follow-up period. There was poor compliance with methods and girls did not follow instructions adequately. Some appeared not to actually want contraception: they were given pills and did not take them; coils fell out and girls did not bother to go back to the clinic—one girl certainly pulled it out herself. Girls did not like barrier methods and they proved ineffective. Depot injections were more the choice of the doctor than their own (Birch 1986).

Why is contraceptive use so poor even after an unwanted pregnancy? Do these girls need to take risks? Are they so used to being unable to control their environment and bodies that the idea of controlling their reproductive capacities is totally alien to them? Unwanted pregnancy is the ultimate form of loss of control over one's body. Is this their subconscious aim? Is there a tendency for professionals to push these girls into using contraception against their true wishes because the concept of young mothers having another child is considered undesirable?

Seen from the young girl's viewpoint, pregnancy may not be so undesirable. Certainly it brings heartache and hardship, the extent of which should not be underestimated, but for underprivileged girls with little education and non-existent job prospects, motherhood is a fulfilment. With the birth of her baby a 'failed' school drop-out, an unemployable misfit, becomes an acceptable member of society with a valued role—that of a mother. She is successful, and out of her loveless world she has created her own baby who will love her.

REFERENCES

Alton I 1979 Nutrition services for pregnant adolescents within a public high school. Journal of the American Dietary Association 74: 667
Anderson E W, Kenna J C, Hamilton M W 1960 A study of extramarital conception in adolescence. Psychiatria et Neurologia 139: 313–362
Ashken I C, Soddy A G 1980 Study of pregnant schoolage girls. British Journal of Family Planning 6: 77–82
Babikian H, Goldman A 1971 A study in teenage pregnancy. American Journal of Psychiatry 128: 111–116
Bewley B R 1984 Smoking in pregnancy. British Medical Journal 288(6415): 424–426
Birch D 1986 Schoolgirl pregnancy in Camberwell, MD thesis, University of London
Blackwell R Q, Chow B F, Chinn K S K, Blackwell B, Hsu S C 1973 Prospective maternal

malnutrition study in Taiwan; Rationale, study design, feasibility and preliminary findings. Nutrition Reports International 7: 517–532

Block R W, Saltzman S, Block S A 1981 Teenage pregnancy, Year Book Medical, Chicago

Blum R W, Resnick M D 1982 Adolescent sexual decision-making: contraception, pregnancy, abortion, motherhood. Pediatric Annals 11(10): 797–805

Bury J 1984 Teenage pregnancy in Britain, Birth Control Trust, London

Christopher E 1978 Sex education. British Journal of Family Planning 4(1): 15–17

Cohen S J 1983 Intentional teenage pregnancies. Journal of School Health 53(3): 210–211

Dean E 1984 Abortion statistics in Camberwell Health Authority, 1982, unpublished work prepared for MFCM course work

Duenhoelter J H, Jiminez J M, Baumann G 1975 Pregnancy performance in patients under fifteen years of age. American Journal of Obstetrics and Gynecology 46(1): 49–52

Dunnell K 1979 Family formation 1976, OPCS HMSO, London

Dwyer J F 1974 Teenage pregnancy. American Journal of Obstetrics and Gynecology 8(3): 373–376

Elliott H R, Beazley J M 1980 A clinical study of pregnancy in younger teenagers in Liverpool. British Journal of Obstetrics and Gynaecology 1: 16–19

Elster A B 1983 Parental behavior of adolescent mothers. Pediatrics 71: 494–503

Elster A B 1984 The effect of maternal age, parity, and prenatal care on perinatal outcome in adolescent mothers. American Journal of Obstetrics and Gynecology 149: 845–847

Farrell C 1978 My mother said . . ., Routledge Kegan Paul, London

Frisancho R, Matos J, Flegel P 1983 Maternal nutritional status and adolescent pregnancy outcome. American Journal of Clinical Nutrition 38: 739–746

Ghishan F K, Greene H L 1983 Fetal alcohol syndrome: failure of zinc supplementation to reverse the effect of ethanol on placental transport of zinc. Pediatric Research 17: 529–531

Gill D, Illesley R, Koplick L 1970 Pregnancy in teenage girls. Social Science and Medicine 3(4): 549–574

Gispert M, Brinich P, Wheeler, Krieger L 1984 Predictors of repeat pregnancies among low income adolescents. Hospital and Community Psychiatry 35(7): 719–723

Gough D 1966 The very young mother. Family Planning 15(2): 42–46

Hansard 1983 Pregnancies, abortions and births in under 15 year olds. 48(44) cols 50–52, 8 Nov 1983

Hassan H M, Falls F H 1964 The young primipara: a clinical study. American Journal of Obstetrics and Gynecology 88: 256–269

Hendricks L E, Montgomery T 1983 A limited population of unmarried adolescent fathers: a preliminary report of their views on fatherhood and the relationship with the mothers of their children. Adolescence XVIII(69): 201–210

Horon I L, Strobino D M, MacDonald H M 1985 Birthweights among infants born to adolescent and young adult women. American Journal of Obstetrics and Gynecology 146(4): 444–449

Jovanovitch D 1972 Pathology of pregnancy and labour in adolescent patients. Journal of Reproductive Medicine 9: 61–66

Ketting E 1982 Second trimester abortion as a social problem. In: (ed) Kierse Second trimester pregnancy termination, Leiden University Press, Leiden, p 16

Lambert P 1976 Perinatal mortality: social and environmental factors. Population Trends 4: 4

Landy S, Schubert J, Cleland J F, Clerk C, Montgomery J S 1983 Teenage pregnancy—family syndrome? Adolescence XVIII(71): 679–694

Lechtig A, Habicht J P, Delgado H, Klein R E, Yarbrough C, Martorell R 1975 Effect of food supplementation during pregnancy on birthweight. Pediatrics 56: 508–520

Marchetti A A, Menaker J S 1950 Pregnancy and the adolescent. American Journal of Obstetrics and Gynecology 59: 1013–1020

Martin J C 1982 An overview: maternal nicotine and caffeine consumption and offspring outcome. Neurobehavioral Toxicology and Teratology 4: 421–427

McEwan J A, Owens C, Newton J R 1974 Pregnancy in girls under 17: a preliminary study in a hospital district in south London. Journal of Biosocial Science 6: 357–381

McKenry P C, Walters L H, Johnson C 1979 Adolescent pregnancy: a review of the literature. The Family Coordinator, Jan

Meadows N J, Smith M F, Keeling P W N et al 1981 Zinc and small babies. Lancet ii: 1135–1137

Miller S H 1984 Childbearing and child rearing among the very young. Children Today, May–June: 26–29

Miller K A, Field C 1984 Adolescent pregnancy: a combined obstetric and pediatric management approach. Mayo Clinic Proceedings 59: 311–317

Morrison J H 1953 The adolescent primigravida. Obstetrics and Gynecology 2: 297–301

Mussio T J 1962 Primigravidas under age 14. American Journal of Obstetrics and Gynecology 84: 442–444

National Birthday Trust and Royal College of Obstetricians and Gynaecologists (1975) British births, 1970, the first week of life. In: British births 1970, vol 1, Heinemann Medical, London

National Center for Health Statistics 1976 Report of the Department of Health Education and Welfare US Department of Health, Education and Welfare, Washington DC

O'Brien M J, Chang A M Z, Esler E J 1982 Antenatal care, obstetric and neonatal outcome of teenage pregnancies. Asia-Oceania Journal of Obstetrics and Gynaecology 8(2): 163–168

OPCS (Office of Population Census and Surveys) 1981 Birth statistics England and Wales 1981, OPCS Series FM1, no 8, HMSO, London

OPCS (Office of Population Census and Surveys) 1983 Birth statistics England and Wales 1983, OPCS Series FM1, no 10, HMSO, London

Osbourne G K, Howat R C L, Jordan M M 1981 The obstetric outcome of teenage pregnancy. British Journal of Obstetrics and Gynaecology 88: 215–221

Parks P, Jenkins L 1983 Mothers of adolescent mothers—letters to the editor. Journal of Adolescent Health Care 4: 137–138

Phipps-Yonas S 1980 Teenage pregnancy and motherhood: a review of the literature. American Journal of Orthopsychiatry 50(3): 403–431

Reichelt P, Werley H 1975 Contraception, abortion and venereal disease: teenagers' knowledge and the effects of education. Family Planning Perspectives 7: 83–88

Rosenstock H A 1980 Recognising the teenager who needs to be pregnant: a clinical perspective. Southern Medical Journal 73: 134–136

Russell J K 1983 School pregnancies—medical, social and educational considerations. British Journal of Hospital Medicine 29: 159–166

Savage W 1985 Requests for late termination of pregnancy; Tower Hamlets, 1983. British Medical Journal 290: 621–623

Schinke S P 1984 Preventing teenage pregnancy. In: Progress in behaviour modification, 16: 13–64

Schofield M 1975 The sexual behaviour of young people, Longman, London

Scholl T O, Decker E, Karp R J, Greene G, De Sales M 1984 Early adolescent pregnancy: a comparative study of pregnancy outcome in young adolescents and mature women. Journal of Adolescent Health Care 5: 167–171

Schoolgirl Mum (October 1985) BBC television production, '40 minutes', producer Jeremy Bennett

Simkins L 1984 Consequences of teenage pregnancy and motherhood. Adolescence XIX(73): 39–54

Simms M, Smith C 1983 Teenage mothers: late attenders at medical and antenatal care. In: Aspects of social medicine, Institute for Social Studies in Medical Care, London

Stanley F J, Straton J A Y 1981 Teenage pregnancies in Western Australia. Medical Journal of Australia 2: 468–469

Straton J A Y, Stanley F J 1983 Medical risks of teenage pregnancy. Australian Family Physician 12(6): 474–480

Surgeon General 1980 The health consequences of smoking for women, US Dept of Health Education and Welfare, Washington DC, pp 211–214

Tobin J 1985 How promiscuous are our teenagers? A study of teenage girls attending a family planning clinic. British Journal of Family Planning 10(4): 107–111

Ulvedal S K, Feeg V D 1983 Pregnant teens who choose childbirth. Journal of School Health 53(4): 229–233

Ventura S J, Hendershott G E 1984 Infant health consequences of childbearing by teenagers and older mothers. Public Health Reports 99(2): 138–146

Zabin L S, Kantner J F, Zelnik M 1979 The risk of adolescent pregnancy in the first months of intercourse. Family Planning Perspectives 11: 215

Zelnik M, Kim Y J, Kantner J F 1979 Probabilities of intercourse and conception among US teenage women, 1971 and 1976. Family Planning Perspectives 11: 177–183

Zongker C E 1977 The self concept of pregnant adolescent girls. Adolescence 12: 477

Zuckerman E 1983 Neonatal outcome: is adolescent pregnancy a risk factor? Pediatrics 71: 489–493

Maternal narcotic addiction

In countries where drug abuse is prevalent, it is inevitable that there will be maternal narcotic addiction. The size of the problem is understated when one examines the available statistics. For example, in New South Wales (predominantly Sydney) there are estimated to be between 5 and 10 thousand narcotic addicts in a population of more than 4 million (i.e. between 1 in 500 and 1 in 1000). Acknowledging the very real problem of certain identification of all affected pregnancies, these authors estimate that about 1 in 400 pregnancies which reach 20 weeks' gestation are complicated by narcotic drug abuse or addiction. However, the adverse obstetric and perinatal effects encountered magnify the problem out of all proportion to those relatively small numbers.

THE PATIENT

Identification

The first problem to be considered is that of identification. Although many addicts present to major centres by self-referral (which accounts for 80% of those attending the drug-dependency antenatal clinic at King George V Hospital, Sydney), this cannot be relied upon. Some addicts will openly advertise their habit with visible 'needle-tracks' in prominent places, although in pregnancy unusual injection sites such as breast veins may be used. Urinary drug screening has been used as part of routine antenatal testing in an effort to identify all addicts (Collins 1982), and this is presently used in Sydney although the cost effectiveness of this approach should be determined.

Patient characteristics

The pregnant addict may be of any age, but in our experience tends to be older than average and likely to be a long-term abuser of heroin. In the most recent series from Sydney the mean duration of drug habit was nearly 7 years, with an average intake of about 1 g of street heroin per day (Ellwood et al 1987). Although many are or have been prostitutes and indulged in petty crime to support their habit, some lead remarkably normal lives and are gainfully employed. If this group can be easily characterised at all it is by their past medical, surgical and obstetric histories. Many problems such as hepatitis B surface antigen (HBSAg) carriage and human immune deficiency virus (HIV) antibody positivity relate directly to the drug-taking habit and particularly to the use of intravenous injections. Unusual past problems are sometimes elicited which are also drug-related, such as bowel obstruction, bacterial endocarditis, fungal endophthalmitis and thrombophlebitis. However, in our recent series the highest incidence of previous problems were in categories of respiratory disease (asthma, pneumonia and bronchitis) and major trauma (motor vehicle incidents and assault), but these are also presumably related to the addicts' life-style (Ellwood et al 1987). Table 6.1 shows

Table 6.1   Past reproductive problems of narcotic addicts compared with non-drug-using clinic patients from the same hospital

	Drug abusers (%) ($n = 182$)	Clinic patients (%) ($n = 182$)
First trimester abortion	51	30
Two or more abortions	24	10
Second trimester abortion	11	1
First trimester miscarriage	14	16
Second trimester miscarriage	7	3

Data adapted from Ellwood et al (1987)

data on past reproductive problems in the same group of Australian addicts. Many have experienced previous termination of pregnancy (both first and second trimester) and previous second-trimester miscarriage.

THE DRUGS

'Street' heroin varies considerably in cost and quality but currently retails in Sydney for approximately $250 (£100) per gram. The concentration of diacetylmorphine in this city is usually between 20 and 30% (Donkin et al 1985), but it should be noted that this figure may be very much less in other countries, so data comparison on drug effects in pregnancy may be hazardous. For example, in the USA, from where the majority of reports on pregnancy outcome have originated, the concentration of diacetylmorphine is usually less than 10% (Perlmutter 1974). More recent data suggest that this international difference persists (Finnegan 1986, personal communication). Contaminants used to 'cut' the pure drug are usually harmless, such as mono-, di- or polysaccharides, sodium bicarbonate, calcium sulphate or milk powder. However, other, active ingredients such as acetylcodeine, quinine and even strychnine have been reported.

Other drugs of abuse should be considered in this group. In our experience nearly all narcotic addicts smoke to excess, and this may have considerable importance when analysing pregnancy outcome effects of the narcotics. Many addicts are 'polydrug abusers', using cannabis, benzodiazepines and other drugs to supplement heroin in times of shortage. Alcohol abuse is very rarely encountered in pregnancy, perhaps because the combined effects of narcotics and alcohol on the gastrointestinal tract are particularly unpleasant! However, it is not unusual for this to be a problem prior to the pregnancy and patients may subsequently resume this in the puerperium.

THE PREGNANCY

Having identified a pregnancy complicated by narcotic addiction, the management options must be considered. Termination of the pregnancy is frequently requested by the patient, and in our practice is recommended for those patients with HIV antibodies present. Unfortunately many terminations will be performed in the second trimester. Oligo- and amenorrhoea are commonly found in narcotic abusers who may not use contraception, believing themselves to be infertile (Gaulden et al 1964). Presentation is often too late for first-trimester termination and even for accurate dating by untrasound, and this is a considerable problem for antenatal care, with dating uncertain in many.

Methadone stabilisation

The basis of modern management of narcotic addition is some form of methadone stabilisation and maintenance linked with a programme of comprehensive antenatal care (Connaughton et al 1977, Newman et al 1975). Indeed, many addicts will present with their first pregnancy having been previously stabilised on a low-dose methadone programme which had the effect of restoring ovulatory menstrual cycles and fertility. The principle of such a management approach is that a regular, orally administered dose of long-acting narcotic will satisfy the patient's addition without the need for any illegal or time-consuming activity required to obtain money for drugs and without the considerable health risks incurred by intravenous drug use.

Loretta Finnegan, whose pioneering work in Philadelphia is a model to all who would manage these patients, describes the problem in a nutshell: 'Since most of her day is engulfed between the two activities of either obtaining drugs or being overcome by drugs she spends most of her time unable to function in the usual activities of daily living' (Finnegan 1979a).

Methadone can be used as a low-dose maintenance drug (usually less than 60 mg per day) or as so-called 'blockade' therapy, using higher doses of 80–180 mg per day. Such high-dose regimens are designed to avoid any narcotic craving and the use of heroin 'tastes' or 'top-ups'. However, in our experience the dose of methadone does not seem to relate to continuing heroin abuse and this is still found in patients on blockade therapy (Fig. 6.1). If the addict presents de novo, the switch from heroin to methadone can be achieved

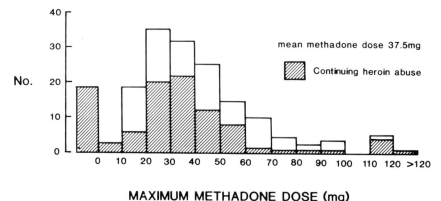

MAXIMUM METHADONE DOSE (mg)

Methadone therapy started :

Pre-pregnancy or 1st trimester-35%

2nd trimester-32%

3rd trimester-24%

No methadone-9%

(49% of patients continued to abuse heroin after stabilisation)

Fig. 6.1 Maximum methadone dosages used during pregnancy in a group of Australian narcotic abusers. The hatched bars in each group represent the proportion who continued to abuse heroin in the pregnancy. The percentages starting methadone in each trimester are shown also (from Ellwood et al 1987)

as an in- or out-patient, but the hospital setting is preferred as it is likely to lead to more rapid stabilisation and a smoother transition from one drug to the other. Patients already on a methadone maintenance programme may need some dose adjustments as the pharmacokinetics of methadone administration are considerably altered by pregnancy necessitating increased doses to continue maintenance (Pond et al 1985).

Detoxification

Acute detoxification of the pregnant addict should not be considered as a management option due to the simultaneous narcotic withdrawal experienced by the fetus, which may lead to intra-uterine death (Neuberg 1970). Slow detoxification in pregnancy using methadone substitution, then gradual withdrawal, through the remainder of the pregnancy has been proposed as a means of obtaining a drug-free mother and fetus at delivery, theoretically avoiding problems of neonatal narcotic withdrawal. However, in practice this is difficult to achieve, perhaps due to the altered methadone pharmacokinetics. It has been proposed that acupuncture therapy be used to aid withdrawal, utilising this technique's known ability to stimulate production of endogenous opiates, and it is hoped that a trial of this therapy in postnatal patients will be started in our unit next year. However, it is unlikely to be an option in pregnancy as it would not overcome the problem of fetal withdrawal in utero and may cause additional fetal stress.

Antenatal care

Because of the highly specialised nature of this work, it is preferable that such patients are managed by an experienced multidisciplinary unit providing comprehensive antenatal care. Whether such a unit should be linked to the methadone maintenance programme is debatable, but this probably makes the management easier and allows for more rational dose adjustments as the pregnancy progresses. Regular urinary drug-screening to watch for continuing heroin abuse may be employed on a random basis. In our experience this is often welcomed by patients who appreciate the continuing surveillance and the objective evidence of abstention from heroin. Because of the high level of care which these patients require, we see all patients at least every 2 weeks throughout the pregnancy. It is also worth noting that the success of a comprehensive care programme depends a lot on the type of trusting relationship which can be built up between the addict and her doctors. For this reason we believe that continuity of care by one or two obstetricians is an ideal for which one should aim.

Antenatal screening

Apart from the usual antenatal screening tests, certain specific additional tests are performed. Because of the past sexual histories of these patients, who may have been highly promiscuous or working as prostitutes, it is to be expected that a high incidence of sexually-transmitted diseases will be found. Although reports from the USA have shown this to be the case (Stone et al 1971, Ostrea & Chavez 1979, Strauss et al 1974), our recent study has not confirmed this for an Australian population (Ellwood et al 1987). Nevertheless, we routinely perform endocervical swabs at booking and this should be repeated in the third trimester. It should be noted that serological tests for syphilis may often show biological false-positives in pregnancy and particularly in intravenous drug users. HbSAg screening is routinely done twice in the pregnancy, and more recently we have introduced testing for HIV antibodies which we also do twice, the final testing being at 36 weeks. Because of the very high rate of uncertain pregnancy dating, an ultrasound scan between 16 and 22 weeks is helpful and is done routinely in this unit.

Antenatal complications

Apart from higher incidences of many of the antenatal complications experienced by the routine clinic patient, there are a number of specific problems which make management of the pregnancy difficult. Hyperemesis gravidarum is a troublesome condition which, in this group, may be very severe and persist throughout the pregnancy. This inevitably leads to repeated difficulties with daily methadone administration and is a reason why stabilisation in the first trimester may be hard to achieve. Whether this is a significant contributing factor in the maternal malnutrition reported by some workers is uncertain (Finnegan 1979b), but disease due to vitamin B_6, folic acid and thiamine deficiencies are common in this group (Wapner & Finnegan 1981). Our recent series of nearly 200 patients showed anaemia (Hb < 10 g/dl) to be present in 12%, and this may also reflect their poor nutritional status (Ellwood et al 1987).

Obstetric problems are increased by the unexplained higher incidences of breech presentation and multiple pregnancy (Ostrea & Chavez 1979, Rementeria et al 1975), although the latter may be the result of multiple ovulations induced by a direct narcotic effect on the ovary leading to dizygotic twinning (see Table 6.2). However, of all the antenatal complications which

Table 6.2 Details of labour and delivery in a group of narcotic drug abusers compared with a group of routine clinic patients from the same hospital

	Drug abusers (%) ($n = 182$)	Clinic patients (%) ($n = 182$)
Time of delivery		
37 weeks	75	87
34–36 weeks	14	9
33 weeks	11	4
Intervention		
Induction	37	15
Epidural analgesia	61	45
Forceps	30	16
Caesarean section	13	10
Breech	9	4
(Twins)	3.5	1

Data adapted from Ellwood et al (1987)

occur, by far the commonest are pre-term labour and intra-uterine growth retardation (IUGR), the former often being associated with abruption, chorioamnionitis and premature rupture of the membranes. In our clinic population, the rates of pre-term delivery and growth retardation have both been approximately 25%, although it should be remembered that many of the small-for-gestational age infants will deliver pre-term either spontaneously or electively (Ellwood et al 1987). These patients rarely 'threaten' to labour pre-term, and if admitted with the diagnosis of pre-term labour they frequently deliver, with attempts at suppression proving futile.

Fetal assessment

With such a high-risk group it is important to have reliable methods of detecting fetal compromise. However, the traditionally used methods are not without problems. Antenatal cardiotocographs (CTGs) are very much affected by methadone, with loss of variability and lack of accelerations being common occurrences. Oestriol excretion is also an unreliable indicator as it is commonly low in this group. It may be that newly developed methods such as Doppler studies of umbilical artery blood flow will be of use in fetal monitoring antenatally, particularly in those pregnancies with IUGR.

THE LABOUR

Certain characteristics of these patients contribute to intrapartum management difficulties that are not often encountered with the average patient. The frequent use of intravenous injections may leave the woman with poor venous access, and as a precautionary measure it is wise to insert an intravenous line when in established labour as this can be difficult when faced with an intrapartum emergency (Perlmutter 1974). Analgesia in labour is also a problem as intramuscular opiates are not particularly desirable and are often ineffective. In our practice epidural anaesthesia is used often and has high patient acceptability. Because of the high prevalence of fetal compromise during these pregnancies and the especially high rate of IUGR, all of our patients are continuously monitored in labour. Meconium staining of the liquor is reported to be more common in these patients (Finnegan 1979b) and may be an unreliable indicator of fetal stress, most likely resulting from episodes of narcotic overdosage and withdrawal prior to labour. In one way the history of narcotic abuse seems to be of benefit to the patient, as it appears that the length of labour is significantly reduced (Finnegan 1986, personal communication). Other obstetric problems faced during intrapartum management are those caused by pre-term labour, breech presentation and multiple pregnancy. Because of these factors, and possibly due to our liberal use of epidural anaesthesia, our recent series showed high rates of operative delivery (see Table 6.2). One further point to note is that labour ward protocols need to be established which clearly define the intrapartum management of patients who are either HBSAg- or HIV-positive.

THE NEONATE

Apart from the neonatal problems caused by pre-term delivery, IUGR and the other pregnancy complications discussed above, the neonate must contend with the problems caused by acute narcotic withdrawal—the neonatal abstinence syndrome. The former problems present the same hazards to these narcotic-dependent neonates as they do to any other except that they are far more frequently encountered, and it is certainly in these areas of prematurity and growth retardation where most of the morbidity and mortality occurs. Although methadone stabilisation and antenatal care seem to have reduced the extremely high perinatal mortality rates seen in uncontrolled heroin addicts (e.g. 174 cases in 1000 quoted by Perlmutter 1967), the rate is still high and in the most recent series was twice that of a comparable drug-free group (Ellwood et al 1987). Many of these deaths are still-births, which have often been excluded from the figures presented by authors writing about this problem in the USA. Of the neonatal deaths in the Sydney group, all were associated with pre-term delivery, and the prevention of this problem is of paramount importance. Although claims have been made that methadone may reduce the incidence of IUGR, there has not been a well-controlled trial and the uncertainty of dating in these patients makes such an analysis difficult (Kandall et al 1976, Zelson et al 1973). Data from our unit would suggest that the earlier the time of methadone stabilisation in pregnancy, the lower the pre-term delivery rate will be (Table 6.3), but it is not possible

Table 6.3   Rates of pre-term delivery and small-for-gestational age (SGA) babies related to the time of methadone stabilisation

	SGA (%)	Pre-term delivery(%)
First trimester	25	20
Second trimester	24	22
Third trimester	25	29
No methadone	25	37.5

Data adapted from Ellwood et al (1987)

from these data to differentiate between an effect of methadone and more comprehensive antenatal care.

Neonatal abstinence syndrome

Narcotic withdrawal in the neonate will occur regardless of the narcotic used in pregnancy. Neonatal abstinence syndrome (NAS) is characterised by signs and symptoms of central nervous system irritation, with gastrointestinal dysfunction, respiratory distress and signs of autonomic dysfunction such as yawning, sneezing and fever. As the syndrome progresses, a high-pitched cry may be heard and hypertonia becomes evident. It has been reported that more than 90% of neonates with NAS will convulse if untreated (Perlmutter 1974) and herein lies the danger, particularly in those neonates from unidentified narcotic-abuser pregnancies. Once the pregnancy has been identified, a rigid surveillance system can be initiated, preferably using a chart such as that designed by Finnegan et al (1975). Many treatments have been tried for the relief of the symptoms of NAS, including benzodiazepines, phenothiazines, and opiates, but one of the most commonly used drugs is phenobarbitone, which can be given intramuscularly at first, then orally. The withdrawal rates quoted in large series vary from 30 to 80%, and in our recent series 46% of neonates showed signs of NAS sufficient to warrant treatment. Claims have been made that methadone control in pregnancy causes less severe withdrawal than heroin (Connaughton et al 1977), but the converse has also been stated (Zelson 1973, Kandall et al 1976). There is no clear evidence that the methadone or heroin dose is realted to the incidence of NAS, although the duration of treatment may be significant (Connaughton et al 1977). Again, the uncertainty of methadone pharmacokinetics in the pregnant woman may be responsible for the apparent lack of correlation of the incidence and severity of NAS with the dose. From a practical point of view it should be remembered that the inadvertent administration of the opiate antagonist, naloxone, to a narcotic-dependent neonate may provoke an instantaneous and severe form of NAS.

Congenital malformations

There is no apparent increase in the risk of severe congenital malformations associated with narcotic abuse in pregnancy, but inguinal herniae and hypospadias have been reported to occur more commonly than would be expected (Perlmutter 1974, Finnegan 1979a). A recent report suggests a reduction in both intracranial hemi-diameter and cerebral ventricular size at birth, but the significance of these findings is unclear (Pasto et al 1985).

THE INFANT

Having safely negotiated the hurdles of prematurity, low birth weight, NAS and the rest, what lies ahead for thcse infants? A more than five-fold increase in the incidence of sudden infant death syndrome (SIDS) has been reported in infants of narcotic-dependent mothers (Rajegouda et al 1978), and this finding has been confirmed in our series from Sydney (Ellwood et al 1987). Maternal death is also not uncommon from overdose, suicide and murder, and combined with the high perinatal death rate and the high incidence of SIDS will mean that a lot of family units are dissolved within 12 months. Developmental delay has been reported in up to 75% of such children studied at various times during the first 10 years of life (Oloffson et al 1983), but detailed follow-up and assessment of infants born to mothers from our clinic have shown more optimistic results (Hogan et al 1986, Di Gusto et al 1986). An important point to make here is that mothers and their infants require continuity of care beyond delivery, which includes social work support and easy access for the mother and child to paediatric services. One practical point worthy of discussion is the place of breast-feeding in mothers who are continuing on a methadone programme. Some units use an arbitrary cut-off of a methadone dose of 50 mg per day, below which breast-feeding is positively encouraged and above which it is not permitted. The effect of continued exposure to narcotics is not clear, but theoretically sudden cessation of breast-feeding by mothers on high methadone doses (or who are continuing to abuse heroin) could precipitate a withdrawal in the infant.

THE FUTURE

It seems likely that the problem of maternal narcotic addiction will be a permanent feature of our society. Narcotic abuse in Sydney is an increasing problem and unless the whole drug scene changes dramatically the future looks bleak, with increasing numbers of drug-dependent pregnancies. It is also likely that other, perhaps more sinister, drugs of abuse will be seen in increasing frequency, such as cocaine and its newer synthetic derivatives which will cause different problems in pregnancy. Combinations of cocaine and heroin may lead to a much higher perinatal mortality rate (Finnegan 1986, personal communication). This population is at considerable risk from AIDS and we are starting to see more and more pregnancies complicated by HIV antibodies.

One of the most important aims for the future should be to explore alternatives to long-term methadone maintenance, particularly as this is still associated with high rates of pre-term delivery and IUGR. It is likely that pre-term delivery in this group has many causes. Some of these are listed in Table 6.4, and since many relate to the addict's previous life-style, methadone main-

Table 6.4   Some of the possible contributing factors leading to pre-term delivery

Narcotic effects on fetal and maternal control of gestation length
Smoking and other drugs
Previous second trimester and repeated first trimester termination
Genital tract microorganism colonisation
Multiple pregnancy
Malnutrition
Previous medical and surgical problems
Acute detoxification

tenance should not be expected to have a major effect. However, comprehensive antenatal care and patient education early in the pregnancy may be more significant. Improvements in methods of identifying such pregnancies are needed, as the failure to identify drug addiction may lead to unexplained neonatal morbidity which is inappropriately diagnosed and treated. In larger maternity units in inner-city areas it may be reasonable to advocate antenatal urinary drug screening, and we would certainly recommend the establishment of at least one specialised drug and alcohol antenatal service in each major city.

Finally, in view of the considerable cost to health services caused by both maternal and neonatal morbidity from these pregnancies, it is vital that there is continuing audit of pregnancy outcome with an emphasis on cost-effectiveness of the management. For example, there has never been a controlled trial comparing pregnancy outcome in patients managed by methadone stabilisation with those in whom continuing heroin abuse is permitted whilst offering the maximum in antenatal health care and support. It may be that medical supervision of the continuing use of a regulated dose of legally prescribed pure heroin would produce the best results of pregnancy outcome, and that any attempt at methadone stabilisation should be left until the puerperium.

REFERENCES

Collins E 1982 A hospital based drug screening program. Australian Alcohol/Drug Review 1: 52–53
Connaughton J F, Reser D, Schut J, Finnegan L P 1977 Perinatal addiction: outcome and management. American Journal of Obstetrics and Gynecology 129: 679–686
Di Gusto J, Collins E, Herbutt S, Hogan M 1986 Children exposed ante-natally to narcotic drugs: developmental status at 18–24 months of age. Australian Paediatric Journal 22: 238
Donkin P, Vilkins B, Beilby V et al 1985 Report on illicit drug analysis statistics 1980 to 1984, Division of Analytical Laboratories, NSW Department of Health, Australia, p 5
Ellwood D A, Sutherland P, Kent C, O'Connor M 1987 Maternal narcotic addiction: pregnancy outcome in patients managed by a specialised drug-dependency antenatal clinic. Australian and New Zealand Journal of Obstetrics and Gynaecology 27: 92–98
Finnegan L P 1979a Pathophysiological and behavioural effects of the transplacental transfer of narcotic drugs to the fetuses and neonates of narcotic-dependent mothers. Bulletin of Narcotics 31 (3 & 4): 1–58
Finnegan L P 1979b Drug dependence in pregnancy: clinical management of mother and child. In: Services Research Monograph Series, US Government Printing Office, Washington, p 34
Finnegan L P, Kron R E, Connaughton J F, Emrich J P 1975 A scoring system for evaluation and treatment of the neonatal abstinence syndrome: a clinical and research tool. In: Morsilli P L, Garatinni S, Sereni F (eds) Basic and therapeutic aspects of perinatal pharmacology, Raven Press, New York, p 139
Gaulden E, Littlefield D, Putoff O, Sievert A 1964 Menstrual abnormalities associated with heroin addiction. American Journal of Obstetrics and Gynecology 90: 155–160
Hogan M, Collins E, DiGusto J, Harbutt S 1986 Children exposed ante-natally to narcotic drugs: health and growth at 18–24 months of age. Australian Paediatric Journal 22: 238
Kandall S R, Albin S, Lowinson J, Berlc B, Eidelman A I, Gartner L M 1976 Differential effects of maternal heroin and methadone use on birthweight. Pediatrics 58: 681–685
Neuberg R 1970 Drug dependence and pregnancy: a review of the problems and their management. Journal of Obstetrics and Gynaecology of the British Commonwealth 77: 1117–1123
Newman R G, Bashkow S, Calko D 1975 Results of 313 consecutive live births of infants delivered to patients in the New York City methadone-maintenance program. American Journal of Obstetrics and Gynecology 120: 895–900
Oloffson M, Buckley W, Andersoen G E, Friis-Hansen B 1983 Investigation of 89 children born by drug-dependent mothers. II. Follow up 1–10 years after birth. Acta Pediatricia Scandinavica 72: 407–410
Ostrea E M, Chavez C J 1979 Perinatal problems (excluding neonatal withdrawal) in maternal drug addiction: a study of 830 cases. Journal of Pediatrics 94: 292–295
Pasto M E, Graziani L J, Tunis S L et al 1985 Ventricular configuration and cerebral growth in infants born to drug-dependent mothers. Pediatric Radiology 15: 77–81
Perlmutter J F 1967 Drug addiction in pregnant women. American Journal of Obstetrics and Gynecology 99: 569–572
Perlmutter J F 1974 Heroin addiction and pregnancy. Obstetrical and Gynecological Survey 29: 439–446
Pond S M, Kreek M J, Tong T G, Raghuntath J, Benowitz N L 1985 Altered methadone pharmacokinetics in methadone-maintained pregnant women. Journal of Pharmacology and Experimental Therapeutics 233: 1–6
Rajegouda B K, Kandal J R, Falcighia H 1978 Sudden infant death in infants of narcotic-dependent mothers. Early Human Development 2: 219–225
Rementeria J L, Jankammal S, Hollander M 1975 Multiple births in drug-addicted women. American Journal of Obstetrics and Gynecology 122: 958–960
Stone M L, Salerno L J, Green M, Zelson C 1971 Narcotic addiction in pregnancy. American Journal of Obstetrics and Gynecology 109: 716–723

Strauss M E, Andresko M, Styker J C, Wardell J N, Dunkel L D 1974 Methadone maintenance during pregnancy: pregnancy, birth and neonate characteristics. American Journal of Obstetrics and Gynecology 120: 895–900

Wapner R J, Finnegan L P 1981 Perinatal aspects of psychotropic drug abuse. In: Bolognese R J, Schwarz R H, Schneider J (eds) Perinatal medicine, Williams & Wilkins, Baltimore

Zelson C 1973 Infant of the addicted mother. New England Journal of Medicine 288: 1393–1395

Zelson C, Lee S J, Casalino M 1973 Neonatal narcotic addiction. New England Journal of Medicine 289: 1216–1220

Fetal heart rate variability

INTRODUCTION

Fetal heart rate variability (FHRV), the irregularity of the heart beat, was originally described as the fluctuations seen on chart recordings of the continuous heart rate during labour (Caldeyro-Barcia et al 1966, Wood et al 1967, Hammacher et al 1968). In 1968, Hon introduced the idea of baseline variability as the degree of irregularity of the heart rate between the periodic changes associated with uterine contractions. This has come to be regarded as long-term FHRV, which does not take into account large departures from the baseline such as accelerations or decelerations. He also described short-term beat-to-beat variability of the fetal heart rate (FHR) as the variation in successive pulse intervals. This may be seen as small, rapid fluctuations superimposed on the longer-term oscillations of the FHR record if the monitor identifies consecutive R waves of the fetal electrocardiogram (ECG) and converts each pulse interval to an instantaneous heart rate. On-line calculation of beat-to-beat variability requires a microprocessor.

FHRV has increasingly come to be regarded as one of the most important features of the continuously recorded FHR. The presence of variability is thought to differentiate physiological from pathological decelerations and bradycardias (Paul et al 1975, Krebs et al 1979b) and is considered to represent fetal reserve by being an indicator of central (cerebral and myocardial) oxygenation (Parer 1983). However, the origins of FHRV remain poorly understood and the distinction between 'asphyxial' and 'non-asphyxial' causes of decreased variability has caused some confusion in clinical obstetrics (Court & Parer 1984).

This chapter will review data concerning the origins of FHRV and will briefly present some of the methods that have been used to quantify and measure it. Factors known to affect FHRV and the significance of FHRV in clinical practice will then be discussed.

THE ORIGINS OF FETAL HEART RATE VARIABILITY

The autonomic nervous system

Blockade of the parasympathetic nervous system using atropine produces a significant reduction in the high frequency, beat-to-beat variability of the FHR in sheep (Kleinhout et al 1977, Zugaib et al 1980, Dalton et al 1983) and in man (Renou et al 1969, Schifferli & Caldeyro-Barcia 1973). Such short-term FHRV is not significantly affected by sympathetic blockade using propranolol, despite a fall in heart rate (de Haan et al 1979, Dalton et al 1983), which would imply that FHRV is not purely the result of a balance between the two components of the autonomic nervous system. However, a decrease in long-term FHRV occurs after sympathetic blockade in exteriorised fetal lambs (Kleinhout et al 1977) and in neonatal lambs (Zugaib et al 1980). Changes in heart rate do not account for the changes in variability during pharmacological blockade in the neonatal lamb (Zugaib et al 1980), although spontaneous changes in FHR do affect the variability (Dalton et al 1977, de Haan et al 1979). There is a progressive increase in variability associated with the progressive fall in FHR during the last third of gestation in fetal lambs (Dalton et al 1977). Long-term changes in FHRV during pregnancy include a diurnal rhythm where both heart rate and variability are higher in the evening (Dalton et al 1977).

After combined parasympathetic and sympathetic blockade in fetal lambs to isolate the heart from all autonomic influence, Dalton et al (1983) found that 35–40% of total variability remained. In other studies long-term variability was either abolished (Kleinhout et al 1977) or decreased significantly (Zugaib et al 1980). Dalton et al (1983) concluded that there is a major non-neuronal component to total FHRV, but this view is at variance with that of others who feel that variability can be explained on the basis of combined autonomic nervous system influences (Kleinhout et al 1977, de Haan et al 1979, Zugaib et al 1980).

The influence of fetal breathing and body movements

Fetal breathing movements occur during episodes of low-voltage, fast electrocortical activity in the fetal sheep (Dawes et al 1976) and are associated with an increase in FHRV (Dalton et al 1977). There are no fetal breathing movements after destruction of the brain stem in the fetal lamb (Robinson et al 1980) and the FHR loses its variability (Martin 1984). Sectioning of the brain stem of the fetal lamb above the pons to separate it from higher centres results in continuous fetal breathing, even during high-voltage electrocortical activity which normally inhibits fetal breathing (Dawes et al 1983), and short-term variability increases (Hofmeyr et al 1985).

The human fetus exhibits a respiratory sinus arrhythmia (Fouron et al 1975, Timor-Tritsch et al 1977, Wheeler et al 1980, Divon et al 1985a). This may be due to discharges from the respiratory centre affecting the cardiovascular centre in the brain stem as it is unlikely that the chest movements are sufficient to stimulate lung reflexes. However, changes in venous return to the heart during fetal breathing may contribute directly to the beat-to-beat variability in heart rate (Kirkpatrick et al 1976, Wheeler et al 1980), and a baroreceptor reflex secondary to rhythmic changes in blood pressure during breathing cannot be excluded (Fouron et al 1975, Divon et al 1985b).

A reduction in variability of the heart rate in the fetal lamb following administration of the neuromuscular blocking agent, gallamine, suggested that much of the FHRV was attributable to fetal movements (Dalton et al 1977). Periods of activity in the human fetus often occur without fetal breathing movements (Junge & Walter 1980) and are associated with increased short-term and long-term variation of the baseline (Wheeler et al 1980). Fetal body movements are also associated with accelerations of the fetal heart rate (Aladjem et al 1977) which further highlight the visual appearance of increased long-term variability on records of the FHR during fetal activity.

Thus long-term variability probably results from the activities of both the parasympathetic and sympathetic systems, whilst short-term, beat-to-beat variability results mainly from small fluctuations in parasympathetic activity (de Haan et al 1979) or the local effects of fetal activities such as movements and breathing (Dalton et al 1977) or both. Because of the number of physiological parameters known to influence short-term FHRV, its true value remains undetermined.

THE MEASUREMENT OF FETAL HEART RATE VARIABILITY

Visual methods

The visual apperance of FHRV was first described by Caldeyro-Barcia et al (1966) in terms of irregularities of the basal rate. Hon (1968) described a template, calculated for different heart rates, to place over the heart rate trace to measure the amplitude of these fluctuations as a percentage of the baseline rate. Hammacher et al (1968) described a value of less than five beats per minute amplitude of fluctuation (silent pattern) as abnormal, and values of between 5 and 10 (narrow undulatory) beats per minute were regarded as the lower limit of normal. Variability above 25 beats per minute (saltatory) was also considered abnormal, and between 10 and 25 beats per minute amplitude the variability was described as normal (undulatory). These values have been perpetuated by subsequent studies (Beard et al 1971, Paul et al 1975) and are still considered the normal limits of visually discernible long-term variability.

Calculated indices of intrapartum FHRV

Quantitative measurement of FHRV began by using the R–R intervals obtained from the scalp ECG during labour, and a large number of derived formulae now exist. The methods of de Haan et al (1971a) and Yeh et al (1973), and Hon's visual index, were compared by Laros et al (1977). They found that the indices of de Haan et al (1971a), derived by plotting consecutive R–R intervals against each other, were the least interdependent, with long-term irregularity measurements being completely insensitive to artificially generated short-term variability. The differential index (DI) of short-term variability (standard deviation of R–R intervals) and the interval index (II) of long-term variability (coefficient of variation of R–R intervals) devised by Yeh et al (1973) exhibited substantial positive interdependence. Hon's visual index was a measure of long-term variability only. Laros et al (1977) derived the interquartile range of the short-term and long-term irregularity of de Haan et al (1971a) and called these the short-term index (STI) and the long-term index (LTI) respectively. Further study of the STI and the DI as measures of short-term variability (Detwiler et al 1980) showed that 30 seconds of data with a mean heart rate of 150 beats per minute could only be measured with 95% confidence to within plus or minus 32% of random error. Five minutes of sampling would be necessary to reduce random error to plus or minus 10% with 95% confidence. They suggested averaging the intervals between several successive contactions so that statistical reliability might be obtained, though with less frequent short-term variability values.

In an attempt to simplify R–R interval analysis in labour, Young et al (1978) described a graphic display of the cumulative percentage of R–R interval changes plotted as interval differences in beats per minute. This method was shown to correlate well with visual descriptions of variability without the need for complex mathematical calculations and provided a simple on-line quantification of fetal heart rate variability from the R wave of the fetal ECG over pre-determined intervals.

Organ et al (1978) described the calculation of instantaneous variability (IV) for short-term variability (average absolute value of instantaneous rate differences over 30 seconds) and band-width variability as a measure of long-term variability (twice the standard deviation of instantaneous rates every 30 seconds). They showed the similarity between continuous recordings of IV, DI and STI calculated over 30-second intervals, and the similarity between band-width variability, II and LTI also calculated over 30-second intervals. A 30-second interval was chosen for sufficient resolution of any changes in variability without the sample size being too small. Wade et al (1976) calculated variability in a manner similar to instantaneous variability as part of a computer program for labour monitoring, and set the alarm criterion for short-term variability as diminished variability in six of the previous eight 30-second segments. Modanlou et al (1977) derived a method of short-term variability quantitation (VQ) in which the summation of consecutive differences in instantaneous heart rate was divided by the number of determinations over a given period (abitrarily chosen as 1 minute). This method was incorporated into an automated on-line analysis system with a modification to give a VQ value for consecutive 10-minute periods (Tromans et al 1982).

A comparison of visual assessment of variability with the DI, II and bandwidth variability showed that there was a high degree of observer agreement on variability content for both short-term and long-term variability (Escarcena et al 1979). However, the calculated indices did not compare well with the clinical estimates and the authors concluded that clinical interpretation of variability (by nine experts in their study) encompasses different information than is found in the calculated indices. Kariniemi (1978) also showed a poor correlation between the II and DI compared with visual assessment of FHRV according to Hammacher et al (1968). He concluded that such visual assessment was inappropriate for evaluating FHRV from records obtained directly from the fetal ECG and showed that a computer could be used to teach obstetric staff to improve their evaluation of the two components of FHRV.

A major drawback of the calculated indices of FHRV is that they are all subject to random sampling fluctuations when computed over a finite number of cardiac cycles (Detwiler et al 1980). These authors showed how the coefficient of variation decreased with increasing sample size. However, Parer et al (1984) reported that, whilst few of the indices related to clinically recognizable long-term variability, most indices of short-term variability were valid measurements of beat-to-beat differences in FHR. As pointed out by Dalton et al (1977), calculated indices which compound quantitative measurements of mean heart rate and variability into a single statistic have relied on the assumption that heart rate variability decreases as heart rate increases, but this is not true in the fetal sheep. Visual evaluation of variability from continuous heart rate records is an assessment of long-term variability (Laros et al 1977, Kariniemi 1978), and the high degree of observer agreement on variability, despite the fact that visual evaluation is undoubtedly subjective, suggests that a specific visually recognizable variability pattern does exist and is evaluated in a similar fashion (Escarcena et al 1979). Thus, in practice, long-term FHRV continues to be visually interpreted from continuous FHR records whilst computations of short-term variability remain the subject of research.

FHRV from the fetal ECG during pregnancy

The fetal ECG may be picked up from electrodes placed on the mother's abdomen and the R waves used to derive an instantaneous or beat-to-beat FHR. The accuracy of this method of deriving the ECG for calculation of the II and the DI has been shown by simultaneous recordings of the fetal ECG from scalp electrodes and maternal abdominal electrodes during early labour (Kariniemi et al 1979, Solum et al 1980). The success rate of recording the fetal ECG from the mother's abdomen decreases significantly between 28 and 34 weeks, thereby limiting the value of the technique at this time (Wheeler et al 1978, Kariniemi et al 1980, Carter et al 1980).

FHRV using Doppler ultrasound

Continuous records of the FHR derived from the Doppler shift of ultrasound signals using external transducers on the maternal abdominal wall appear similar to records derived from the ECG. However, ultrasound signals are less reliable, so averaging techniques are used by the fetal monitors to calculate the FHR from more than one pulse interval. Thus true beat-to-beat variability cannot be determined from ultrasound-derived signals, but long-term variability of the baseline is adequately displayed and can be assessed visually or by using a perspex grid (Wheeler & Guerard 1974). As true beat-to-beat variation encompasses only the components of highest frequency, which amount to less than one-tenth of the total FHR variation (Dawes et al 1981a), these authors have questioned the value of beat-to-beat variation as an indicator of fetal well-being because it is influenced by so many physiological variables. They have developed a computerized analysis system for ultrasound-derived FHR signals (Dawes et al 1981b, Wickham et al 1983) and conclude that the most useful measures of FHR analysis are medium-term variations and accelerations (Dawes et al 1985).

Ultrasound signal loss and FHRV measurement

The main problem with ultrasound as a technique for recording the fetal heart is that movement—both maternal and fetal—interferes with signal pick-up. Wheeler & Guerard (1974) found that only 30% of antenatal records were complete, whilst in 12% of cases there was more than 20% of the record missing. Continuous-wave Doppler ultrasound monitors have a mean signal loss of 23% (Dawes et al 1981b), and the missing data occur to a great extent during episodes of increased baseline variability associated with an increase in fetal activity. Pulsed Doppler ultrasound with autocorrelation was introduced with the new generation of microprocessor-based fetal monitors and has reduced signal loss during pregnancy to less than 5% (Dawes et al 1985). Increased loss of the ultrasound signal significcnatly reduces the calculated FHR variation when compared with that from the simultaneously recorded fetal scalp ECG in labour (Spencer et al 1987).

FACTORS AFFECTING FETAL HEART RATE VARIABILITY

Behavioural state changes

High-voltage electrocortical activity in the fetal sheep is associated with increased sympathetic activity and produces a rise in FHR (Clapp et al 1980, Hofmeyr et al 1985) and a fall in long-term variability (van der Wildt 1982). This differs from the human fetus at term in that a decrease in heart rate and a reduction in oscillation band-width (long-term variability) occur during quiet sleep (Nijhuis 1984). In the human neonate both heart rate and variability were increased during activity and reduced in quiet sleep (de Haan et al

1977, van Geijn et al 1980a). Such discrepancies between the sheep and human fetus reflect species differences in the interaction between central nervous system activity, fetal breathing, fetal body movements and their effects on the FHR and its variability.

The mature human fetus undergoes cyclical changes in behavioural state, alternating between active periods with frequent episodes of body movements, and rest periods with little fetal activity (Timor-Tritsch et al 1978, Nijhuis et al 1982). The influence of such changes on the FHR in late pregnancy has been well described (Wheeler & Murrills 1978, Dawes et al 1982) and is seen as consecutive episodes of high- and low-FHR variability. Episodes of fetal rest with reduced FHR variability and no fetal movements or FHR accelerations are therefore interpreted as non-reactive unless either the period of recording is extended until spontaneous change to the active state occurs (Merkur 1979, Brown & Patrick 1981) or a change in state is induced such as by vibratory-acoustic stimulation (Ohel et al 1986). Only 5% of recordings needed to be continued after 40 minutes, and only 1% remained unreactive for up to 120 minutes (Brown & Patrick 1981).

Fetal rest–activity cycles continue into labour as indicated by the persistence of episodic changes in FHRV despite the reduction in fetal body and breathing movements (Richardson et al 1979, Greene et al 1980). Consecutive episodes of low and high FHRV consistent with cycles of quiet and active fetal behaviour could be identified in 38% of spontaneous and 68% of induced labours (Spencer & Johnson 1986). The mean duration of quiet episodes (with low FHRV) was 25 minutes, but the range was up to 90 minutes. However, only 5% of quiet episodes lasted for longer than 46 minutes, which is in broad agreement with the antenatal findings of Brown & Patrick (1981). In 48% of labours exhibiting rest–activity cycles, the quiet episodes had a FHRV of less than five beats per minute. First quiet episodes with such a low FHRV lasted for longer than 20 minutes in 28% of cases and for longer than 30 minutes in 9% of cases (Spencer & Johnson 1986).

Fetal stimulation

External physical stimulation is not effective in terminating a period of fetal rest and inducing activity (Visser et al 1983), and does not reduce the number of non-reactive FHR records (Druzin et al 1985). Several workers have shown the value of assessing the response of the FHR to sound stimulation. An impaired response, in terms of a failure to induce fetal movements with their associated FHR acceleration, was more predictive of subsequent perinatal morbidity than a non-reactive FHR record alone (Trudinger & Boylan 1980, Jensen 1984). Sound stimulation reduces the number of equivocal FHR records during pregnancy (Davey et al 1984). Leader et al (1982) studied fetal habituation to a repeated vibrotactile stimulus and showed highly significant differences between high-risk and normal fetuses.

Fetal stimulation in the presence of a worrying FHR record during labour was suggested by Clark et al (1984) who showed that a FHR acceleration in response to scalp stimulation (tissue forceps or scalpel) indicated an absence of significant acidosis.

Hypoxaemia and acidosis

The primary response of the healthy sheep fetus to acute hypoxaemia is profound stimulation of the vagus nerve secondary to the hypertension and peripheral vasoconstriction (Rudolph & Heymann 1974). FHRV increases (Stange et al 1977, Dalton et al 1977) despite the cessation of fetal breathing movements (Dalton et al 1977). In addition, a stimulation of catecholamine secretion occurs (Jones & Robinson 1975) and the percentage of the cardiac output directed to the brain and myocardium is increased. Blood flow to the adrenals is also maintained or even increased, and the abundant stores of catecholamines play a critical role in maintaining ventricular contractility (Cohn et al 1974). Fetal cardiac muscle relies on its glycogen stores for continued glycolysis during oxygen deprivation, and spontaneous atrial contraction in the fetus is maintained for substantially longer periods of time than in the adult during profound hypoxaemia (Friedman & Kirkpatrick 1977). Severe hypoxaemia results in a fall in cardiac output presumably due to decreased myocardial performance secondary to the reduced delivery of oxygen to the heart (Cohn et al 1980).

Hypoxaemia in sheep produced a rise in FHRV even after inhibition of fetal breathing and body movements by the neruomuscular blocking agent, gallamine (Dalton et al 1977). Hypercarbia increased FHRV in association with an increase in fetal breathing movements. An infusion of adrenaline to achieve plasma levels similar to those produced during hypoxaemia (Jones & Robinson 1975) also resulted in an increase in FHRV. This effect was not altered by the administration of 60% oxygen to the maternal ewe. Thus the rise in FHRV seen with experimentally produced hypoxaemia in the sheep may result from the increased levels of catecholamines which slowly overcome the initial vagal bradycardia (Jones & Robinson 1975, Jones & Know Ritchie 1983). A raised level of fetal scalp plasma noradrenaline has also been found to be associated with increased FHRV in normal human labour (Bistoletti et al 1983).

The effects of drugs on FHRV

Diazepam significantly reduces visually assessed long-term variability (Scher et al 1972) and beat-to-beat interval differences (Yeh et al 1974). The administration of diazepam in late pregnancy and labour reduces neonatal heart rate variability as measured by the long-term irregularity index (de Haan et al 1971a) and the II (van Geijn et al 1980b). Using the DI and II of Yeh et al (1973) to assess the effects of pethidine on FHRV in labour, Petrie et al (1978) found a clinically meaningful but statistically insignificant reduction in variability with 50 mg given intravenously. However, Kariniemi and Ammala (1981a) showed a significant reduction in long-term variability (II) and a downward trend in the DI—both maximal at 40 minutes—after 75 mg of pethidine intramuscularly. Bistoletti et al (1983) found that pethidine produced a significant reduction in a modification of the DI performed on-line by the Corometrics 112 fetal monitor (the DI was calculated over 2 minutes of heart rate sampled between uterine contactions). This effect was not accompanied by a change in fetal scalp catecholamine levels and they concluded that the effect of pethidine was not mediated by a depression of sympathoadrenal activity.

Different local anaesthetic agents used for epidural analgesia have produced different effects on FHRV. Lignocaine 2% reduced variability (Hehre et al 1969, Boehm et al 1975), possibly by crossing the placenta and directly depressing the fetal myocardium. Chloroprocaine has a much shorter plasma half-life and has significantly less vasoconstrictive effect on the uterine arteries, which may explain the lack of effect on FHRV (Lavin et al 1981). Bupivacaine crosses the placenta less readily and has a variable effect on FHRV (Lavin et al 1981). These authors showed that the effects on the FHR were due to the drugs and not to volume distension of the epidural space.

The effect of oxytocin on DI and II has been studied (Kariniemi et al 1981), and no trend or correlation with dose was found for the II. However, a decrease in DI with time and with decreasing dose was found. These findings showed that the influence of oxytocin would need to be excluded if the effect of other drugs on FHRV were to be tested.

THE CLINICAL SIGNIFICANCE OF FETAL HEART RATE VARIABILITY

Intrapartum FHRV

Caldeyro-Barcia et al (1966) found no relationship between the incidence and amplitude of the 'rapid fluctuations of fetal heart rate' during labour and the Apgar score of the newborn. In contrast, Hammacher et al (1968) found a correlation between a lower Apgar score and FHRV with oscillations of less than 10 beats per minute amplitude in a group of high-risk pregnancies. Subsequent studies in labour have suggested that a loss of long-term FHRV (five beats per minute or less), particularly when accompanied by tachycardia above 160 beats per minute or late decelerations (Hon 1968), is indicative of fetal hypoxaemia and acidosis (Beard et al 1971, Schifrin & Dame 1972, Bissonnette 1975, Liu et al 1975, Paul et al 1975, Thomas & Blackwell 1975, Gaxiano 1979). Paul et al (1975) showed that, irrespective of the FHR pattern in the last 20 minutes of labour, normal variability (amplitude greater than five beats per minute) was associated with significantly higher 1- and 5-minute Apgar scores after delivery. Krebs et al (1979a) also showed that no single abnormal pattern allowed determination of fetal prognosis and suggested that

FHRV was more an indicator of fetal 'reserve', which would allow classification of FHR changes into compensated and decompensated patterns (Krebs et al 1979b). Cibils (1976) showed an association between low variability in labour and placental insufficiency. Martin et al (1974) found a significant increase in the death rate of low birthweight babies who had shown decreased heart rate variability prior to delivery, but this was not confirmed for growth-retarded fetuses (Odendall 1976).

Sinusoidal FHRV

A sinusoidal FHR pattern in labour has been associated with fetal hypoxia (Baskett & Koh 1974) and fetal death (Sibai et al 1980, Sacks et al 1980), such that operative intervention has been recommended if pH measurements are not possible (Ayromlooi et al 1979). However, the necessity to base management on fetal blood sampling was stressed by Young et al (1980a), who found a poor association between sinusoidal variability and fetal acidosis. They suggested that whilst a sinusoidal pattern may well be due to mild hypoxaemia, this may be transitory and may have no effect on the fetus. The aetiology of sinusoidal FHRV remains unexplained and controversy exists in the literature as to its significance.

Computer analysis of FHRV during labour

Computer analysis of the FHR during labour has not so far contributed significantly to an understanding of FHRV during labour. de Haan et al (1971b) showed the presence of a fixed heart rate in anencephalics, and that administration of sedatives to the mother with a normal fetus produced a similar variability. Kariniemi & Hukkinen (1977) found that the range of values for the DI and the II widened during labour. They ascribed this to sedation and stronger external stimuli, which tended to reduce and increase the values respectively, and they concluded that such measurements might be of more value for the detection of fetal hypoxia prior to labour.

FHRV and scalp oxygen tension measurements

Decreased FHRV was not associated with reduced fetal scalp transcutaneous oxygen tension ($TcPo_2$) measurements during labour (Huch et al 1977, Stange 1979, Willcourt et al 1981, Sykes et al 1984), although there was some correlation between low fetal $TcPo_2$ and a reduced frequency of variability (Huch et al 1977). It seems likely that Willcourt et al (1981) studied changes in the long-term variability of the FHR related to behavioural cycles, as they described reductions lasting from 10 to 50 minutes in duration. During such episodes of low FHRV they found that the $TcPo_2$ rose by 4–12 mmHg. Exaggerated short-term variability, seen visually as a superimposition on the long-term variability, was always associated with a fall in $TcPo_2$ to levels of

3–9 mmHg. They concluded that changes in $TcPo_2$ were related to changes in the heart rate variability but that the presence or absence of FHRV did not reflect baseline levels of fetal oxygenation.

Predictive value of reduced FHRV in labour

The rate of fetal scalp sampling for reduced variability alone varies in incidence from 5 to 28% but the incidence of fetal acidosis (scalp pH 7.20 or less) is only 1–7% (Table 7.1). Using data from six studies reported in the literature over the last 15 years, the significance of reduced FHRV alone in labour is shown in Table 7.2 Calculation of the positive predictive value (Grant 1984) of reduced variability alone for fetal acidosis was 32% at best and varied to as low as 2%. However, the chance of acidosis in the presence of 'normal' variability was also very low, as indicated by the high negative predictive value (Table 7.2). From two of these studies the loss of variability could be differentiated into 'uncomplicated' and 'complicated' (presence of a tachycardia and/or late or variable declerations). The sensitivity and the positive predictive value both increased (Table 7.3) when the loss of variability was complicated, but the positive predictive value was still only around 30%. It should be noted that the majority of women in the study of Beard et al (1971) had been given diazepam in labour, and this may have reduced the sensitivity. Nevertheless, the similarity between the positive predictive values from these two studies is striking.

Table 7.1 Fetal scalp sampling for reduced FHRV alone

Reference	Incidence of fetal sampling		Incidence of fetal acidosis $(=/<7.2)$	
	n	%	n	%
Clark et al (1984)	26	26	1	3.8
Young et al (1980b)	24	10	1	4.2
Zalar & Quilligan (1979)	73	28.3	1	1.4
Thomas & Blackwell (1975)	16	6.3	1	6.3
Beard et al (1971)	15	5.4	1	7.1
Mean		15.2		4.6
SD		11.1		2.2

FHR changes prior to fetal death

Hon (1959) reported that the pattern of the FHR prior to intra-uterine death at 25 weeks could appear normal for periods of time between the episodes of prolonged bradycardia characteristic of impending fetal death. Despite this, it was expected that the FHR would undergo a specific sequence of changes prior to death, and that recognition of the early stages of such a sequence would result in timely intervention. In particular, loss of visually

Table 7.2   Prediction of fetal acidosis by reduced FHRV

Reference	Sensitivity (%)	Specificity (%)	Positive predictive value (%)	Negative predictive value (%)	Prevalence (%)
Scalp pH 7.20 or less					
Clark et al (1984)	7	29	21	79	21
Scalp pH 7.25 or less					
Beard et al (1971)	28	10	32	89	14
Thomas & Blackwell (1975)	57	33	22	91	14
Zalar & Quilligan (1979)	3	18	2	86	12
Young et al (1980b)	5	11	4	91	7
Spencer & Johnson (1986)			32	93	42

Table 7.3   Prediction of fetal acidosis (pH 7.20 or less) with uncomplicated and complicated loss of FHRV

	Beard et al (1971)		Clark et al (1984)	
	Uncomplicated	Complicated	Uncomplicated	Complicated
Sensitivity (%)	2.6	13	5	67
Specificity (%)	94	94	68	61
Positive predictive value (%)	7	26	4	31
Negative predictive value (%)	86	87	72	87

assessed long-term variability has become the key feature of the 'terminal' FHR pattern, both during (Hon & Lee 1963, Cetrulo & Schifrin 1976, Cibils 1977) and before labour (Langer et al 1982).

The value of antepartum FHR variability

The visual assessment of long-term baseline variability has become an integral component of antepartum FHR interpretation. Most scoring systems give reduced values if the baseline variability is less than five beats per minute in amplitude (Fischer et al 1976, Krebs & Petres 1978, Lyons et al 1979). Descriptive classifications have used five beats per minute (Flynn & Kelly 1977) or 10 beats per minute (Visser & Huisjes 1977) as lower levels of normal. Most workers agree that loss of baseline variability is an ominous feature of the antepartum FHR.

The characteristic changes in the FHR (usually recorded by ultrasound) associated with the progressive effects of chronic placental failure and fetal growth retardation include loss of accelerations associated with a reduction in fetal movements, a baseline variability below five beats per minute and, later, the onset of recurrent decelerations (Emmen et al 1975, Rochard et al 1976, Visser & Huisjes 1977, Flynn et al 1979, Keirse & Trimbos 1980, Weingold et al 1980). Such evidence of 'critical fetal reserve' requires delivery, usually by caesarean section, if the fetus is viable, because the quality of survival of such infants was found to be satisfactory (Beischer et al 1983). At delivery there was a significantly higher incidence of metabolic acidosis associated with FHR patterns showing the above features (Visser et al 1980, Chew et al 1985), but when delivery was expedited prior to such 'ominous' or 'terminal' appearances, then fetal decompensation into metabolic acidaemia had not occurred (Henson et al 1983). Cardiotocography has become an indispensable aid in the management of pregnancies complicated by fetal growth retardation and is particularly useful in governing the timing of delivery.

A proportion of antenatal FHR records cannot be called either normal or abnormal. Such patterns have been labelled doubtful (Fischer et al 1976), non-reactive (Rochard et al 1976, Flynn & Kelly 1977), sub-optimal (Visser & Huisjes 1977), suspicious (Trimbos & Keirse 1978), suspect or flat (Flynn et al 1979) and prepathological (Lyons et al 1979). The combination of reduced baseline variability and absence of accelerations accounts for more than 80% of these patterns, and such a record was found on at least one occasion in 37% and twice or more in 9% of normal pregnancies (Trimbos & Keirse 1978). The incidence of a suspicious record in normal pregnancies is about 7%, whereas in high-risk pregnancies it is 17% and the recurrence rate was much higher in high-risk pregnancy (Keirse & Trimbos 1981). They showed that adequate follow-up of such records allowed the majority of cases which did not need intervention to be distinguished from those which did.

A number of studies have evaluated the DI and II (Yeh et al 1973) as an index of fetal well-being during pregnancy. Kariniemi & Ammala (1981b) showed that the DI was a more sensitive indicator of developing fetal acidosis if IUGR was suspected (64%) or if postmature (54%) with predictive values of 80% and 58% respectively. They subsequently showed that the sensitivity of the DI during hypertensive pregnancy in predicting fetal distress in labour was 46%, with a specificity of 97% and a predictive value of 88% (Ammala & Kariniemi 1983).

SUMMARY

FHRV derives from intrinsic beat-by-beat changes in stroke volume as well as from longer-term fluctuations resulting from the influence of the autonomic nervous system. Short-term variability due to fluctuations in venous return is influenced predominantly by respiratory movements. The larger fluctuations of approximately 2–6 cycles per minute, together with accelerations, represent the combined effects of both the sympathetic and parasympathetic nervous systems in maintaining normal blood pressure and peripheral perfusion through reflex pathways which depend upon an intact and adequately oxygenated central nervous system. The ability to change the circulation in response to variations in body function, such as the different behavioural states, means that control must be both sensitive and effective. The parasympathetic nervous pathway via the vagus nerves has the ability to slow the heart rate very quickly in response to baroreceptor stimulation during hypertension. Cardiac acceleratory activity associated with fetal movements also occurs rapidly and is the result of brain stem influences on cardiac control. Conversely, the sympathetic adrenergic receptors in the heart respond to the slower and longer-lasting effects of changes in catecholamine levels, seen particularly in the sheep fetus during induced hypoxaemia as a gradual return to normal of the heart rate following the initial bradycardia. The fetal sheep demonstrates increased FHRV in association with increased catecholamine levels during acutely induced hypoxaemia. Such changes have not been documented in the human fetus but it is interesting to note the increased FHRV associated with raised levels of catecholamines during human labour.

Chronic placental failure, with fetal growth retardation secondary to reduced maternal placental perfusion, is also associated with elevated fetal levels of catecholamines which determine the circulatory changes to maintain cerebral oxygenation. As fetal adaptation reaches its limit, the fetus becomes metabolically acidaemic, and these circumstances are associated with specific changes in FHR which include a loss of variability. However, other causes of reduced FHRV, such as a quiet behavioural state and drugs like diazepam, do not relate to fetal problems and so contribute to the false positivity of reduced FHRV alone as an indicator of fetal compromise. Various means to improve the specificity of the FHR as a means of assessing fetal well-being have included the effect of acoustic-vibratory stimulation through the maternal abdomen, combined assessment with other factors in the biophysical profile, the effect of oxytocin-induced contractions, and direct stimulation of the fetal scalp in labour. Changes in the FHR during labour are still used to indicate the necessity for measurement of fetal scalp blood pH, although this is not universally accepted. Blood gas measurement from the fetal scalp during labour is still under research.

Measurement of short-term, beat-to-beat variability requires accurate identification of cardiac events, usually from the R wave of the ECG. Many computer-based numerical analysis systems have been developed, but the value of short-term variability has yet to be determined. Long-term variability is still assessed visually from graphic records of the FHR. However, long-term FHRV lends itself to numerical analysis because a major degree of data reduction is possible. Some correlation exists between changes in long-term variability and fetal condition. Normal variability has greater predictive value for fetal well-being than does reduced variability for fetal compromise.

REFERENCES

Ammala P, Kariniemi V 1983 Short-term variability of fetal heart rate during pregnancies complicated by hypertension. British Journal of Obstetrics and Gynaecology 90: 705–709

Aladjem S, Feria A, Rest J, Stojanovic J 1977 Fetal heart rate responses to fetal movements. British Journal of Obstetrics and Gynaecology 84: 487–491

Ayromlooi J, Berg P, Tobias M 1979 The significance of sinusoidal fetal heart rate pattern during labour and its relation to fetal status and neonatal outcome. International Journal of Gynaecology and Obstetrics 16: 341–344

Baskett T F, Koh K S 1974 Sinusoidal fetal heart rate pattern. A sign of fetal hypoxia. Obstetrics and Gynecology 44: 379–382

Beard R W, Filshie G M, Knight C A, Roberts G M 1971 The significance of the changes in the continuous fetal heart rate in the first stage of labour. Journal of Obstetrics and Gynaecology of the British Commonwealth 78: 865–881

Beischer N A, Drew J H, Ashton P W et al 1983 Quality of survival of infants with critical fetal reserve detected by antenatal cardiotocography. American Journal of Obstetrics and Gynecology 146: 662–670

Bissonnette J M 1975 Relationship between continuous fetal heart rate patterns and Apgar score in the newborn. British Journal of Obstetrics and Gynaecology 82: 24–28

Bistoletti P, Lagercrantz H, Lunell N-O 1983 Fetal plasma catecholamine concentrations and fetal heart-rate variability during first stage of labour. British Journal of Obstetrics and Gynaecology 90: 11–15

Boehm F H, Woodruff L F, Growdan J H 1975 The effect of lumbar epidural anesthesia on fetal heart rate baseline variability. Anesthesia and Analgesia 54: 779–782

Brown R, Patrick J 1981 The nonstress test: how long is enough? American Journal of Obstetrics and Gynecology 141: 646–651

Caldeyro-Barcia R, Mendez-Bauer C, Poseiro J J et al 1966 Control of the human fetal heart rate during labour. In: Cassels D E (ed) The heart and circulation in the newborn and infant, Grune & Stratton, New York, pp 7–35

Carter M C, Gunn P, Beard R W 1980 Fetal heart rate monitoring using the abdominal fetal electrocardiogram. British Journal of Obstetrics and Gynaecology 87: 396–401

Cetrulo C L, Schifrin B S 1976 Fetal heart rate patterns preceding death in utero. Obstetrics and Gynecology 48: 521–527

Chew F T, Drew J H, Oats J N, Riley S F, Beischer N A 1985 Nonstressed antepartum cardiotocography in patients undergoing elective cesarean section. American Journal of Obstetrics and Gynecology 151: 318–321

Cibils L A 1976 Clinical significance of fetal heart rate patterns during labour. 1. Baseline patterns. American Journal of Obstetrics and Gynecology 125: 290–305

Cibils L A 1977 Clinical significance of fetal heart rate patterns during labour. IV. Agonal patterns. American Journal of Obstetrics and Gynecology 129: 833–844

Clapp III J F, Szeto H H, Abrams R, Larrow R, Mann L I 1980 Physiologic variability and fetal electrocortical activity. American Journal of Obstetrics and Gynecology 136: 1045–1050

Clark S L, Gimovsky M L, Miller F C 1984 The scalp stimulation test: a clinical alternative to fetal blood sampling. American Journal of Obstetrics and Gynecology 148: 274–277

Cohn H E, Sacks E J, Heymann M A, Rudolph A M 1974 Cardiovascular responses to hypoxaemia and acidaemia in fetal lambs. American Journal of Obstetrics and Gynecology 120: 817–824

Cohn H E, Piasecki G J, Jackson B T 1980 The effect of fetal heart rate on cardiovascular function during hypoxemia. American Journal of Obstetrics and Gynecology 138: 1190–1199

Court D J, Parer J T 1984 Experimental studies of fetal asphyxia and fetal heart rate interpretation. In: Nathanielsz P W, Parer J T (eds) Research in perinatal medicine (1), Perinatology Press, Ithaca, New York, pp 113–169

Dalton K J, Dawes G S, Patrick J E 1977 Diurnal, respiratory, and other rhythms of fetal heart rate in lambs. American Journal of Obstetrics and Gynecology 127: 414–424

Dalton K J, Dawes G S, Patrick J E 1983 The autonomic nervous system and fetal heart rate variability. American Journal of Obstetrics and Gynecology 146: 456–462

Davey D A, Dommisse J, Macnab M, Dacre D 1984 The value of an auditory stimulatory test in antenatal fetal cardiotocography. European Journal of Obstetrics, Gynecology, and Reproductive Biology 18: 273–277

Dawes G S, Fox H E, Leduc B M, Liggins G C, Richards R T 1976 Respiratory movements and rapid eye movement sleep in the foetal lamb. Journal of Physiology 220: 119–143

Dawes G S, Visser G H A, Goodman J D S, Levine D H 1981a Numerical analysis of the human fetal heart rate: modulation by breathing and movement. American Journal of Obstetrics and Gynecology 140: 535–544

Dawes G S, Visser G H A, Goodman J D S, Redman C W G 1981b Numerical analysis of the human fetal heart rate: the quality of ultrasound records. American Journal of Obstetrics and Gynecology 141: 43–52

Dawes G S, Houghton R S, Redman C W G, Visser G H A 1982 Pattern of the normal human fetal hesart rate. British Journal of Obstetrics and Gynaecology 89: 276–284

Dawes G S, Gardner W N, Johnston B M, Walker D W 1983 Breathing in fetal lambs: the effect of brain stem section. Journal of Physiology 335: 535–553

Dawes G S, Redman C W G, Smith J H 1985 Improvements in the registration and analysis of fetal heart rate records at the bedside. British Journal of Obstetrics and Gynaecology 92: 317–325

de Haan J, van Bemmel J H, Versteeg B et al 1971a Quantitative evaluation of fetal heart rate patterns. I. Processing methods. European Journal of Obstetrics, Gynecology, and Reproductive Biology 3: 95–102

de Haan J, van Bemmel J H, Stolte L A M et al 1971b Quantitative evaluation of fetal heart rate patterns. II. The significance of the fixed heart rate during pregnancy and labour. European Journal of Obstetrics, Gynecology, and Reproductive Biology 3: 103–110

de Haan R, Patrick J, Chess G F, Jaco N T 1977 Definition of sleep state in the newborn infant by heart rate analysis. American Journal of Obstetrics and Gynecology 127: 753–758

de Haan J, Martin C B, Evers J L H, Jongsma H W 1979 Pathophysiologic mechanisms underlying fetal heart rate patterns. In: Thalhammer O, Baumgarten K, Pollak A (eds) Perinatal medicine. Proceedings of the VIth European Congress of Perinatal Medicine, Georg Thieme, Stuttgart, pp 200–216

Detwiler J S, Jarisch W, Caritis S N 1980 Statistical fluctuations in heart rate variability indices. American Journal of Obstetrics and Gynecology 136: 243–248

Divon M Y, Yeh S-Y, Zimmer E Z, Platt L D, Paldi E, Paul R H 1985a Respiratory sinus arrhythmia in the human fetus. American Journal of Obstetrics and Gynecology 151: 425–428

Divon M Y, Zimmer E Z, Platt L D, Paldi E 1985b Human fetal breathing: associated changes in heart rate and beat-to-beat variability. American Journal of Obstetrics and Gynecology 151: 403–406

Druzin M L, Gratacos J, Paul R H, Broussard P, McCart D, Smith M 1985 Antepartum fetal heart rate testing. XII. The effect of manual manipulation of the fetus on the nonstress test. American Journal of Obstetrics and Gynecology 151: 61–64

Emmen L, Huisjes H J, Aarnoudse J G, Visser G H A, Okken A 1975 Antepartum diagnosis of the 'terminal' fetal state by cardiotocography. British Journal of Obstetrics and Gynaecology 82: 353–359

Escarcena L, McKinney R D, Depp R 1979 Fetal baseline heart rate variability estimation. I. Comparison of clinical and stochastic quantification techniques. American Journal of Obstetrics and Gynecology 135: 615–621

Fischer W M, Stude I, Brandt H 1976 Proposal for a new evaluation score of the antepartum cardiotocogram. In: Abstracts of free communications. 5th European Congress of Perinatal Medicine, Uppsala, Sweden, Almqvist & Wiksell, Stockholm

Flynn A M, Kelly J 1977 Evaluation of fetal wellbeing by antepartum fetal heart monitoring. British Medical Journal 1: 936–939

Flynn A M, Kelly J, O'Conor M 1979 Unstressed antepartum cardiotocography in the management of the fetus suspected of growth retardation. British Journal of Obstetrics and Gynaecology 86: 106–110

Fouron J-C, Korcaz Y, Leduc B 1975 Cardiovascular changes associated with fetal breathing. American Journal of Obstetrics and Gynecology 123: 868–876

Friedman W F, Kirkpatrick S E 1977 Fetal cardiovascular adaptation to asphyxia. In: Gluck L (ed) Intrauterine asphyxia and the developing fetal brain, Year Book Medical, Chicago, pp 149–165

Gaziano E P 1979 A study of variable decelerations in association with other heart rate patterns during monitored labour. American Journal of Obstetrics and Gynecology 135: 360–363

Grant A 1984 Principles for clinical evaluation of methods of perinatal monitoring. Journal of Perinatal Medicine 12: 227–230

Greene K R, Natale R, Harrison C Y 1980 Heart period variation and gross body and breathing movements after amniotomy in the human fetus. In: Rolfe P (ed) Fetal and neonatal physiological mesurements, Pitman Medical, London, pp 250–255

Hammacher K, Huter K A, Bokelmann J, Werners P H 1968 Foetal heart frequency and perinatal condition of the foetus and newborn. Gynaecologia 166: 349–360

Hehre F W, Hook R, Hon E H 1969 Continuous lumbar peridural anesthesia in obstetrics. VI. The fetal effects of transplacental passage of local anesthetic agents. Anesthesia and Analgesia 48: 909–913

Henson G L, Dawes G S, Redman C W G 1983 Antenatal fetal heart-rate variability in relation to fetal acid–base status at Caesarean section. British Journal of Obstetrics and Gynaecology 90: 516–521

Hofmeyr G J, Bamford O S, Dawes G S, Parkes M J 1985 High frequency heart rate variability in the fetal lamb. In: Jones C T, Nathanielz P W (eds) The physiological development of the fetus and newborn, Academic Press, London, pp 440–444

Hon E H 1959 The fetal heart rate patterns preceding death in utero. American Journal of Obstetrics and Gynecology 78: 47–56

Hon E H 1968 An atlas of fetal heart rate patterns, Harty Press, New Haven, Connecticut

Hon E H, Lee S T 1963 Electronic evaluation of the fetal heart rate. VIII. Patterns preceding fetal death, further observations. American Journal of Obstetrics and Gynecology 87: 814–826

Huch A, Huch R, Schneider H, Rooth G 1977 Continuous transcutaneous monitoring of fetal oxygen tension during labour. British Journal of Obstetrics and Gynaecology 84 (suppl 1)

Jensen O H 1984 Fetal heart rate response to a controlled sound stimulus as a measure of fetal well-being. Acta Obstetricia et Gynecologica Scandinavica 63: 97–101

Jones C T, Knox Ritchie J W 1983 The effects of adrenergic blockade on fetal response to hypoxia. Journal of Developmental Physiology 5: 211–222

Jones C T, Robinson R O 1975 Plasma catecholamines in foetal and adult sheep. Journal of Physiology 248: 15–33

Junge H D, Walter H 1980 Behavioral states and breathing activity in the fetus near term. Journal of Perinatal Medicine 8: 150–157

Kariniemi V 1978 Evaluation of fetal heart rate variability by a visual semiquantitative method and by a quantitative statistical method with the use of a microcomputer. American Journal of Obstetrics and Gynecology 130: 588–590

Kariniemi V, Ammala P 1981a Effects of intramuscular pethidine on fetal heart rate variability during labour. British Journal of Obstetrics and Gynaecology 88: 718–720

Kariniemi V, Ammala P 1981b Short-term variability of fetal heart rate during pregnancies with normal and insufficient placental function. American Journal of Obstetrics and Gynecology 139: 33–37

Kariniemi V, Hukkinen K 1977 Quantification of fetal heart rate variability by magnetocardiography and direct electrocardiography. American Journal of Obstetrics and Gynecology 128: 526–530

Kariniemi V, Hukkinem K, Katila T, Laine H 1979 Quantification of fetal heart rate variability by abdominal electrocardiography. Journal of Perinatal Medicine 7: 27–32

Kariniemi V, Katila T, Laine H, Ammala P 1980 On-line quantification of fetal heart rate variability. Journal of Perinatal Medicine 8: 213–216

Kariniemi V, Paatero H, Ammala P 1981 The effects of oxytocin on fetal heart rate variability during labour. Journal of Perinatal Medicine 9: 251–254

Keirse M J N C, Trimbos J B 1980 Assessment of antepartum cardiotocograms in high-risk pregnancy. British Journal of Obstetrics and Gynaecology 87: 261–269

Keirse M J N C, Trimbos J B 1981 Clinical significance of suspicious antepartum cardiotocograms: a study of normal and high-risk pregnancies. British Journal of Obstetrics and Gynaecology 88: 739–746

Kirkpatrick S E, Pitlick P T, Naliboff J, Friedman W F 1976 Frank-Starling relationship as an important determinant of fetal cardiac output. American Journal of Physiology 231: 495–500

Kleinhout J, Stolte L A M, Janssens J, Knoop A A 1977 The fetal autonomic nervous system, the fetal heart rate and the beat-to-beat irregularity. European Journal of Obstetrics, Gynecology, and Reproductive Biology 7: 373–376

Krebs H B, Petres R E 1978 Clinical application of a scoring system for evaluation of antepartum fetal heart rate monitoring. American Journal of Obstetrics and Gynecology 130: 765–772

Krebs H B, Petres R E, Dunn L J, Jordaan H V F, Segreti A 1979a Intrapartum fetal heart rate monitoring. I. Classification and progress of fetal heart rate patterns. American Journal of Obstetrics and Gynecology 133: 762–772

Krebs H B, Petres R E, Dunn L J, Jordaan H V F, Segreti A 1979b Intrapartum fetal heart rate monitoring. II. Multifactorial analysis of intrapartum fetal heart rate tracings. American Journal of Obstetrics and Gynecology 133: 773–780

Langer O, Sonnendecker E W W, Jacobson M J 1982 Categorization of terminal fetal heart-rate patterns in antepartum cardiography. British Journal of Obstetrics and Gynaecology 89: 179–185

Laros R K, Wong W S, Heilbron D C et al 1977 A comparison of methods for quantitating fetal heart rate variability. American Journal of Obstetrics and Gynecology 128: 381–392

Lavin J P, Samuels S V, Miodovnik M, Holroyde J, Loon M, Joyce T 1981 The effects of bupivacaine and chloroprocaine as local anesthetics for epidural anesthesia on fetal heart rate monitoring parameters. American Journal of Obstetrics and Gynecology 141: 717–722

Leader L R, Baillie P, Martin B, Vermeulen E 1982 Fetal habituation in high-risk pregnancies. British Journal of Obstetrics and Gynaecology 89: 441–446

Liu D T Y, Thomas G, Blackwell R J 1975 Progression in response patterns of fetal heart rate throughout labour. British Journal of Obstetrics and Gynaecology 82: 943–951

Lyons E R, Bylsma-Howell M, Shamsi S, Towell M E 1979 A scoring system for nonstressed antepartum fetal heart rate monitoring. American Journal of Obstetrics and Gynecology 133: 242–246

Martin C B 1984 Fetal heart rate variability—regulatory mechanisms. In: Nathanielsz P W, Parer J T (eds) Research in perinatal medicine (1), Perinatology Press, Ithaca, New York, pp 179–204

Martin C B, Siassi B, Hon E H 1974 Fetal heart rate patterns and neonatal death in low birthweight infants. Obstetrics and Gynecology 44: 503–510

Merkur H 1979 Normal and abnormal antenatal ultrasonic cadiographic patterns. British Journal of Obstetrics and Gynaecology 86: 533–539

Modanlou H D, Freeman R K, Braly P, Rasmussen S B 1977 A simple method of fetal and neonatal heart rate beat-to-beat variability quantitation: preliminary report. American Journal of Obstetrics and Gynecology 127: 861–868

Nijhuis J G 1984 Behavioural states in the human fetus, thesis, University of Nijmegen, Netherlands

Nijhuis J G, Prechtl H F R, Martin C B, Bots R S G M 1982 Are there behavioural states in the human fetus? Early Human Development 6: 177–195

Odendall H 1976 Fetal heart rate patterns in patients with intrauterine growth retardation. Obstetrics and Gynecology 48: 187–190

Ohel G, Birkenfeld A, Rabinowitz R, Sadovsky E 1986 Fetal response to vibratory acoustic stimulation in periods of low heart rate reactivity and low activity. American Journal of Obstetrics and Gynecology 154: 619–621

Organ L W, Hawrylyshyn P A, Goodwin J W, Milligan J E, Bernstein A 1978 Quantitative indices of short- and long-term heart rate variability. American Journal of Obstetrics and Gynecology 130: 20–27

Parer J T 1983 Handbook of fetal heart rate monitoring, W B Saunders, Philadelphia

Parer W J, Parer J T, Holbrook R H, Block B S B 1984 Comparison of mathematical indices of fetal heart rate variability (oscillation frequency, short term and long term variability). Abstracts of the XIth Annual Conference of the Society for the Study of Fetal Physiology, Oxford

Paul R H, Suidan A K, Yeh S-Y, Schifrin B S, Hon E H 1975 Clinical fetal monitoring. VII. The evaluation and significance of intrapartum baseline FHR variability. American Journal of Obstetrics and Gynecology 123: 206–210

Petrie R H, Yeh S-Y, Murata Y et al 1978 The effect of drugs on fetal heart rate variability. American Journal of Obstetrics and Gynecology 130: 294–299

Renou P, Newman W, Wood C 1969 Autonomic control of fetal heart rate. American Journal of Obstetrics and Gynecology 105: 949–953

Richardson B, Natale R, Patrick J 1979 Human fetal breathing activity during electively induced labour at term. American Journal of Obstetrics and Gynecology 133: 247–255

Robinson J S, Kingston E J, Thorburn G D 1980 Increased fetal breathing activity after fetal hypophysectomy. American Journal of Obstetrics and Gynecology 137: 729–734

Rochard F, Schifrin B S, Goupil F, Legrand H, Blottiere J, Sureau C 1976 Nonstressed fetal heart rate monitoring in the antepartum period. American Journal of Obstetrics and Gynecology 126: 699–706

Rudolph A M, Heymann M A 1974 Fetal and neonatal circulation and respiration. Annual Review of Physiology 36: 187–207

Sacks D A, Bell K E, Schwimmer W B, Schifrin B S 1980 Sinusoidal fetal heart rate pattern with intrapartum fetal death. Journal of Reproductive Medicine 24: 171–173

Scher J, Hailey D M, Beard R W 1972 The effects of diazepam on the fetus. Journal of Obstetrics and Gynaecology of the British Commonwealth 79: 635–638

Schifferli P-Y, Caldeyro-Barcia R 1973 Effects of Atropine and beta-adrenergic drugs on the heart rate of the human fetus. In: Boreus L O (ed) Fetal pharmacology, Raven Press, New York, pp 259–279

Schifrin B S, Dame L 1972 Fetal heart rate patterns. Prediction of Apgar score. Journal of the American Medical Association 219: 1322–1325

Sibai B M, Lipshitz J, Schneider J M, Anderson G D, Morrison J C, Dilts P V 1980 Sinusoidal fetal heart rate pattern. Obstetrics and Gynecology 55: 637–642

Solum T, Ingemarsson I, Nygren A 1980 The accuracy of abdominal ECG for fetal electronic monitoring. Journal of Perinatal Medicine 8: 142–149

Spencer J A D, Johnson P 1986 Fetal heart rate variability changes and fetal behavioural cycles during labour. British Journal of Obstetrics and Gynaecology 93: 314–321

Spencer J A D, Belcher R, Dawes G S 1987 The influence of signal loss on the comparison between computer analyses of the fetal heart rate in labour using pulsed doppler ultrasound (with autocorrelation) and simultaneous scalp electrocardiogram. European Journal of Obstetrics, Gynaecology and Reproductive Biology 25: 29–34

Stange L 1979 Fetal TcpO2 and fetal heart rate variability. In: Huch A, Huch R, Lucey J F (eds) Continuous transcutaneous blood gas monitoring, Alan R Liss, New York, pp 209–216

Stange L, Rosen K G, Hokegard K-H et al 1977 Quantification of fetl heart rate variability in relation to oxygenation of the sheep fetus. Acta Obstetricia et Gynecologica Scandinavica 56: 205–209

Sykes G S, Molloy P M, Wollner J C et al 1984 Continuous, noninvasive measurement of fetal oxygen and carbon dioxide levels in labor by use of mass spectrometry. American Journal of Obstetrics and Gynecology 150: 847–858

Thomas G, Blackwell R J 1975 The analysis of continuous fetal heart rate traces in the first and second stages of labour. British Journal of Obstetrics and Gynaecology 82: 634–642

Timor-Tritsch I, Zador I, Hertz R H, Rosen M G 1977 Human fetal respiratory arrhythmia. American Journal of Obstetrics and Gynecology 127: 662–666

Timor-Tritsch I E, Dieker L J, Hertz R H, Deagan N C, Rosen M G 1978 Studies on antepartum behavioural state in the fetus at term. American Journal of Obstetrics and Gynecology 132: 524–528

Trimbos J B, Keirse M J N C 1978 Significance of antepartum cardiotocography in normal pregnancy. British Journal of Obstetrics and Gynaecology 85: 907–913

Tromans P M, Sheen M A, Beazley M 1982 Feto-maternal surveillance in labour: a new approach with an on-line microcomputer. British Journal of Obstetrics and Gynaecology 89: 1021–1030

Trudinger B J, Boylan P 1980 Antepartum fetal heart rate monitoring: value of sound stimulation. Obstetrics and Gynecology 55: 265–268

van der Wildt B 1982 Heart rate, breathing movements and brain activity in fetal lambs, thesis, University of Nijmegen, Netherlands

van Geijn H P, Jongsma H W, de Haan J, Eskes T K A B, Prechtl H F R 1980a Heart rate as an indicator of the behavioural state. American Journal of Obstetrics and Gynecology 136: 1061–1066

van Geijn H P, Jongsma H W, Doesburg W H, Lemmens W A J G, de Haan J and Eskes T K A B 1980b The effect of diazepam administration during pregnancy or labour on the heart rate variability of the newborn infant. European Journal of Obstetrics, Gynecology, and Reproductive Biology 10: 187–201

Visser G H A, Huisjes H J 1977 Diagnostic value of the unstressed antepartum cardiotocogram. British Journal of Obstetrics and Gynaecology 84: 321–326

Visser G H A, Redman C W G, Huisjes H J, Turnbull A C 1980 Nonstressed antepartum heart rate monitoring: implications of decelerations after spontaneous contractions. American Journal of Obstetrics and Gynecology 138: 429–435

Visser G H A, Zeelenberg H J, de Vries J I P, Dawes G S 1983 External physical stimulation of the human fetus during episodes of low heart rate variation. American Journal of Obstetrics and Gynecology 145: 579–584

Wade M E, Coleman P J, White S C 1976 A computerized fetal monitoring system. Obstetrics and Gynecology 48: 287–291

Weingold A B, Yonekura M L, O'Kieffe J 1980 Nonstress testing. American Journal of Obstetrics and Gynecology 138: 195–202

Wheeler T, Guerard P 1974 Fetal heart rate during late pregnancy. Journal of Obstetrics and Gynaecology of the British Commonwealth 84: 348–356

Wheeler T, Murrills A 1978 Patterns of fetal heart rate during normal pregnancy. British Journal of Obstetrics and Gynaecology 85: 18–27

Wheeler T, Murrills A, Shelley T 1978 Measurement of the fetal heart rate during pregnancy by a new electrocardiographic technique. British Journal of Obstetrics and Gynaecology 85: 12–17

Wheeler T, Gennser G, Lindvall R, Murrills A J 1980 Changes in the fetal heart rate associated with fetal breathing and fetal movement. British Journal of Obstetrics and Gynaecology 87: 1068–1079

Wickham P J D, Dawes G S, Belcher R 1983 Development of methods for quantitative analysis of the fetal heart rate. Journal of Biomedical Engineering 5: 302–308

Willcourt R J, King J C, Indyk L, Queenan J T 1981 The relationship of fetal heart rate patterns to the fetal transcutaneous pO2. American Journal of Obstetrics and Gynecology 140: 760–769

Wood C, Ferguson R, Leeton J, Newman W, Walker A 1967 Fetal heart rate and acid–base status in the assessment of fetal hypoxia. American Journal of Obstetrics and Gynecology 98: 62–70

Yeh S-Y, Forsythe A, Hon E H 1973 Quantification of fetal heart beat-to-beat interval differences. Obstetrics and Gynecology 41: 355–363

Yeh S-Y, Paul R H, Cordero L, Hon E H 1974 A study of diazepam during labour. Obstetrics and Gynecology 43: 363–373

Young B K, Weinstein H N, Hochberg H M, George M E D 1978 Observations in perinatal heart rate monitoring. 1. A quantitative method of describing baseline variability of the fetal heart rate. Journal of Reproductive Medicine 20: 205–212

Young B K, Katz M, Wilson S J 1980a Sinusoidal fetal heart rate. 1. Clinical significance. American Journal of Obstetrics and Gynecology 136: 587–593

Young D C, Gray J H, Luther E R, Peddle L J 1980b Fetal blood pH sampling: its value in an active obstetric unit. American Journal of Obstetrics and Gynecology 136: 276–281

Zalar R W, Quilligan E J 1979 The influence of scalp sampling on the Cesarean section rate for fetal distress. American Journal of Obstetrics and Gynecology 135: 239–246

Zugaib M, Forsythe A B, Nuwahid B et al 1980 Mechanisms of beat-to-beat variability in the heart rate of the neonatal lamb. 1. Influence of the autonomic nervous system. American Journal of Obstetrics and Gynecology 138: 444–452

Cordocentesis

During the last 20 years the techniques and indications for fetal blood sampling have changed (Figs 8.1 and 8.2). Access to the fetal circulation was achieved originally by hysterotomy (Freda & Adamsons 1964). Subsequently, with the development of fibreoptics, transabdominal fetoscopy was used to visualise and sample vessels of the umbilical cord (Rodeck & Campbell 1979). More recently, improvements in imaging by ultrasonography have made fetoscopic guidance unnecessary. Ultrasound-guided puncture of the umbilical cord (cordocentesis) is the current method of fetal blood sampling (Daffos et al 1983, Nicolaides et al 1986a).

The indications for fetal blood sampling have evolved from primarily the prenatal diagnosis of hereditary disorders, to the prenatal diagnosis of fetal hypoxia and the prenatal treatment of fetal anaemia. Placental biopsy ('chorionic villous sampling') and recombinant-DNA techniques can now be used in the first trimester of pregnancy to diagnose the majority of those genetic conditions that previously required second-trimester fetal blood sampling (Nicolaides et al 1985a). Similarly, fetal karyotyping, which is at present the main indication for blood sampling (Nicolaides et al 1986b), can now be carried out throughout pregnancy by cytogenetic analysis of the placenta (Nicolaides et al 1986c). Therefore, placental biopsy, which is easier to do and gives faster results, will soon replace fetal blood sampling for karyotyping.

TECHNIQUE

Cordocentesis is performed as an out-patient procedure (Nicolaides et al 1986a). The site and direction of the umbilical cord at its insertion into the placenta are identified by ultrasound scanning with a curvilinear transducer. This transducer makes orientation and guidance easier by combining the advantages of sector scanners, which enlarge the visual field, and linear array transducers, which allow visualisation of the whole path of the needle. With the transducer in one hand, held parallel to the intended course of the needle (Fig. 8.3), the chosen site of entry on the maternal abdomen is cleaned with

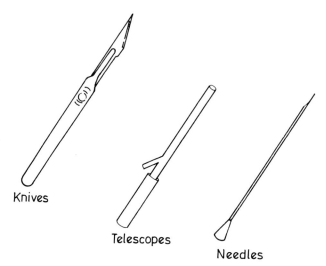

Fig. 8.1   Instruments used in fetal blood sampling

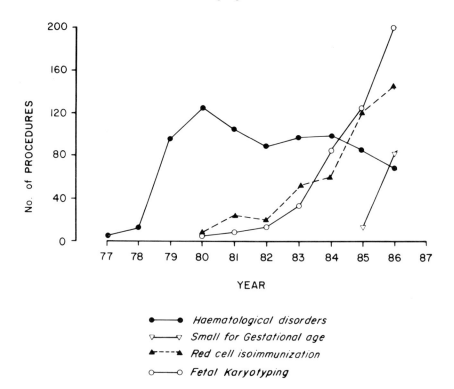

Fig. 8.2   Indications for fetal blood sampling at King's College Hospital from 1977 to 1986

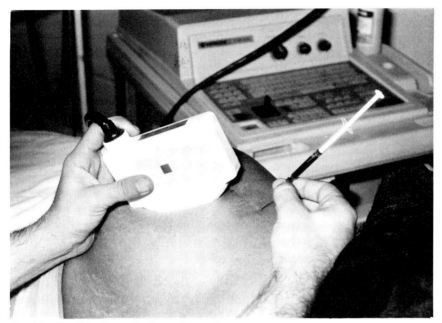

Fig. 8.3 Fetal blood sampling by cordocentesis

antiseptic solution and local anaesthetic is infiltrated down to the myo-metrium. Where the placenta is anterior or lateral, a 20-gauge needle is intro-duced transplacentally into the umbilical cord. When the placenta is posterior, the needle is introduced trans-amniotically and the cord punctured close to its placental insertion. The umbilical cord vessel sampled is identified as artery or vein by the turbulence seen ultrasonically when sterile saline (0.2 ml) is injected via the sampling needle. In addition, when the needle is inserted transplacentally, as in approximately 60% of cases, intervillous maternal blood can be aspirated during withdrawal of the needle, thus enabling the study of placental transfer. When the placenta is posterior, intervillous blood may be obtained by advancing the needle through the cord, or by placental punc-ture, after fetal blood sampling.

Training

Many obstetricians are now developing skills in ultrasound-guided needle techniques for amniocentesis, placental biopsy or oocyte recovery. Therefore, should cordocentesis prove to be of clinical value for the assessment of fetal well-being in the management of high-risk pregnancy, it need not be restricted to a few specialised centres. An operator skilled at avoiding the placenta during amniocentesis will require minimal training to hit the placenta and avoid the amniotic membrane in transabdominal placental biopsy (Fig. 8.4). Similarly, when skill is obtained at placental biopsy it is relatively easy to guide the needle through the placenta into the umbilical cord for cordocentesis.

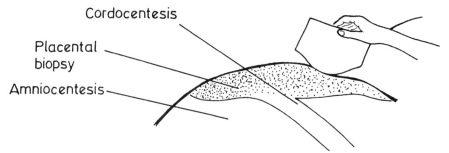

Fig. 8.4 Amniocentesis, placental biopsy and cordocentesis are performed in the same way

Risks

The risk of fetal death after cordocentesis depends on the indication for sampling and the skills of the operator. For example, 8 out of 10 fetuses with non-immune hydrops that we sampled died 1–6 weeks after the procedure. In contrast, in a series of 406 cases sampled for prenatal diagnosis of genetic disease (e.g. thalassaemia), or for karyotyping in cases of minor fetal malformations (e.g. hydronephrosis), the procedure-related fetal loss rate was <1% (3 out of 346 pregnancies that did not undergo elective abortion). These three losses occurred as a result of chorio-amnionitis or fetal haemorrhage. In addition, these were 4 intrauterine deaths at 8–18 weeks after cordocentesis. Similarly, Daffos et al (1985), in a series of 562 cases sampled primarily for diagnosis of toxoplasmosis, reported seven fetal losses. The procedure-related risk would be even lower than 0.5–1% should cordocentesis be undertaken at a gestational age at which the fetus is mature enough to be delivered if fetal bradycardia or premature labour occur.

PRENATAL DIAGNOSIS OF FETAL HYPOXIA

Knives

The first fetal blood gas measurements before labour or delivery were made in samples obtained from the umbilical cord at the time of hysterectomy for second-trimester abortion (Rudolph et al 1971). The umbilical venous pH (7.40) and Po_2 (55 mmHg) were much higher and the Pco_2 (26 mmHg) lower than after delivery at term.

Telescopes

In 1957, Westin studied human fetal oxygenation by inspection of the colour of the fetus and umbilical cord vessels through a telescope that was introduced into the uterus transcervically before elective abortion at 14–18 weeks' gestation (hystero-photography). Fetuses were not cyanosed and the cord vessels were much pinker than after delivery. He concluded that the second-trimester human fetus was not as hypoxic as was suggested by post-delivery studies. More recently, transabdominal uterine endoscopy (fetoscopy) was used to obtain umbilical cord blood samples from second-trimester fetuses (Soothill et al 1986a). The data confirmed the results of Rudolph et al (1971) and the observation of Westin (1957).

Needles

The current method of fetal blood sampling for the assessment of fetal well-being is cordocentesis (Nicolaides et al 1986a).

Normal fetuses

Reference ranges of blood gas and acid–base parameters in umbilical venous, umbilical arterial and intervillous blood have been established from the analysis of blood obtained for prenatal diagnosis from fetuses that were subsequently shown to be unaffected by the condition under investigation (Soothill et al 1986b). The Po_2 decreases linearly with advancing gestation in each compartment (Fig. 8.5). Since the maternal arterial Po_2 and uterine blood

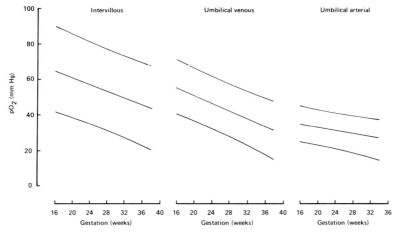

Fig. 8.5 Reference ranges (mean and 95% confidence intervals) of Po_2 in intervillous, umbilical venous and umbilical arterial blood. The Po_2 falls significantly with gestational age in all three compartments

flow (ml/kg/min) are unchanged with advancing gestation (Huch & Huch 1984, Assali et al 1960), the decrease in the fetal Po_2 implies increased oxygen consumption by the fetoplacental unit or worsening placental transfer. The latter is unlikely because the fall in umbilical venous Po_2 is accompanied by a decrease in intervillous Po_2. Since the rate of decrease is greater in the umbilical vein than in the artery, it is likely that the major site of increased oxygen consumption is the placenta and not the fetus. This suggestion is supported by measurements in pregnancies at hysterotomy and hysterectomy (Assali et al 1960). Despite the decrease in fetal Po_2 with gestational age, the umbilical venous blood oxygen content remains the same because the fetal haemoglobin concentration rises with gestational age. This is probably mediated by erythropoietin since its concentration is higher in the cord blood of normal term than in that of premature infants (Finne 1966).

Fetal blood Pco_2 rises with advancing gestation, but the pH remains the same (Figs 8.6 and 8.7).

Small-for-gestational-age (SGA) fetuses

Blood gases

SGA fetuses can be (a) constitutionally small, due to racial or familial differences and are therefore at no increased risk of perinatal mortality or morbidity, or (b) growth retarded, either due to (1) 'fetal insufficiency'—the result of genetic disease or environmental damage, or (2) 'utero-placental insufficiency'—the result of inadequate maternal blood supply. Uteroplacental insufficiency leads to a spectrum of fetal damage, including growth retardation, death before or during labour, distress in labour, neonatal asphyxia and long-term brain damage (Pasamanick & Lilienfeld 1955). Distinguishing between normal small fetuses and growth-retarded fetuses remains one of the major challenges of antenatal management.

Analysis of blood samples obtained by cordocentesis from SGA fetuses has shown that a substantial proportion are chronically hypoxic (Fig. 8.8) and that the degree of hypoxia correlates well with acidosis (Fig. 8.9), hypercapnia, hyperlacticaemia and erythroblastosis (Soothill et al 1987a). These findings demonstrate that asphyxia manifested at birth may not be due to the process of birth itself, but may exist antenatally. Furthermore, hypoxic growth-retarded fetuses are hypoglycaemic (Fig. 8.10), indicating that 'neonatal hypoglycaemia' is not necessarily of neonatal origin. The association could be due to poor uteroplacental perfusion leading to reduced placental transfer of both glucose and oxygen. Alternatively, the low glucose could be the result of hypoxia. In fetal anaemia, plasma lactate concentration rises in the umbilical artery before it does in the umbilical vein, indicating that lactate is cleared from fetal blood by the placenta (Soothill et al 1987b). This supports the suggestion that placental clearance of lactate might 'repay' a fetal oxygen debt (Huckabee 1962). The hypoxic fetus and placenta may be analogous to muscle and liver respectively in the exercising adult, and the fetus could obtain energy by anaerobic metabolism of glucose to lactate. Provided the glucose supply is maintained and the lactate is removed, the fetus could continue to survive with very little oxygen. This could explain the hypoglycaemia of hypoxic SGA fetuses and the low glycogen stores of small-for-dates neonates.

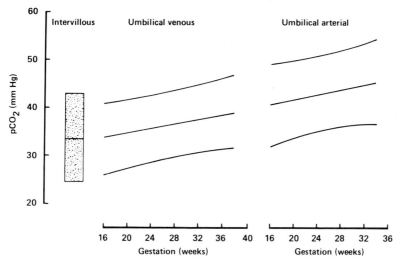

Fig. 8.6   Reference ranges (mean and 95% confidence intervals) of P_{CO_2} in intervillous, umbilical venous and umbilical arterial blood. The P_{CO_2} rises with gestational age in fetal blood

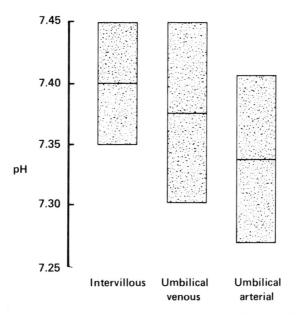

Fig. 8.7   Reference ranges (mean and 95% confidence intervals) of pH in intervillous, umbilical venous and umbilical arterial blood. There is no significant change with gestational age in any of the three compartments

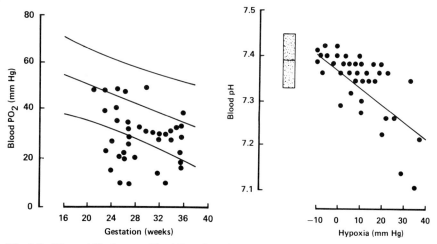

Fig. 8.8   The umbilical venous blood Po_2 of 38 small-for-gestational-age fetuses plotted against the reference range

Fig. 8.9   The relationship between umbilical venous blood pH and the severity of hypoxia (normal mean for gestational age—observed Po_2) in small-for-gestational-age fetuses

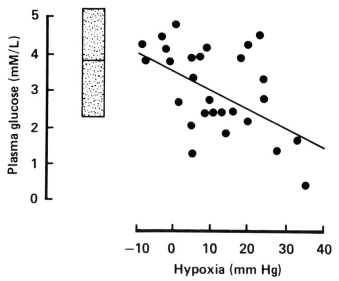

Fig. 8.10   The relationship between umbilical venous blood glucose and the severity of hypoxia (normal mean for gestational age—observed Po_2) in small-for-gestational-age fetuses

Evidence for uteroplacental insufficiency

The uteroplacental blood velocity resistance index, determined by Doppler ultrasound scanning (Campbell et al 1983), correlates significantly with the parameters of hypoxia (Fig. 8.11), in blood obtained by cordocentesis from SGA fetuses (Soothill et al 1986c). This supports both the findings from histopathological studies that in some pregnancies with SGA fetuses there is failure of the normal development of maternal placental bed arteries into low resistance vessels (Brosens et al 1977, Sheppard & Bonnar 1981), and also the concept that one of the causes of fetal growth retardation is poor maternal blood supply leading to fetal malnutrition.

Haemodynamic responses to fetal hypoxia

Mean velocity of blood in the fetal aorta. The use of a combined linear array and pulsed Doppler ultrasound system allows visualisation of the fetal descending aorta and calculation of the mean velocity of blood in this vessel. In SGA fetuses, decrease in aortic blood velocity is associated with fetal hypoxia (Fig. 8.12), acidosis, hypercapnia and hyperlacticaemia (Soothill et al 1986d). The reduction in the blood velocity within the aorta is probably secondary to the compensatory redistribution of blood flow which occurs in response to hypoxia. For example, when the inspired oxygen of pregnant sheep is reduced, fetuses are made hypoxic and when fetal blood oxygen content falls below 2 mmol/l, blood is diverted to the most vital organs, such as the brain and the heart, and the supply to the rest of the body falls, producing tissue hypoxia and lactate production (Peeters et al 1979). Evidence that a similar mechanism operates in the human fetus was obtained from patients with rhesus disease in which fetal hyperlacticaemia occurred when the oxygen content was 2 mmol/l or less (Soothill et al 1987b).

Absence of blood flow at the end of diastole in the umbilical artery. There is an association between the absence of Doppler shift frequencies at the end of diastole in the umbilical artery and fetal hypoxia and acidosis. Thus, umbilical venous blood Po_2 and pH were measured in samples obtained by cordocentesis, and the umbilical artery blood velocity waveforms were recorded, using continuous wave Doppler ultrasound, in 39 small-for-gestational age fetuses. In 22 fetuses Doppler frequencies were not detected at the end of diastole; of these, 21 (95%) were hypoxic and/or acidotic. In contrast, of the 17 fetuses with Doppler frequencies at the end of diastole, only 2 were hypoxic and none were acidotic. The equipment required to record umbilical arterial blood velocity waveforms is relatively cheap, and this screening test of fetal condition is relatively easy to learn.

Maternal hyperoxygenation

The ability to diagnose hypoxia when the fetus is too immature for delivery has already stimulated attempts at therapy. In an investigation of the effect of long-term maternal hyperoxygenation on the hypoxic growth-retarded fetus, humidified oxygen (55%) was administered continuously through a face mask to five patients whose pregnancies were complicated by the follow-

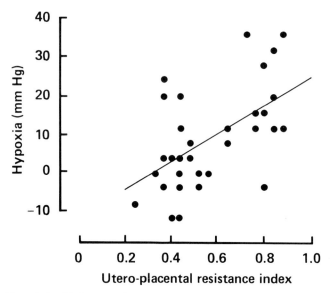

Fig. 8.11   The relationship between the uteroplacental resistance index and umbilical venous hypoxia (normal mean for gestational age—observed P_{O_2}) in small-for-gestational-age fetuses

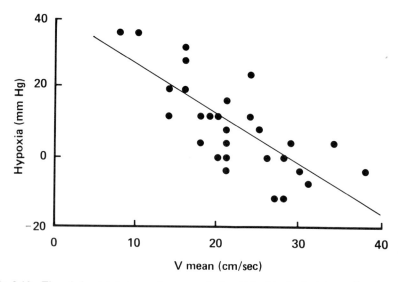

Fig. 8.12   The relationship between the mean velocity of blood in the fetal descending thoracic aorta (V mean) and umbilical venous hypoxia (normal mean for gestational age—observed P_{O_2}) in small-for-gestational-age fetuses

ing features: severe fetal growth retardation, oligohydramnios, high blood flow impedance in the fetal aorta and umbilical artery, and low mean blood velocity in the fetal thoracic aorta (Nicolaides et al 1987a). Maternal hyperoxygenation for 10 minutes raised the fetal Po_2 to within or near the normal range (Fig. 8.13). Furthermore, prolonged hyperoxygenation resulted in a sustained rise in the mean blood velocity in the fetal thoracic aorta (Fig. 8.14). Five of the six fetuses survived with minimal neonatal morbidity. These

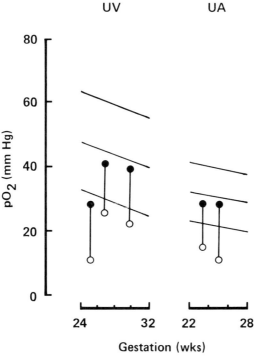

Fig. 8.13 The effect of 10 minutes of maternal hyperoxgenation on the Po_2 of hypoxic fetuses (○ = pre- and ● = post-hyperoxygenation) (UV = umbilical vein, UA = umbilical artery)

preliminary observations suggest that if a hypoxic or acidotic fetus is too immature for delivery, maternal hyperoxygenation may prevent fetal death and allow the pregnancy to continue long enough for the fetus to be viable after delivery. Similarly, fetal hypoglycaemia might be improved by maternal hyperglycaemia. Alternatively, the improved Po_2 might reduce the anaerobic metabolism of glucose, reverse the hypoglycaemia and allow the fetus to replace its glycogen stores.

Implications for obstetrics

The major causes of perinatal mortality are fetal hypoxia, congenital abnormalities and premature labour. The widespread application of ultrasound scan-

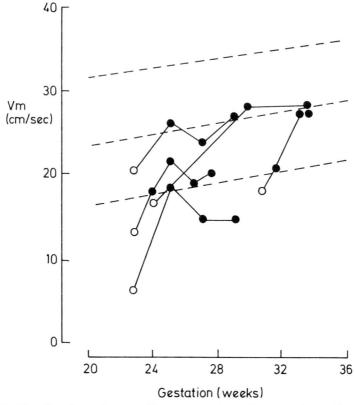

Fig. 8.14   The effect of chronic maternal hyperoxygenation on the mean velocity of blood in the fetal descending thoracic aorta (Vm)

ning and ultrasound-guided invasive techniques can potentially diagnose all fetal abnormalities and, through abortion, fetal therapy or improved perinatal management, can eliminate these as a cause of perinatal mortality. In the majority of cases of premature labour there is no obvious underlying cause. The value of attempts at prevention by measures such as bed rest, insertion of cervical sutures or chronic maternal administration of uterine muscle relaxants is doubtful.

Hypoxia is the common end-pathway of fetal death in conditions such as pre-eclampsia, fetal growth retardation, abruptio placentae, the so-called 'unexplained' mature stillbirths, red cell isoimmunisation, maternal diabetes mellitus and other maternal diseases. Indeed, it is likely that the first four of these conditions are different manifestations of the same disease. For example, failure of trophoblastic invasion of the maternal spiral arteries is observed in both pre-eclamptic and normotensive fetal growth retardation, and abnormal uteroplacental blood velocity waveforms (Campbell et al 1986) and fetal hypoxia (Nicolaides et al 1987a) precede the development of maternal hypertension by several weeks. Similarly, fetal growth retardation and maternal hypertension are observed commonly in abruptio placentae (Hibbart & Jeffcoate 1966, Pritchard et al 1970). Furthermore, in diabetic pregnancies, fetuses have a significantly lower umbilical venous blood Po_2 than normal (Bradley et al 1988, unpublished observations), indicating that chronic fetal hypoxia may be the cause of the associated polycythaemia and high erythropoietin levels of diabetic neonates (Finne 1966), and may explain the 'unexplained' death of fetuses of diabetic mothers.

In the antenatal prediction of fetal hypoxia, measurement of haemodynamic responses to hypoxia has distinct advantages over measurement of fetal size. Therefore, maternal weighing, abdominal palpation, symphysis fundal height measurement and fetal abdominal circumference determination may give way to Doppler ultrasound study of the uteroplacental and fetal circulations. The majority of SGA fetuses are not growth retarded but are constitutionally small, and the majority of growth-retarded fetuses are not SGA but have birthweights that are in the normal range for gestational age. Should the study of aorta or umbilical artery blood velocity, with the back-up of fetal blood gas analysis, prove to be as reliable in predicting prenatal asphyxia in apparently well-grown fetuses, as has been demonstrated for the SGA fetuses, 'unexplained' stillbirth and handicap may be explained and prevented, the incidence of unexpected fetal distress in labour may be reduced, and emergency caesarean sections may be turned into elective procedures. The responsibility for hypoxic fetal damage is moving from the labour ward to the antenatal clinic.

PRENATAL TREATMENT OF FETAL ANAEMIA

Knives

The first fetal intravascular blood transfusions for severe rhesus disease were performed in the 1960s by cannulation of the fetal femoral artery (Freda & Adamsons 1964), saphenous vein (Asensio et al 1966) or a chorionic plate vessel (Seelen et al 1966), which were exposed by hysterotomy. These techniques of open fetal transfusion were associated with high rates of fetal mortality, mainly due to pre-term delivery, and were subsequently abandoned in favour of the less invasive percutaneous intraperitoneal route (Liley 1961). Nonetheless, they had the advantage of providing accurate data regarding the degree of fetal anaemia and the severity of the disease.

Telescopes

During the next two decades, various refinements in the technique of intraperitoneal transfusion contributed to a dramatic improvement in survival rates (Harman et al 1983). However, the outlook for fetuses developing hydropic changes at an early gestational age remained extremely poor (Frigoletto et al 1981), possibly because of the ascites preventing adequate resorption of erythrocytes. This stimulated renewed interest in the intravascular route and the development of a fetoscopic technique for transfusion through an umbilical cord vessel (Rodeck et al 1981, 1984).

Needles

More recently, cordocentesis has been used for fetal 'top-up' (Nicolaides et al 1986d, Berkowitz et al 1986) and exchange intravascular blood transfusion (Grannum et al 1986).

How to transfuse

A fetal blood sample is obtained by cordocentesis and the haematocrit determined using the Coulter Channelizer. If this is less than 2 SD below the normal mean for gestation, the tip of the needle is kept in the lumen of the umbilical cord vessel and fresh, packed blood compatible with that of the mother is infused through a 10 ml syringe into the fetal circulation (Fig. 8.15, Nicolaides et al 1986d). The fetal heart rate and the flow of the infused blood are monitored continuously throughout the procedure by ultra-

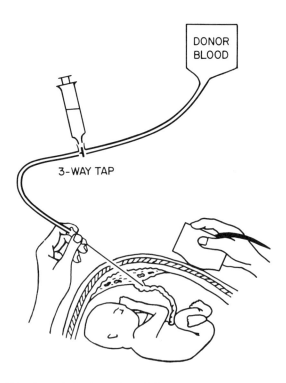

Fig. 8.15   Fetal blood transfusion by cordocentesis

sonography. At the end of the transfusion a further fetal blood sample (2–3 ml) is aspirated and the final haematocrit determined.

Who needs to be transfused?

The severity of fetal haemolysis has traditionally depended on: (1) the history of previous affected pregnancies, (2) the levels of maternal haemolytic antibodies, (3) the amniotic fluid delta optical density at 450 nm (AOD450), and (4) ultrasonographic findings of fetal hydrops.

For patients with a previous red cell isoimmunisation affected pregnancy, the first amniocentesis should be aimed to be performed at approximately 10 weeks before the time of the earliest previous fetal or neonatal death, fetal transfusion or birth of a severely affected baby, but not before 17–18 weeks' gestation. In our experience, from the management of more than 100 rhesus isoimmunised patients, fetal death or the development of hydrops does not occur before this gestation, presumably because the fetal reticulo-endothelial system is too immature to result in the destruction of antibody-coated erythrocytes.

In patients that had no, or mildly affected, previous pregnancies, the maternal haemolytic antibody levels are measured at 2–3 weekly intervals from 17 weeks onwards. When the antibody concentrations are persistently below 4 iu/ml, the degree of fetal haemolysis is insignificant or mild, and delivery can be allowed to occur spontaneously at term (Bowell et al 1982). For antibody levels of 4–20 iu/ml there is mild fetal haemolysis. If the antibody levels are 20 iu/ml or higher, the disease may be severe and the extent of the haemolytic process in the fetus should be determined by cordocentesis and measurement of the fetal haemoglobin concentration (Fig. 8.16). Alternatively, amniocentesis may be performed. For the third trimester of pregnancy, interpretation of amniotic fluid AOD450 values by the Liley method (Liley 1961) has proved to be reliable. However, in the second trimester the only accurate method of assessing the severity of fetal anaemia is by fetal blood sampling (Nicolaides et al 1986e).

Ultrasonographic evaluation of the fetus at weekly intervals is an integral part of the modern management of these pregnancies. Hydrops fetalis and fetal acidosis occur when the fetal haemoglobin concentration is less than one-third of the normal mean for gestation (Nicolaides et al 1985b, Soothill et al 1987c). Visualisation of both sides of the fetal bowel wall may be the earliest evidence of fetal ascites (Benacerraf & Frigoletto 1985). However, in the absence of ascites, ultrasonographic measurements of placental thickness, umbilical vein diameter, fetal abdominal circumference, head-to-abdomen circumference ratio or intraperitoneal volume cannot reliably distinguish mild from severe fetal disease (Nicolaides et al 1988). Preliminary studies suggest that Doppler ultrasound measurements of blood velocity in the fetal thoracic aorta may be helpful, although this is unlikely to provide

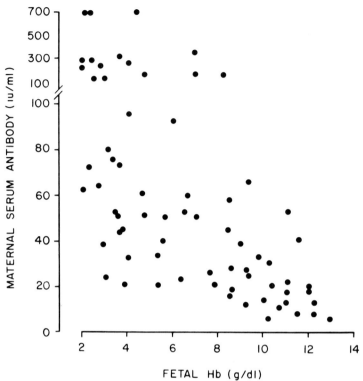

Fig. 8.16 The relationship between maternal haemolytic antibodies and fetal haemoglobin concentration in pregnancies complicated by red cell isoimmunisation

a sufficiently precise estimate of the fetal haemoglobin concentration (Rightmire et al 1986).

When to transfuse

Blood transfusions are timed on the basis of, first, the fetal haematocrit achieved at the end of the previous transfusion and, second, the observation that following a transfusion the rate of decrease in the fetal haematocrit is approximately 1% per day. However, although this figure is useful in timing the next transfusion, the wide range of results indicates the need for additional criteria, such as weekly ultrasound scans to detect early ascites (Benacerraf & Frigoletto 1985) and blood velocity measurements (Rightmire et al 1986), if fetal hydrops and intra-uterine death are to be avoided. It is aimed to prevent the development of hydrops by maintaining the fetal haematocrit above the critical level of one-third of the normal mean for gestation (Nicolaides et al 1985b). Cordocentesis and measurement of the fetal haematocrit is undertaken when the estimated fetal haematocrit falls to 20–25%; if the fetus is found not to be anaemic, no transfusion is given. In contrast, transfusions are given earlier than the predicted time if fetal hydrops is detected at the ultrasonographic examinations that are performed at weekly intervals.

The umbilical cord vessel and transfusion

It has been suggested that the umbilical artery should be the preferred route for intravascular fetal blood transfusion (1) to achieve oxygenation and buffering of the acidotic donor blood in the placenta before it enters the fetus, and (2) because thrombotic occlusion of one of the two umbilical arteries rather than the single umbilical vein may not be fatal (Rodeck et al 1984). Unlike fetoscopy, accurate selection of the umbilical cord vessel may not be possible with cordocentesis; the vein is punctured more commonly, presumably because of its larger diameter. The advantages of transfusing into the vein are as follows: (1) the sonographic observation of the intravascular flow of blood provides constant reassurance that the tip of the needle has not slipped into the Wharton's jelly, where injection of even 0.5 ml of blood could lead to cord tamponade and fetal death, and (2) fetal bradycardias occur more often when transfusing into an artery than a vein, presumably as a result of procedure-related spasm of the more muscular umbilical artery.

Volume of transfusion

The quantity of blood transfused is determined by consideration of the estimated fetoplacental blood volume (Nicolaides et al 1987b), the pre-transfusion fetal haematocrit and the haematocrit of the transfused blood, as shown in Figure 8.17. After transfusion of the calculated volume of donor blood, the fetal haematocrit is assessed, and further blood transfused as necessary to bring the final value to the normal range for gestation.

Rate of transfusion

Transfusions can be performed at a rate of 10–15 ml/min without adverse effects on the fetal heart rate (Fig. 8.18). This is the maximum rate possible for manual injection of packed donor blood through a 15 cm long 20-gauge needle. Therefore, fetal anaemia can be corrected by 'top-up' blood transfusion, and intra-uterine exchange transfusions are unnecessary. An extended duration of transfusion may increase the risks of procedure-related complications such as infection, or cord accidents as a result of fetal movements (tamponade, vasospasm or haemorrhage).

Gestation and mode of delivery

Transfusions need not be restricted to the second and early third trimesters of pregnancy but can be given until term. This may reduce the need for caesarean section and prolonged, expensive neonatal hospitalisation. Indeed,

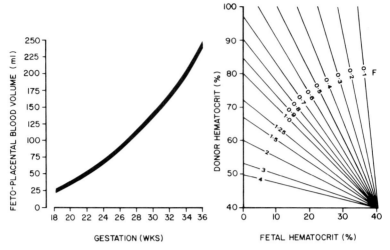

Fig. 8.17   To calculate the volume of donor blood necessary to achieve a post-transfusion fetal haematocrit of 40%, the estimated fetoplacental blood volume (left), e.g. 100 ml at 27 weeks, is multiplied by F (right), e.g. 0.8 for a pre-transfusion fetal haematocrit of 10% and a donor haematocrit of 80%

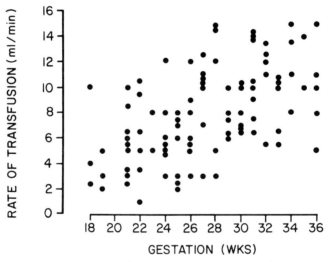

Fig. 8.18   The rate of fetal blood transfusions plotted against the gestation at which the transfusions were performed. In the first part of the series transfusions were given slowly, but they were subsequently increased by up to 15 ml/min without any obvious adverse effects

transfusion by cordocentesis becomes technically easier with advancing gestation due to the increasing diameter of the umbilical cord vessels.

Prognosis

In a series of 21 patients, including 11 with fetal hydrops, a total of 96 transfusions were given by cordocentesis and 20 (95%) survived (Nicolaides et al 1986d).

CONCLUSIONS

The example of red cell immunisation shows that better understanding of the pathophysiology of a fetal disease can lead to successful antenatal diagnosis and therapy. Should the same process achieve a similar success in the management of conditions associated with fetal hypoxia, the impact on perinatal mortality and morbidity would be even greater.

REFERENCES

Asensio S H, Figueroa-Longo J G, Pelegrina I A 1966 Intrauterine exchange transfusion. American Journal of Obstetrics and Gynecology 95: 1129–1133
Assali N S, Rauramo L, Peltonen T 1960 Measurement of uterine blood flow and uterine metabolism. American Journal of Obstetrics and Gynecology 79: 86–98
Benacerraf B R, Frigoletto F D 1985 Sonographic sign for the detection of early fetal ascites in the management of severe isoimmune disease without intrauterine transfusion. American Journal of Obstetrics and Gynecology 152: 1039–1041
Berkowitz R L, Chitkara U, Goldberg J D, Wilkins I, Chervenak F A 1986 Intrauterine transfusion in utero: the percutaneous approach. American Journal of Obstetrics and Gynecology 154: 622–627
Bowell P, Wainscoat J S, Peto T E A, Gunson H H 1982 Maternal anti-D concentrations and outcome in rhesus haemolytic disease of the newborn. British Medical Journal 2: 327–329
Brosens I, Dixon H G, Robertson W B 1977 Fetal growth retardation and the arteries of the placental bed. British Journal of Obstetrics and Gynaecology 84: 656–664
Campbell S, Griffin D R, Pearce J M et al 1983 New doppler technique for assessing uteroplacental blood flow. Lancet i: 675–677
Campbell S, Pearce J M F, Hackett G, Cohen-Overbeek T, Hernandez C 1986 Qualitative assessment of utero-placental blood flow: early screening test for high-risk pregnancy. Obstetrics and Gynecology 68: 649–653
Daffos F, Cappella-Pavlovsky M, Forestier F 1983 Fetal blood sampling via the umbilical cord using a needle guided by ultrasound. Report of 66 cases. Prenatal Diagnosis 3: 271–277
Daffos F, Capella-Pavlovsky M, Forestier F 1985 Fetal blood sampling during pregnancy with use of a needle guided by ultrasound: a study of 606 consecutive cases. American Journal of Obstetrics and Gynecology 153: 655–660
Finne P H 1966 Erythropoietin levels in cord blood as an indicator of intrauterine hypoxia. Acta Paediatrica Scandinavica 55: 478–489
Freda V J, Adamsons K 1964 Exchange transfusion in utero. American Journal of Obstetrics and Gynecology 89: 817–821
Frigoletto F D, Umanski I, Birnholz J et al 1981 Intrauterine fetal transfusion in 365 fetuses during fifteen years. American Journal of Obstetrics and Gynecology 139: 781–790
Grannum P A, Copel J A, Plaxe S C, Scioscia A L, Hobbins J C 1986 In utero exchange transfusion by direct intravascular injection in severe erythroblastosis fetalis. New England Journal of Medicine 314: 1431–1434

Harman C R, Manning F A, Bowman J M, Lange I R 1983 Severe Rh disease—poor outcome is not inevitable. American Journal of Obstetrics and Gynecology 145: 823–829

Hibbart B M, Jeffcoate T N A 1966 Abruptio placentae. Obstetrics and Gynecology 27: 155–161

Huch R, Huch H 1984 Maternal and fetal acid base balance and blood gas measurements. In: Beard R, Nathanielsz P (eds) Fetal physiology and medicine, 2nd edn, Marcel Dekker, New York

Huckabee W E 1962 Uterine blood flow. American Journal of Obstetrics and Gynecology 84: 1623–1633

Liley A W 1963 Intrauterine transfusion of foetus in haemolytic disease. British Medical Journal 2: 1107–1109

Nicolaides K H, Rodeck C H, Mibashan R S 1985a Obstetric management and diagnosis of haematological disorders. Clinics in Haematology 14: 775–786

Nicolaides K H, Rodeck C H, Millar D S, Mibashan R S 1985b Fetal haematology in rhesus isoimmunisation. British Medical Journal 290: 661–663

Nicolaides K H, Soothill P W, Rodeck C H, Campbell S 1986a Ultrasound-guided sampling of umbilical cord and placental blood to assess fetal wellbeing. Lancet i: 1065–1067

Nicolaides K H, Rodeck C H, Gosden C M 1986b Rapid karyotyping in non-lethal malformations. Lancet i: 283–286

Nicolaides K H, Soothill P W, Rodeck C H, Warren R C, Gosden C M 1986c Why confine chorionic villus (placental) biopsy to the first trimester? Lancet i: 543–544

Nicolaides K H, Soothill P W, Rodeck C H, Clewell W 1986d Rh disease: intravascular fetal blood transfusion by cordocentesis. Fetal Therapy 1(4): 179–185

Nicolaides K H, Rodeck C H, Mibashan R S, Kemp J 1986e Have Liley charts outlived their usefulness? American Journal of Obstetrics and Gynecology 155: 90–94

Nicolaides K H, Campbell S, Bradley R J, Bilardo C M, Soothill P W, Gibb D 1987 Oxygen therapy for intrauterine growth retardation. Lancet i: 942–944

Nicolaides K H, Clewell W H, Rodeck C H 1987b Measurement of human fetoplacental blood volume in erythroblastosis fetalis. American Journal of Obstetrics and Gynecology 157: 50

Nicolaides K H, Gabbe S G, Fontanarosa M, Rodeck C H 1988 Failure of ultrasonographic parameters to predict the severity of fetal anemia in Rhesus isoimmunization. American Journal of Obstetrics and Gynecology 158: 920

Pasamanick B, Lilienfeld A M 1955 Association of maternal and fetal factors with development of mental deficiency. Journal of the American Medical Association 159: 155–160

Peeters L L H, Sheldon R F, Jones M D, Makowski E L, Meschia G 1979 Blood flow to fetal organs as a function of arterial oxygen content. American Journal of Obstetrics and Gynecology 135: 639–646

Pritchard J, Mason R, Corley M, Pritchard S 1970 Genesis of severe placental abruption. American Journal of Obstetrics and Gynecology 108: 22–28

Rightmire D A, Nicolaides K H, Rodeck C H, Campbell S 1986 Midtrimester fetal blood flow velocities in rhesus isoimmunization: relationship to gestational age and to fetal hematocrit in the untransfused patient. Obstetrics and Gynecology 68: 233–236

Rodeck C H, Campbell S 1979 Umbilical cord insertion as a source of pure fetal blood for prenatal diagnosis. Lancet i: 1244–1245

Rodeck C H, Holman C A, Karnicki J, Kemp J R, Whitmore D N, Austin M A 1981 Direct intravascular fetal blood transfusion by fetoscopy in severe Rhesus isoimmunisation. Lancet i: 625–628

Rodeck C H, Nicolaides K H, Warsof S L, Fysh W J, Gamsu H R, Kemp J R 1984 The management of severe rhesus isoimmunization by fetoscopic intravascular transfusions. American Journal of Obstetrics and Gynecology 150: 769–773

Rudolph A M, Heymann M A, Teramo K A W, Barrett C T, Raiha N C R 1971 Studies on the circulation of the previable human fetus. Pediatric Research 5: 452–465

Seelen J, Van Kessel H, Eskes T et al 1966 A new method of exchange transfusion in utero. Cannulation of vessels on the fetal side of the human placenta. American Journal of Obstetrics and Gynecology 95: 872–876

Sheppard B L, Bonnar J 1981 An ultrastructural study of the utero-placental spiral arteries in hypertensive and normotensive pregnancy and fetal growth retardation. British Journal of Obstetrics and Gynaecology 88: 695–705

Soothill P W, Nicolaides K H, Rodeck C H, Gamsu H 1986a Blood gas and acid–base status of the human second trimester fetus. Obstetrics and Gynecology 68: 173–176

Soothill P W, Nicolaides K H, Rodeck C H, Campbell S 1986b The effect of gestational age on blood gas and acid–base values in human pregnancy. Fetal Therapy 1: 168–175

Soothill P W, Nicolaides K H, Bilardo C, Hackett G, Campbell S 1986c Utero-placental blood velocity resistance index and umbilical venous pO_2, pCO_2, pH, lactate and erythroblast count in growth retarded fetuses. Fetal Therapy 1: 176–179

Soothill P W, Nicolaides K H, Bilardo C, Campbell S 1986d The relationship of fetal hypoxia in growth retardation to the mean velocity of blood in the fetal aorta. Lancet ii: 1118–1120

Soothill P W, Nicolaides K H, Campbell S 1987a Prenatal asphyxia, hyperlacticaemia and erythroblastosis in growth retarded fetuses. British Medical Journal 294: 1051–1053

Soothill P W, Nicolaides K H, Rodeck C H, Clewell W, Lindridge J 1987b The relationship of fetal haemoglobin and oxygen content to lactate concentration in rhesus isoimmunized pregnancies. Obstetrics and Gynecology 69: 268–271

Soothill P W, Nicolaides K H, Rodeck C H 1987c The effect of anaemia on fetal acid–base status. British Journal of Obstetrics and Gynaecology 94: 880

Westin B 1957 Technique and estimation of oxygenation of the human fetus in utero by means of hystero-photography. Acta Paediatrica Scandinavica 46: 117–124

The fetal biophysical profile

As maternal risk in pregnancy has diminished, obstetrical care has focused on the fetus and neonate. Correspondingly, as parents feel more secure about maternal safety, they increasingly expect a perfect outcome for their infant. Approximately half of all stillbirths are due to asphyxia, often complicating intra-uterine growth retardation (Chamberlain et al 1975, Morrison 1985). In addition, perinatal asphyxia jeopardises intact neonatal survival. Clinical management has stressed the recognition of the fetus at risk, with intervention based on broad and imprecise factors, e.g. the routine induction of labour in all pregnancies reaching 42 weeks' gestation. In the 1960s and 1970s biochemical assays—most commonly oestriol and human placental lactogen—were widely used to assess placental function and predict fetal asphyxia. While these assays have a general association with fetal well-being, and may possibly have a role in screening programmes, they have been of limited clinical value. The wide range of normal values and poor sensitivity and specificity limit their usefulness in individual cases and they have been largely supplanted by biophysical assessment. Other than maternal perception of fetal movement and auscultation of the fetal heart, it was the advent of fetal heart rate monitors that first allowed fetal biophysical assessment. This developed into the now widely used non-stress test (Keegan & Paul 1980) and cardiotocography (Pearson & Weaver 1978). The contraction stress test, or oxytocin challenge test, is now used less commonly. The development of real-time ultrasound stimulated a more comprehensive study of fetal behaviour, allowing the observation of several fetal biophysical events.

FETAL BIOPHYSICAL ACTIVITIES

The central nervous system (CNS) function of the fetus is reflected in its biophysical activities. The function and activity of the fetal CNS are not constant but exhibit a cyclical rhythmicity. The two main patterns are low activity, or quiet sleep, and high activity, or active (rapid eye movement) sleep. These two types of altered sleep state influence the biophysical activities of the fetus. Fetal breathing movements, fetal movements and the associated

145

fetal heart rate accelerations tend to be absent or diminished during quiet sleep. Patrick et al (1978) showed that fetal breathing movements and fetal movements have a short-term (20–40 min) cyclicity and a longer-term diurnal rhythm. The fetus responds to hypoxia with attempts to reduce oxygen consumption and conserve energy. These may include a reduction, or cessation, of fetal breathing movements, fetal movements and the loss of fetal tone. Other factors may suppress fetal biophysical activities, such as drugs (tranquillisers, narcotics, alcohol and smoking) and hypoglycaemia. These factors must be considered when observation of fetal biophysical activities is used in the detection of hypoxia.

Antepartum fetal heart rate assessment

Following work by Hammacher (1969), unstressed cardiotocography has become the most widely used biophysical test of fetal oxygenation. Known in Europe as cardiotocography and in North America as the non-stress test (NST), the principle involved is observation of the characteristics of the baseline fetal heart rate. Accelerations of the fetal heart rate associated with fetal movement, representing a well-oxygenated fetal CNS, is the most commonly used index of fetal health.

Lavery, in 1982, reviewed eleven series and calculated a false-negative rate for perinatal death of 6.8 per 1000 following a normal reactive NST. The predictive accuracy of the test may be improved by adding assessment of baseline variability and decelerations (Phelan & Lewis 1981, Dawes et al 1982), or increasing the frequency of testing (Boehm et al 1986). One practical drawback to the NST is the relatively high frequency of falsely abnormal test results—about 10–15% in the mature fetus and 20–40% in the early third trimester. The vast majority of the abnormal test results are due to the fetal sleep cycle; this can be verified by prolonging the test for up to 120 minutes (Brown & Patrick 1981). An extension of non-stress testing involves observation of periodic fetal heart rate changes in response to spontaneous or induced uterine contractions—the contraction stress test. The false-positive rate for perinatal death with this method of testing is about 90% (Baskett & Sandy 1977). The false-negative rate, however, is low—0.3 per 1000 for stillbirth in one large multicentre trial (Freeman et al 1982).

Another drawback of fetal assessment, using fetal heart rate testing alone, is the correlation of major fetal anomalies with an abnormal test result (Powell et al 1980), which may lead to inappropriate intervention for a 'distressed' but lethally malformed fetus. The use of ultrasound during fetal assessment may detect up to 90% of major structural anomalies in utero and thus may influence clinical management (Manning et al 1982).

Fetal breathing movements

The healthy human fetus performs breathing movements about 30–40% of the time (Patrick et al 1980, Roberts et al 1980). The time spent making breathing movements increases from 12% at the start to 50% at the end of the third trimester (Fox et al 1979). Fetal breathing movements are initiated by impulses from the brain stem but are influenced and modulated by the higher cortical centres. The periodicity of fetal breathing movements is related to the sleep state of the fetus, with most breathing activity occurring during rapid eye movement sleep. The observation that hypoxaemia in the sheep fetus abolished breathing movements (Boddy et al 1974) sparked hope that observations of fetal breathing movements may be a useful clinical tool. Although there is a correlation with reduced fetal breathing movement activity over a 30-minute observation period, and poor perinatal outcome (Platt et al 1978, Calvert & Richards 1979), the low predictive value is probably explained by the need for 100–120 minutes of observation to cover a whole cycle of fetal breathing movement incidence (Campbell 1980). Indeed, Patrick et al (1980) have shown that the healthy human fetus may exhibit episodes of absent breathing movements that last for up to 120 minutes. Such a long period of observation is not feasible in clinical practice.

Fetal movement

Maternal perception of fetal movement is the most readily available monitor of fetal biophysical activity. Sadovsky & Yaffe, in 1973, suggested that the loss of maternally perceived fetal movement presaged imminent fetal death. Further work has supported this principle (Pearson & Weaver 1976, Liston et al 1982). Neldam (1980) has shown that application of maternal counting of fetal movement has the potential to reduce antepartum fetal death. Although, in general, maternal perception of fetal movements correlates well with objective ultrasound observation, the mother may not feel smaller movements (Hertogs et al 1979). Ultrasound allows a more accurate and objective appraisal of fetal movement and confirms the relationship with perinatal outcome (Manning et al 1979a).

Fetal tone

The tone of the fetus is the most subjective of the biophysical observations. Normal tone of fetal movement is exemplified by prompt return to flexion after extension of the limbs or trunk. When at rest, the fetus with normal tone tends to hold its limbs and trunk in flexion. The rationale for including tone as a biophysical observation is that asphyxia tends initially to blunt the most differentiated and co-ordinated movements. In addition, the asphyxiated newborn is hypotonic, with deflexed limbs. The inclusion of tone in antepartum fetal assessment correlated as well as, or better than, other biophysical variables (Manning et al 1980).

Amniotic fluid volume

A reduction in the volume of amniotic fluid may reflect fetal health structurally, as in congenital anomalies, or functionally as a result of chronic hypoxia reducing blood flow to the fetal lungs and kidneys—two of the main contributors to amniotic fluid production. If the hypoxia is chronic and intermittent, the other biophysical variables may be normal when tested. In more acute hypoxia the amniotic fluid volume will not be reduced, while the other variables may all be affected. In addition to chronic hypoxia reducing the volume of amniotic fluid, the loss of cushioning may make the umbilical cord more susceptible to compression, resulting in superimposed acute hypoxia during uterine contractions (Baskett & Sandy 1979).

DEVELOPMENT OF THE BIOPHYSICAL PROFILE

Single biophysical variable assessment has a high predictive value for good perinatal outcome when the result is normal. This holds for the NST, the contraction stress test (CST), fetal breathing movements or fetal movement counting. However, the predictive value of an abnormal NST or fetal breathing movements is poor, with a false-positive rate of more than 80% for poor perinatal outcome (fetal distress in labour, intra-uterine growth retardation or low 5-minute Apgar score) and more than 95% for perinatal death (Baskett et al 1987). Most of the false-positive results are due to an altered fetal sleep state and require repeat or prolonged testing or other assessment methods to differentiate the fetal behavioural state from hypoxia. The rationale for testing several biophysical variables when seeking fetal hypoxaemia is based on the principle that different sites in the fetal brain control different biophysical events. The sensitivity of these different sites to hypoxia may vary so that the subsequent biophysical manifestations may be diverse and inconsistent. Assessing and combining several biophysical variables may provide an advantage in fetal surveillance if such graded responses to hypoxia exist.

Manning et al (1979b) found that combining the NST and fetal breathing movements lowered the false-positive rate. In addition, the same author (Manning et al 1979c) showed that the number of false-positive CSTs was reduced when fetal breathing movements were present. With this background Manning developed a fetal profile by assessing five biophysical variables. With his co-workers (Manning et al 1980) he reported results in 216 high-risk pregnancies by evaluating: the NST, fetal breathing movements, fetal movements, fetal tone and amniotic fluid volume. The method and criteria for assessing each of these variables are shown in Table 9.1. In order to interpret the different combinations of variables, each was assigned an arbitrary score of 2 when normal and 0 when abnormal. In this way the biophysical profile score was developed, with a range of 0–10, in an attempt to focus attention on the fetus as a patient, rather like the newborn Apgar score. In this study the results, other than the NST, were blinded and not used in patient management. The predictive accuracy of each variable alone, and in different combinations with the other variables, was compared to fetal distress in labour, low 5-minute Apgar scores and perinatal death. Both the negative and positive predictive accuracy of each variable was improved by combination with other

Table 9.1 Biophysical profile score: variables and interpretation

Biophysical variable	Normal criteria
Non-stress test	Two or more fetal heart rate accelerations of at least 15 beats per minute and 15 seconds duration within a 20-minute observation period
Fetal breathing movements	At least one episode of 30 seconds sustained fetal breathing movements within a 30-minute observation period
Fetal movements	At least three separate fetal limb or trunk movements within a 30-minute observation period
Fetal tone	At least one episode of extension with return to flexion of a limb or the trunk within a 30-minute observation period
Amniotic fluid volume	A pocket of amniotic fluid that measures more than 1 cm in two perpendicular planes
Scoring	Each variable for which the criteria are fulfilled, score 2, if not, score 0 (potential scores: 0, 2, 4, 6, 8 or 10).
Scores	Normal: 8–10, equivocal: 6, abnormal: 0–4

variables. Furthermore, the more variables used in combination the greater the predictive accuracy, being greatest when all five variables were combined. These results were confirmed in a larger series of 1184 patients (Manning et al 1981). Others have modified the biophysical profile, excluding fetal tone (Shime et al 1984) and including placental grading (Vintzileos et al 1983). However, the essential principles of fetal biophysical assessment remain the same.

CLINICAL APPLICATION OF THE BIOPHYSICAL PROFILE

It is important to apply fetal biophysical assessment in a consistent and efficient manner. The means of achieving this will depend on the type of hospital and the size of population served. Our hospital has approximately 5500 deliveries each year and serves as the tertiary care centre for a population of about 850 000. Biophysical fetal assessment is carried out by two specially trained nurses in one area that is easily accessible to both in- and outpatients. In view of the possible influence of the blood glucose levels and smoking on fetal biophysical events (Gennser et al 1975, Natale et al 1978, Thaler et al 1980), one should try and standardise conditions, as far as possible in a busy clinical service. Patients are thus instructed not to smoke in the 2 hours before testing and to have a meal 1–2 hours before their appointment. Access to testing and results must be readily available when demanded by clinical pressures. In this way many patients can be managed on an outpatient basis. In our antepartum assessment unit about two-thirds of the fetal biophysical assessments are performed on outpatients. In the 2 years following the establishment of this unit, antepartum inpatient admissions fell by 20% and the use of biochemical tests of fetal assessment by 90%. Similar findings were noted by Manning et al (1982). The frequency of testing depends on the clinical situation and may vary from daily to weekly testing. It is most commonly done twice weekly and can be allied to daily maternal fetal movement counting. The average time taken for testing is about 20 minutes—10 minutes each for the NST and ultrasound component of the profile. Along with appropriate discussion and documentation, the average patient spends about 30 minutes in the unit.

The NST is performed in the usual manner with the patient in the semi-Fowler position with a lateral tilt to avoid aorto-caval compression. The real-time ultrasound is used initially to screen the fetus for gross anomalies. Placental grading is also performed but is not included as part of the profile score. The fetus is then viewed in the longitudinal plane to allow observation of the fetal thorax, abdomen and upper limbs. In this way fetal breathing movements as well as upper limb and trunk movements can be seen. Fetal tone is a rather subjective observation and really represents the vigour of fetal movement. In addition to extension and flexion of the whole limb or trunk, opening and closing of the fetal hand is regarded as normal tone. Amniotic fluid volume is taken as the largest pocket of fluid and is usually found among the fetal limbs. It is important to keep the ultrasound transducer at right angles to the contour of the uterine wall and to measure the fluid pocket in two perpendicular planes. The five variables making up the biophysical profile score are summarised in Table 9.1.

The interpretation of results has been, to some extent, arbitrary. If the score is normal (8–10), intervention is not indicated, unless for other clinical reasons. For an equivocal score (6), intervention is advised if the fetus is mature and conditions are suitable for induction; if not, re-testing within 24 hours is advised. Following this policy in 66 patients with equivocal scores, 34 were delivered, with two perinatal deaths—one lethal anomaly and one due to twin-to-twin transfusion. In the 32 in whom re-testing was done: 5 (16%) became abnormal and were delivered with no perinatal deaths, 3 (9%) remained equivocal, with one asphyctic perinatal death, and 25 (75%) became normal, with one perinatal death due to a lethal anomaly. In patients with an abnormal score (0–4) and a mature fetus, delivery is indicated. If the fetus is immature, further management may be immediate delivery, delivery preceded by steroid-induced lung maturation or further fetal assessment in the form of prolonged cardiotocography (Brown & Patrick 1981), contraction stress testing or a repeat biophysical profile. Which of these options is chosen will depend on the clinical situation and the degree of fetal immaturity. Of 39 fetuses with an abnormal score: perinatal death occurred in three with a score of 0, three out of 12 with a score of 2, and five out of 24 with a score of 4. In four patients in whom an abnormal BPS was repeated, two remained abnormal and two became normal (Baskett et al 1987).

THE BIOPHYSICAL PROFILE AND GESTATIONAL AGE

The physiological functions of the neonate develop in utero and these may be reflected in the biophysical behaviour of the maturing fetus. With advanc-

Table 9.2 Biophysical profile score (BPS) and gestational age (Grace Maternity Hospital, Halifax, 1981–1985)

Gestation (weeks)	26–30	31–33	34–36	37–44	Total
No of tests	287	890	2642	8969	12 788
Abnormal result (%)					
Non-stress test	101 (35.2)	181 (20.3)	367 (13.9)	922 (10.3)	1571 (12.3)
Fetal breathing movements	14 (4.9)	62 (7.0)	110 (4.2)	389 (4.3)	575 (4.5)
Fetal movement	0	3 (0.3)	5 (0.2)	32 (0.4)	40 (0.3)
Fetal tone	2 (0.7)	7 (0.8)	17 (0.6)	128 (1.4)	154 (1.2)
Amniotic fluid vol.	0	3 (0.3)	4 (0.2)	46 (0.5)	53 (0.4)
Abnormal BPS	0	6 (0.7)	5 (0.2)	21 (0.2)	32 (0.3)
Equivocal BPS	5 (1.7)	10 (1.1)	16 (0.6)	75 (0.8)	106 (0.8)
Normal BPS	282 (98.3)	874 (98.2)	2623 (99.2)	8873 (98.9)	12 650 (98.9)

ing gestational age, the number of fetal heart accelerations rises progressively (Dawes et al 1982), as does the incidence of fetal breathing mvoements (Fox et al 1979). As the fetus develops, movements become more complex, although the incidence of fetal movements has been found to be the same from 28 weeks' gestation to term (Roberts et al 1980).

Antepartum fetal assessment should begin when demanded by the clinical situation and when the fetus is mature enough to consider acting on the result. Thus, the earliest we begin testing is at 26 weeks' gestation and only very rarely before 28 weeks. Because the biophysical performance of the fetus may be linked to maturation, it is wise to be cautious in the interpretation of the biophysical profile in early gestation. A 5-year experience with 12 788 biophysical profiles performed on 4680 fetuses, in whom there were no perinatal deaths, is shown in Table 9.2. The only variable significantly affected by gestational age is the NST, which is known to often be falsely non-reactive in the late second and early third trimester. The other variables are largely unaffected by gestational age and certainly not to a statistically significant degree. Thus the four variables assessed by real-time ultrasound can be useful in clarifying the falsely abnormal NST.

THE BIOPHYSICAL PROFILE SCORE (BPS)

Perinatal mortality and morbidity

The relationship of the biophysical profile to perinatal mortality in seven published series is summarised in Table 9.3. The collective false-negative rate is 0.8 per 1000, but the false-positive rate ranges from 42.6 to 100%. Two of the series involve special high-risk groups: prolonged pregnancy (Shime et al 1984) and insulin-dependent diabetics (Golde et al 1984). The rest involve the usual mixture of high-risk pregnancies. The two largest series, which came from Canadian hospitals, were performed in an identical fashion and comprise 95% of the reported experience with biophysical profile scoring (Manning et al 1985, Baskett et al 1987). The corrected perinatal mortality

Table 9.3 The relationship of biophysical profile scoring to perinatal death

Author	No of patients	No of tests	Perinatal mortality (per 1000)		False-negative rate (per 1000)	False-positive rate (%)
			Total	Corrected*		
Manning et al (1985)	12620	26257	93 (7.4)	24 (1.9)	8 (0.6)	—
Baskett et al (1987)	4184	9624	45 (8.6)	13 (3.1)	4 (1.0)	71.8
Platt et al (1983)	286	1112	4 (14.0)	2 (7.0)	2 (7.0)	71.4
Shime et al (1984)	274	274	0	0	0	100.0
Schifrin et al (1981)	158	240	7 (44.3)	2 (12.7)	1 (6.3)	42.6
Vintzileos et al (1983)	150	342	5 (33.3)	4 (26.6)	0	60.0
Golde et al (1984)	107	459	2 (18.7)	0	0	75.0
Total	17779	38308	156 (8.8)	45 (2.5)	15 (0.8)	42.6–100

*Lethal anomalies excluded

in these two series involving 16 804 patients was 2.2 per 1000, with a false-negative rate of 0.7 per 1000 when testing was done within a week of death or delivery.

Perinatal mortality is an unarguable end-point, albeit an undesirable one. Obviously, a method of fetal assessment in which abnormal test results correlate with a high perinatal morality is too late to be of clinical value. It is acknowledged that using the results of the BPS in clinical management weakens the validity of the test, in particular its relationship to perinatal mortality (Thacker & Berkelman 1986). The association between biophysical profile scoring and perinatal morbidity is stronger. Table 9.4 shows the relationship

Table 9.4. The biophysical profile score (BPS) and perinatal morbidity (Grace Maternity Hospital, Halifax, 1981–1985)—4184 fetuses tested within 7 days of delivery or death

	Test result		Fetal*† Distress (%)	Apgar score <7 at 5 min (%)	IUGR <3rd percentile (%)
	Normal (%)	Abnormal (%)			
NST	3644 (87.1)		257 (7.8)	35 (1.0)	168 (4.6)
		540 (12.9)	78 (16.5)	19 (3.5)	71 (13.1)
FBM	3936 (94.0)		301 (8.4)	45 (1.1)	192 (4.8)
		248 (6.0)	34 (16.5)	9 (3.6)	48 (19.4)
FM	4147 (99.1)		326 (8.7)	43 (1.0)	227 (5.5)
		37 (0.9)	9 (33.3)	11 (29.7)	12 (32.4)
FT	4067 (97.2)		306 (8.3)	40 (1.0)	208 (5.1)
		117 (2.8)	39 (29.9)	14 (11.9)	32 (26.5)
AFV	4138 (98.9)		319 (8.6)	49 (1.2)	226 (5.5)
		46 (1.1)	16 (40.0)	5 (10.9)	13 (28.3)
Normal BPS		4079 (97.5)	303 (8.2)	38 (0.9)	200 (4.9)
Equivocal BPS		66 (1.6)	15 (27.8)	5 (7.6)	20 (30.3)
Abnormal BPS		39 (0.9)	17 (63.0)	11 (28.2)	19 (48.7)

* Calculated for the 3770 fetuses who underwent labour
† Fetal distress in labour: repeated late decelerations or repeated profound variable decelerations (<70 beats per minute for ≥60 seconds) or repeated prolonged decelerations or persistent bradycardia

between normal and abnormal single biophysical variables, the BPS and perinatal morbidity being represented by fetal distress in labour, low 5-minute Apgar scores and intra-uterine growth retardation (IUGR). Of the single variables the strongest predictors of perinatal morbidity are fetal movements (FM), fetal tone (FT) and (AFV) amniotic fluid volume, while the combination of all five variables in the BPS is superior.

In an earlier study (Baskett et al 1984) we correlated biophysical variables with abnormal perinatal outcome, which included any of the following: perinatal death, fetal distress in labour, low 5-minute Apgar scores and IUGR. The positive predictive value of an abnormal test result for abnormal perinatal outcome was as follows: NST 24.9%, fetal breathing movements (FBM) 28.0%, FM 50.0%, FT 43.1%, AFV 59.3% and abnormal BPS 79.2%. The FM, FT and AFV variables were all statistically better than the NST and FBM, and the abnormal BPS was statistically superior ($P < 0.01$) to the NST, FBM and FT.

The main aim of fetal biophysical assessment is to detect hypoxia, and in this respect the combination of biophysical variables improves the predictive ability. In the 150 patients assessed by Vintzileos et al (1983), there were 11 hypoxic fetuses (low 5-minute Apgar score and/or cord pH <7.20) without lethal anomaly, 4 of whom died in the early neonatal period. None had a normal profile score, with the lowest scores being found in the neonatal deaths. They compared the ability of the CST and the BPS to predict the hypoxic fetus and found the BPS to be abnormal in 71.4% and equivocal in 28.6%. In contrast, the CST was abnormal in 16% (all the neonatal deaths), suspicious in 50% and normal in 34%. In our series (Baskett et al 1987) with eight asphyctic perinatal deaths, the variables of the profile were abnormal as follows: NST 7/8, FBM 3/8, FM 4/8, FT 6/8, AFV 2/8 and the full BPS abnormal 6/8, equivocal 1/8 and normal 1/8. In contrast to the study of Vintzileos in which all hypoxic fetuses had absent FBM, we had absent FBM in only three of eight asphyctic perinatal deaths. Benacerraf & Frigoletto (1986) also noted the inconsistency of FBM associated with hypoxia. They found perinatal asphyxia in five neonates of post-term pregnancies with normal FBM but absent FM and FT and reduced AFV within 24 hours of delivery. Manning et al (1985), with 12 asphyctic perinatal deaths, had five abnormal and seven normal BPSs within 1 week of death or delivery. This must be considered in the context of a very low false-negative rate (0.6 per 1000). In a prospective blinded study Manning et al (1984) compared the ability of the NST and BPSs to predict low 5-minute Apgar scores. They found a significant improvement in the positive predictive value with the BPS (56.5% versus 13.1%), but no improvement in the negative predictive value (98.8% versus 98.0%). Likewise, all the series listed in Table 9.3 have shown no improvement in the negative predictive ability of the BPS over single biophysical variable assessment.

It is acknowledged that the assignment of equal weight to each of the biophysical variables is arbitrary. For example, an equivocal score due to a non-reactive NST and absent FBM is more likely to be innocent than one due to absent FM and FT. Oligohydramnios, even when all other variables are normal, demands the exclusion of a fetal anomaly and/or severe IUGR (Bastide et al 1986). The particular role of oligohydramnios in prolonged pregnancy is referred to below. Fetal tone is the most subjective of all the variables and is really just an expression of the vigour and co-ordination of fetal movement, yet it has one of the better correlations with perinatal death, being absent in six of the eight perinatal deaths due to asphyxia in our series.

Prolonged pregnancy

Prolonged pregnancy is one of the commonest indications for fetal assessment and one in which careful application and interpretation of the biophysical profile is required. Although the risk of asphyctic perinatal death doubles for each week past the forty-second week, it is still quite small (McClure Brown, 1963). Routine induction of labour in all patients reaching 42 weeks' gestation increases maternal morbidity due to failed induction, dystocia and caesarean section, without an improvement in perinatal outcome (Gibb et al 1982, Shime et al 1984, Johnson et al 1986, Cardozo et al 1986). On the other hand, the potential for increased perinatal morbidity and mortality is real. Fetal assessment with non-stressed cardiotocography in 125 prolonged pregnancies was associated with a falsely normal test result in 8% of patients in whom there was a poor perinatal outcome, including four antepartum deaths (Miyazaki & Miyazaki 1981). Johnson et al (1986), using twice weekly biophysical testing, found that those with normal assessment and spontaneous labour had a caesarean section rate of 15%, versus 42% for those with normal assessment but induced for dates only. There were no deaths in the 307 patients, but the main neonatal morbidity was in those cases with oligohydramnios. Using ultrasound assessment of amniotic fluid volume, Crowley et al (1984) followed 335 patients delivered after 42 weeks' gestation without perinatal death. Selective induction was performed if the largest pocket of fluid measured less than or equal to 3 cm, which was the case in 19.4% of their patients. In our unit we have followed 555 patients with otherwise uncomplicated prolonged pregnancy using twice weekly biophysical profile testing. The incidence of various degrees of oligohydramnios was as follows: ≤1 cm (1.6%), ≤2 cm (8.6%) and ≤3 cm (23.1%). When patients with normal fetal biophysical assessment were followed and allowed to come into spontaneous labour, the caesarean section rate was 17.4%. Those with normal assessment, but induced for dates only, had a caesarean section rate of 28.2%. We agree with other authors (Crowley et al 1984, Shime et al 1984, Johnson et al 1986) that AFV is the dominant feature of the biophysical profile in prolonged pregnancy. Induction of labour should be considered when the AFV falls below 3 cm, and we regard less than or equal to 2 cm as an absolute indication for induction and delivery, even when all other biophysical variables are normal. In virtually all cases labour is induced by 44 weeks' gestation, even if all the variables are normal. Fetal assessment should take place at least twice weekly. Biophysical fetal assessment and selective induction in prolonged pregnancy will reduce the caesarean section rate and concomitant maternal morbidity; however, very careful application is required if one is to avoid inflicting the family with the tragedy of an antepartum death and the obstetrician with the guilt of having fiddled while Rome burned.

Twin pregnancy

In two published series, twin pregnancies were included but not analysed separately (Baskett et al 1984, Manning et al 1985). Lodeiro et al (1986) reported biophysical assessment of 49 twin pregnancies and concluded that it had a role comparable to that in the singleton fetus. In our hospital, for the 4-year period 1981–1984 we assessed 280 fetuses, alive at initial testing,

Table 9.5 The biophysical profile score (BPS) and twin pregnancies (Grace Maternity Hospital, Halifax, 1981–1984)

BPS	Fetuses (%)	Stillbirths	Neonatal deaths	Perinatal* mortality (per 1000)
Normal (8–10)	272 (97.1)	0	3	3 (11.0)
Equivocal (6)	5 (1.8)	0	0	0 (0)
Abnormal (0–4)	3 (1.1)	1	1	2 (666.6)
Total	280	1	4	5 (17.9)

* ≥500 g, 0–28 days

from 141 twin pregnancies. All were tested within 7 days of delivery, which occurred at or beyond 28 weeks' gestation. The results are shown in Table 9.5 The percentage of normal, equivocal and abnormal scores was the same as for singleton pregnancies. The one stillbirth occurred in a severely growth retarded fetus, with a score of 0, secondary to twin-to-twin transfusion, which died prior to emergency caesarean section. The neonatal death with an abnormal score (4) was severely growth retarded, weighing 470 grams when delivered at 29 weeks' gestation. Of the three neonatal deaths with normal scores, two were due to lethal anomalies and one was a severely hydropic recipient of a twin-to-twin transfusion. Thus, it seems reasonable to apply this type of fetal biophysical assessment to both twin and singleton pregnancies.

SUMMARY

- The BPS improves the positive predictive value for abnormal perinatal outcome, compared with single biophysical variable testing.
- The false-negative rate for BPS is low (<1 per 1000) and comparable to the CST, but superior to the NST. The BPS is less time-consuming than the CST (20 min versus 90 min), can be used when oxytocin is contraindicated and, compared with fetal heart rate testing alone, adds valuable information on fetal anomalies, IUGR and placental grading.
- In high-risk pregnancies the likelihood of a normal BPS result is higher (97.5%) than either a normal NST result (85–90%) or a normal CST result (80–85%). This leads to less anxiety and reduces the need for prolonged, repeat or alternative fetal assessment. This different range of test results suggests that the BPS is better able to differentiate altered fetal behavioural states from hypoxia.
- As the perinatal mortality falls in high-risk pregnancies upon which good management is focused, the relative contribution of perinatal deaths from low-risk pregnancies increases. Many of these deaths are 'unexplained', and presumably hypoxic, in normally grown and formed infants. It is thus logical to consider routine fetal assessment in normal pregnancies, provided that a reliable and practical test can be found. Our experience with biophysical assessment supports maternal fetal movement counting

as a practical and rational screening test for fetal hypoxia. Indeed it may be that fetal movement, as assessed in the biophysical profile, is a late sign of fetal hypoxia and that maternal perception of fetal movement might be a more sensitive test. Maternal fetal movement could therefore be used as a screening test in normal pregnancies, with the BPS used to clarify an abnormal result as well as to provide an initial and more comprehensive assessment of the fetus at risk.

- A weakness of all current methods aimed to detect the early onset of fetal asphyxia is the high false-positive rate which may lead to unnecessary intervention, with potential risks to the mother and infant. However, when the abnormal test result is due to asphyxia it is often too late to avoid serious perinatal morbidity or death. Using a profile of biophysical observations reduces the number of abnormal test results and improves the predictive accuracy. However, it still falls short of the ideal test; as Pearson (1985) stated, 'There are no early warning signs of perinatal asphyxia only late ones'. Refinement of biophysical assessment and the addition of other variables such as eye movements, sucking and urine production may improve the predictive value. It seems likely, however, that we will need to ally our current biophysical assessment to other tests aimed at more accurately evaluating the fetal environment, including uteroplacental and umbilical blood flow and, when safely feasible, fetal blood sampling.
- At present the BPS offers a reasonable and practical guide to clinical management and has helped to produce good perinatal results in high-risk pregnancies. By involving the obstetrician in the assessment of several fetal biophysical responses, it also helps to underline the important principle of treating the fetus as a patient within a patient.

REFERENCES

Baskett T F, Sandy E A 1977 The oxytocin challenge test and antepartum fetal assessment. British Journal of Obstetrics and Gynaecology 84: 39–43
Baskett T F, Sandy E A 1979 The oxytocin challenge test: an ominous pattern associated with severe fetal growth retardation. Obstetrics and Gynecology 54: 365–366
Baskett T F, Gray J H, Prewett S J, Young L M, Allen A C 1984 Antepartum fetal assessment using a fetal biophysical profile score. American Journal of Obstetrics and Gynecology 148: 630–633
Baskett T F, Allen A C, Gray J H, Young D C, Young L M 1987 Fetal biophysical profile and perinatal death. Obstetrics and Gynecology 70: 357–360
Bastide A, Manning F A, Harman C H, Lange I R, Morrison I 1986 Ultrasound evaluation of amniotic fluid: outcome of pregnancies with severe oligohydramnios. American Journal of Obstetrics and Gynecology 154: 895–900
Benacerraf B R, Frigoletto F D 1986 Fetal respiratory movements: only part of the biophysical profile. Obstetrics and Gynecology 67: 556–557
Boddy K, Dawes G S, Fisher R, Robinson J S 1974 Foetal expiratory movements, electrocortical and cardiovascular responses to hypoxaemia and hypercapnia in sheep. Journal of Physiology 243: 599–604
Boehm F H, Salyer S, Shah D M, Vaughn W K 1986 Improved outcome of twice weekly non-stress testing. Obstetrics and Gynecology 67: 566–568
Brown R, Patrick J 1981 The non-stress test: how long is enough? American Journal of Obstetrics and Gynecology 141: 645–648

Calvert J P, Richards C J 1979 Fetal breathing movements and fetal distress. British Journal of Obstetrics and Gynaecology 86: 607–611

Campbell K 1980 Ultradian rhythms in the human fetus during the last ten weeks of gestation: a review. Seminars in Perinatology 4: 301–309

Cardozo L, Fysh J, Pearce J M 1986 Prolonged pregnancy: the management debate. British Medical Journal 293: 1059–1063

Chamberlain R, Chamberlain G, Howlett B, Claireaux A 1975 British births 1970. I: The first week of life, Heinemann, London, p 249

Crowley P, O'Herlihy C, Boylan P 1984 The value of ultrasound measurement of amniotic fluid volume in the management of prolonged pregnancies. British Journal of Obstetrics and Gynaecology 91: 444–448

Dawes G S, Houghton C R S, Redman C W G, Visser G H A 1982 Pattern of the normal human fetal heart rate. British Journal of Obstetrics and Gynaecology 89: 276–284

Fox H E, Inglis J, Steinbrecher M 1979 Fetal breathing movements in uncomplicated pregnancies. I. Relationship to gestational age. American Journal of Obstetrics and Gynecology 134: 544–546

Freeman R K, Anderson G, Dorchester W 1982 A prospective multi-institutional study of antepartum fetal heart rate monitoring. Risk of perinatal mortality and morbidity according to antepartum fetal heart rate test results. American Journal of Obstetrics and Gynecology 143: 771–777

Gennser F, Marsal K, Brantmark B, 1975 Maternal smoking and fetal breathing movements. American Journal of Obstetrics and Gynecology 123: 861–867

Gibb D M F, Cardozo L D, Studd J W W, Cooper J 1982 Prolonged pregnancy: is induction of labour indicated? A prospective study. British Journal of Obstetrics and Gynaecology 89: 292–295

Golde S H, Montero M, Anderson B G et al 1984 The role of nonstress tests, fetal biophysical profile and contraction stress tests in the outpatient management of insulin requiring diabetic pregnancies. American Journal of Obstetrics and Gynecology 148: 269–273

Hammacher K 1969 The clinical significance of cardiotocography. In: Huntingford P J, Huter K A, Saling E (eds) Perinatal medicine, Academic Press, New York, pp 80–93

Hertogs K, Roberts A B, Cooper D, Griffin D R, Campbell S 1979 Maternal perception of fetal motor activity. British Medical Journal 2: 1183–1186

Johnson J M, Harman C R, Lange I R, Manning F A 1986 Biophysical profile scoring in the management of the post-term pregnancy: an analysis of 307 patients. American Journal of Obstetrics and Gynecology 154: 269–273

Keegan K A, Paul R H 1980 Antepartum fetal heart rate testing. IV. The nonstress test as a primary approach. American Journal of Obstetrics and Gynecology 136: 75–80

Lavery J P 1982 Non-stress fetal heart rate testing. Clinical Obstetrics and Gynecology 25: 689–698

Liston R M, Cohen A W, Mennuti M T, Gabbe S G 1982 Antepartum fetal evaluation by maternal perception of fetal movement. Obstetrics and Gynecology 60: 424–426

Lodeiro J G, Vintzileos A M, Feinstein S J, Campbell W A, Nochimson D J 1986 The fetal biophysical profile in twin gestations. Obstetrics and Gynecology 67: 824–827

Manning F A, Platt L D, Sipos L 1979a Fetal movements in human pregnancies in the third trimester. American Journal of Obstetrics and Gynecology 54: 699–703

Manning F A, Platt L D, Sipos L, Keegan K A 1979b Fetal breathing movements and the nonstress test in high-risk pregnancies. American Journal of Obstetrics and Gynecology 135: 511–515

Manning F A, Platt L D 1979c Fetal breathing movements and the abnormal contraction stress test. American Journal of Obstetrics and Gynecology 133: 590–594

Manning F A, Platt L D, Sipos L 1980 Antepartum fetal evaluation: development of a fetal biophysical profile. American Journal of Obstetrics and Gynecology 136: 787–795

Manning F A, Baskett T F, Morrison I, Lange I 1981 Fetal biophysical profile scoring: a prospective study in 1184 high-risk patients. American Journal of Obstetrics and Gynecology 140: 289–294

Manning F A, Morrison I, Lange I R, Harman C R 1982 Antepartum determination of fetal health: composite biophysical profile scoring. Clinics in Perinatology 9: 285–296

Manning F A, Lange I R, Morrison I, Harman C R 1984 Fetal biophysical profile score and the nonstress test: a comparative trial. Obstetrics and Gynecology 64: 326–331

Manning F A, Morrison I, Lange I R, Harman C R, Chamberlain P F 1985 Fetal assessment based on fetal biophysical profile scoring: experience in 12,620 referred high-risk pregnancies. I. Perinatal mortality by frequency and etiology. American Journal of Obstetrics and Gynecology 151: 343–350

McClure Browne J C 1963 Post maturity. American Journal of Obstetrics and Gynecology 85: 573–576

Miyazaki F S, Miyazaki B A 1981 False reactive nonstress test in post-term pregnancies. American Journal of Obstetrics and Gynecology 140: 269–276

Morrison I 1985 Perinatal mortality: basic considerations. Seminars in perinatology 9: 144–150

Natale R, Patrick J, Richardson B 1978 Effects of human maternal venous plasma glucose concentrations on fetal breathing movements. American Journal of Obstetrics and Gynecology 132: 36–41

Neldam S 1980 Fetal movements as an indicator of fetal well-being. Lancet 1: 1222–1224

Patrick J, Fetherson W, Vick H, Voegelin R 1978 Human fetal breathing and gross body movements at 34–35 weeks of gestation. American Journal of Obstetrics and Gynecology 130: 693–699

Patrick J, Campbell K, Carmichael L 1980 Patterns of human fetal breathing during the last 10 weeks of pregnancy. Obstetrics and Gynecology 65: 24–30

Pearson J F 1985 Assessment of fetal health in pregnancy. In: Studd J (ed) The management of labour, Blackwell Scientific, Oxford, p 103

Pearson J F, Weaver J B 1976 Fetal activity and fetal wellbeing: an evaluation. British Medical Journal i: 1305–1307

Pearson J F, Weaver J B 1978 A six-point scoring system for antenatal cardiotocographs. British Journal of Obstetrics and Gynaecology 85: 321–327

Phelan J P, Lewis P E 1981 Fetal heart decelerations during a non-stress test. Obstetrics and Gynecology 57: 228–232

Platt L D, Manning F A, Lemay M, Sipos L 1978 Human fetal breathing: relationship to fetal condition. American Journal of Obstetrics and Gynecology 132: 514–518

Platt L D, Eglinton G S, Sipos L, Broussard P M, Paul R H 1983 Further experience with the fetal biophysical profile. Obstetrics and Gynecology 61: 480–485

Powell Phillips W D, Towell M E 1980 Abnormal fetal heart rate associated with congenital abnormalities. British Journal of Obstetrics and Gynaecology 87: 270–274

Roberts A B, Griffin D, Mooney R, Cooper D J, Campbell S 1980 Fetal activity in 100 normal third trimester pregnancies. British Journal of Obstetrics and Gynaecology 87: 480–484

Sadovsky E, Yaffe H 1973 Daily fetal movement recording and fetal prognosis. Obstetrics and Gynecology 41: 845–850

Schifrin B S, Guntes V, Gergley R C, Eden R, Roll K, Jacobs J 1981 The role of real-time scanning in antenatal surveillance. American Journal of Obstetrics and Gynecology 140: 525–530

Shime J, Gare J D, Andrews J, Bertrand M, Salgado J, Whillans G 1984 Prolonged pregnancy: surveillance of the fetus and the neonate and the course of labor and delivery. American Journal of Obstetrics and Gynecology 148: 547–552

Thacker S B, Berkelman R L 1986 Assessing the diagnostic accuracy and efficacy of selected antepartum fetal surveillance techniques. Obstetrical and Gynecological Survey 4: 121–141

Thaler J, Goodman J D S, Dawes G S 1980 Effects of maternal cigarette smoking on fetal breathing and fetal movements. American Journal of Obstetrics and Gynecology 138: 282–287

Vintzileos A M, Campbell W A, Ingardia C J, Nochimson D J 1983 The fetal biophysical profile and its predictive value. Obstetrics and Gynecology 62: 271–278

The problems of being born too soon

INTRODUCTION

It is over 10 years since Gerald Neligan and his colleagues wrote the mono-graph 'Born Too Soon or Born Too Small' based on babies born between 1960 and 1962. A great deal of progress has been made since then and the outlook for the small baby has never been better than it is today. However, every problem solved has been matched by the emergence of a new difficulty and the future seems as difficult to chart as ever. The objectives of this review are, first, to outline the present state of neonatal medicine in terms of survival, with special regard to survival without handicap, second, to discuss some areas where major changes in the care of the preterm baby are taking place and, finally, to pose some questions regarding future strategy in terms of neonatal intensive care. Since improvements in care have already resulted in largely uneventful neonatal survival in larger preterm babies, this review concentrates almost entirely upon very low birthweight babies (<1500 g) and those born at 32 weeks' gestation or less.

MORTALITY

Major referral centres have achieved spectacular results with 72% first-year survival at 28 weeks' gestation, 56% survival at 26 weeks and even 33% survival at 24 weeks (Yu et al 1986b). Unfortunately, this information is not representative of the outcome in the UK. The data from a recent, large, geographically defined regional survey in Mersey, UK, from 1979 to 1981 (Powell et al 1986) is a better source from which to judge representative UK survival rates, even though there may have been an excess of growth-retarded babies in the sample. However, the data are published in weight groups and would be more relevant to obstetricians if expressed in terms of gestational age. Neonatal mortality rates for each week of gestation from 24 to 32 weeks have been calculated from the original data (Pharoah 1986, personal communication). Although the confidence limits are wide, these figures can be arithmetically smoothed to allow a reasonable prediction of expected neonatal mortality for very immature babies in the UK (Fig. 10.1).

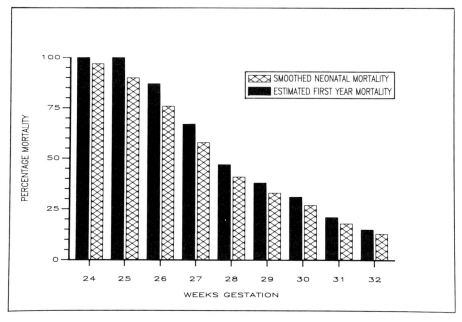

Fig. 10.1   Neonatal mortality by week of gestation derived from Mersey data (Powell et al 1986). Estimated additional first year mortality from Yu et al (1984) and Gerard et al (1985)

POST-NEONATAL MORTALITY

Neonatal (<28 days) mortality is not the only relevant index on which to judge the chances of success in terms of obstetric intervention. First year post-neonatal mortality is high in babies of less than 30 weeks' gestation, with an additional 15% of deaths occurring equally before and after discharge from hospital (Yu et al 1984, Gerard et al 1985). Deaths occur due to problems related to preterm birth, and broncho-pulmonary dysplasia accounts for the majority. Necrotising enterocolitis and sudden infant death syndrome are also common. Obstetricians should add this 15% weighting to the figures given in Figure 10.1 when contemplating intervention.

HANDICAP

With survival below 28 weeks' gestation becoming commonplace as a result of complex neonatal intensive care, fears have been expressed about the possibility of an increased prevalence of mental and physical handicap. The number of very low birthweight survivors is now higher than ever before. Unless increased survival is matched by a decrease in the proportion of survivors with handicap, the total number of handicapped children entering a community will rise. In the era before intensive care the outlook was horrifying. Drillien (1961), referring to babies of less than 1500 g birthweight born between 1948 and 1956, reported that 50% required placement in special schools because of physical or mental handicap, whilst a further 25% required special educational services because of poor function. Nickel et al (1982) showed that 64% of survivors with a birthweight of less than 1000 g born between 1960 and 1972 were, or had been, in special education at a mean age of 10.6 years. A major reduction in the proportion of low birthweight infants with neurodevelopmental sequelae following the introduction of neonatal intensive care was first identified by the University College Hospital group (Stewart et al 1978). 76% of babies with a birthweight of less than 1500 g born between 1966 and 1976 were appropriately placed at normal school when they were 8 years old. In Kentucky (Eilers et al 1986) 30 out of 33 survivors born between 1974 and 1978 at birthweights below 1250 g were in normal education at 5–8 years. When these children were match-paired with their own full-term siblings, the difference in their educational needs was not significant. Melborne data (Orgill et al 1982) showed that of 117 surviving babies weighing less than 1500 g at birth between 1979 and 1980, 92% functioned within the normal range when assessed at 12 months. The more recent Mersey data (Powell et al 1986) showed that 85% of children weighing less than 1000 g at birth between 1979 and 1981 were considered at 2 years of age to be suitable for later normal schooling; this figure rose to 90% for children weighing 1000–1500 g and to 96% for those weighing 1501–2000 g. The proportion of survivors with handicap—mostly cerebral palsy—was highest in the lower gestational age groups, with 15.3% of survivors at 25–30 weeks, 6.1% at 31–34 weeks and 2.1% after 34 weeks showing evidence of major deficit at 2-year follow-up. Whilst there had been a reduction in mortality and also a reduction in the proportion of handicapped survivors since 1963, there had been no apparent increase in the total number of handicapped children entering the community.

Handicap may be of prenatal as well as perinatal origin. The prevalence of prenatally-acquired handicap may be expected to rise with an increased quality of perinatal care. Thus, babies with various congenital malformations may now survive. Such babies exert a disproportionate influence on figures relating to the quality of survival in the bigger and more mature babies (Alberman et al 1985). Cerebral palsy, long thought of as the major sequel of preterm birth, may not be solely due to perinatal factors. Associations with maternal mental retardation and severe proteinuria as well as central nervous system malformations were as important as low birthweight and perinatal asphyxia in the American Collaborative Perinatal Project (Nelson & Ellenberg 1986).

Cerebral palsy is not, of course, the only problem encountered in low birthweight babies at follow-up. The list is long and includes blindness, sensorineural deafness, developmental delay, reduced growth potential, an increased frequency of respiratory infections, inguinal hernias, child abuse and learning difficulties. Sudden infant death syndrome is particularly common, especially in blacks in the USA (Black et al 1986). At school, visual motor integration problems, reading delays and abnormalities of balance are seen. The magnitude of these problems is hard to ascertain. The selection of appropriate controls against which to assess very low birthweight babies has not been properly addressed. Siblings of normal birthweight may be best, but are rarely used. Confusion also arises when comparisons between studies are attempted because of the potential for selection bias in some centres and the varying methods of assessment at different follow-up times. Differences between populations in terms of health and education of the families and social background are also important. Most follow-up workers would prefer to assess children on their school performance. This, of course, leads to long delays between the birth and the reporting of the results of assessment. The suggestion that there may be useful consistency in test results between the age of 1 and 3 years (Ross et al 1985) and between 1 and 7 years (Vohr & Coll 1985) may add validity to the earlier reporting of results. Long-term regionally based follow-up projects (Davies 1984) will continue to be necessary as long as further advances are made.

PREDICTION OF HANDICAP

A major advance in neonatal medicine came with the introduction of ultrasound examination of the neonatal brain (Pape et al 1979). When further studies of brain anatomy and intraventricular haemorrhage (Levene et al 1981) became widely appreciated, the technique became widely used. Most workers now use a 5 or 7.5 MHz sector scanner, imaging through the anterior fontanelle in the coronal and parasagittal planes. Haemorrhages, both within and around the ventricles, can be readily seen and most occur soon after birth. Cerebral ischaemic lesions can be identified as echo-dense areas within the brain and carry a poorer prognosis (Sinha et al 1985). The evolution of both types of lesion can be observed in the neonatal period. Many of the abnormalities seen in the first week resolve spontaneously. The later development of ventricular dilatation (Levene & Starte 1981), transient in about half and progressive in less than a quarter, can be monitored (Baerts & Meradji 1985). Both haemorrhage and ischaemia may lead to later cystic change and periventricular leukomalacia (Levene et al 1983). Unilateral and bilateral cystic lesions seen on ultrasound at 1–3 months correlate well with developmental delay and the later development of cerebral palsy. Conversely, normal cerebral ultrasound appearances on discharge from the neonatal unit are an effective predictor of a satisfactory later outcome (Cooke 1985).

PERIVENTRICULAR HAEMORRHAGE (PVH)

Haemorrhage arising within the subependymal germinal matrix of brain cells in the walls of the lateral cerebral ventricles occurs in 30–50% of preterm babies weighing less than 1500 g at birth (Levene et al 1981). The exact cause of such bleeding is uncertain, but venous congestion (Pape & Wigglesworth 1979), arteriolar hypertension (Hambleton & Wigglesworth 1976), hypoxia and hypercarbia (Wigglesworth & Pape 1978), increased blood flow (Cooke et al 1979) and defects in haemostasis (Beverley et al 1984) have all been implicated. It seems likely that the problem is multifactorial and a number of efforts at intervention have yielded interesting, if as yet inconclusive, results. Phenobarbitone was initially found to be helpful (Donn et al 1986), but the largest and most recent study of phenobarbitone therapy shows no such benefit (Kuban et al 1986). Ethamsylate, a drug which reduces capillary bleeding time, was thought to reduce by half the frequency of PVH (Morgan et al 1981). Intramuscular vitamin E administration (Chiswick et al 1983) appeared to prevent the extension of subependymal haemorrhage into the ventricles and may have prevented subependymal haemorrhage in babies of less than 32 weeks' gestation. The use of fresh frozen plasma appeared to convey considerable advantage, even though no improvement in coagulation variables could be detected as a result of therapy (Beverley et al 1985). In a randomised trial, indomethacin also appeared to convey significant protection from bleeding into the ventricles (Ment et al 1985). The use of heparin to maintain the patency of intravascular catheters has been questioned (Lesko et al 1986) since a significant increase in PVH was associated with routine use of heparin. At the same time various changes in neonatal practice in order to minimise known predisposing factors, without the use of drugs, coincided with a marked reduction in PVH (Szymonowicz et al 1986). Clearly, this is an area where there is a major potential for further investigation and possible change in practice.

BRONCHO-PULMONARY DYSPLASIA (BPD)

This condition represents a major problem in contemporary neonatal medicine. It was first described in 1967 (Northway et al) as a chronic lung condition developing in certain infants who survive long-term mechanical ventilation. Developing in up to a quarter of susceptibles, the disease is defined as a need for supplemental oxygen in order to maintain an arterial Po_2 of greater than 7 kPa for 28 days or more after birth. It is still not clear whether high inspiratory pressure, high oxygen concentration or intrathoracic air leak (Stahlman et al 1979) is the primary cause. Because the disease affects the smaller and sicker babies it is not surprising that the mortality is high, both within and without the neonatal period, and even after discharge from hospital (Yu et al 1983). Similarly, the long-term morbidity associated with the condition is considerable. Cerebral palsy, mental retardation (Northway 1979) and disturbances of growth (Markestad & Fitzharding 1981) are important problems. Few studies have compared the outcome of babies with BPD with controls, but Sauve & Singhal (1985) did so and were able to illustrate an increased frequency of disturbances of speech and vision as well as more frequent respiratory illnesses. A further controlled study indicated a seven-fold increase in the risk of sudden infant death syndrome in preterm infants with BPD (Werthammer et al 1982).

RESPIRATORY DISTRESS SYNDROME (RDS)

Mechanical ventilation has improved the prognosis for babies with RDS enormously. It is now rare for babies to die of uncomplicated disease. However, there are many adverse effects of treatment. Complications arising from ventilation include broncho-pulmonary dysplasia, subglottic stenosis, sepsis and pulmonary air leak. Air leak is associated with considerable morbidity and mortality, even in the most developed centres. In Melbourne, of 230 ventilated infants with a birthweight of less than 1000 g, 35% had pulmonary interstitial emphysema and 20% had pneumothoraces (Yu et al 1986a). Pneumothorax occurred in 36% of 59 very low birthweight babies ventilated in Cambridge (Greenough & Roberton 1985). Pneumothorax may be devastating where staffing levels are inadequate. Consequently, a number of initiatives have been taken to attempt to reduce the frequency of air leak. These include the selective paralysis of babies who expire against positive pressure ventilation (Greenough et al 1984), the use of fast ventilation rates (Greenough et al 1985), manipulations of ventilator settings (Field et al 1985), patient-triggered ventilation (Mehta et al 1986) and high-frequency jet ventilation (Pagani et al 1985). The interesting possibility of supplementing mechanical ventilation by percutaneous oxygenation in very immature babies (Evans & Rutter 1986) has not yet been evaluated clinically. There remains a great deal of scope for improvement in the techniques of mechanical ventilation.

Prevention of RDS by exogenous surfactant has been attempted successfully using natural surface-active agents in rabbits, lambs and monkeys (Morley 1983). Surfactant produced artificially gave encouraging initial results in humans (Morley et al 1981). Recently, a prospective, double-blind clinical trial of calf lung surfactant extract (CLSE) was performed in babies born between 24 and 28 weeks' gestation in Buffalo. Of 14 babies who received intratracheal CLSE before the first breath, only 2 (14%) developed RDS, whereas 7 out of 13 controls (54%) developed the disease (Kwong et al 1985). A similar study was performed nearby in Rochester, New York. At 12 and 24 hours of age, CLSE-treated babies of 25–29 weeks' gestation had less severe RDS than controls, but these differences were not maintained at 48 and 72 hours (Shapiro et al 1985). Further investigations using different dosage schedules may show promise in the future.

Antenatal steroid therapy in order to prevent RDS has recently been reviewed in a large Australian controlled study (Doyle et al 1986). In contrast to earlier work (Liggins & Howie 1972, Collaborative Group on Antenatal Steroid Therapy 1981), reasonable numbers of very low birthweight infants at a single institution were included. After exclusion of babies with lethal malformations and those thought too immature to receive intensive care, a series of advantages were reported. These included a marked reduction in mortality and a significantly reduced incidence of RDS. The incidences of BPD and patent ductus arteriosus were reduced when compared with controls. No adverse affects at all were detected. It appears that there is still good reason to treat mothers with steroids for the purpose of accelerating lung maturity prior to very preterm delivery.

NUTRITION

Immature infants take longer to regain birth weight than full-term newborns. There are obvious difficulties in achieving an adequate energy balance in the first weeks of life in babies who are small and sick. Subsequently, many infants show poor later growth, remaining on the lower centiles for many years. Recently, these observations have been confirmed in terms of a large number of babies born before 30 weeks' gestation (Gill et al 1986). Poor initial growth may adversely affect later head growth and development (Georgieff et al 1985). The use of routine intravenous nutrition is supported by a controlled trial (Yu et al 1979) and is now widely used. Central venous catheterisation is becoming safer (Mactier et al 1986), although silicon catheters inserted through peripheral veins are preferred when possible. However, even when energy is provided in this manner, full 'catch up' growth is rare. Deficiencies in the provision of calcium and phosphate may be implicated (Aiken & Lenney 1986) and trace elements are rarely provided at estimated intra-uterine accretion rates. Very low birthweight infants form a very special population with special needs. Standard parenteral feeding regimens, suitable for adults and older children, may not be appropriate.

Breast milk has long been favoured for enteral feeding for reasons which include its potential ability to aid digestion, its bacteriostatic qualities and because it assists in host defence and gut maturation. It is now clear that expressed and drip-collected breast milk are inadequate in energy for the preterm baby. Preterm infants fed on expressed breast milk grew poorly when compared with infants fed a commercial formula (Lucas et al 1984). Supplementation of mother's milk with the fat from mature human milk (Schanler et al 1985a, b) resulted in growth which was similar to that in formula-fed babies, although deficiencies in calcium and phosphate were identified. Supplementation with nitrogen, glucose polymers and minerals (Tonz & Schubiger 1985) appeared to be effective. Modification of expressed breast milk is a practical possibility, retaining some of the biological advantages of human milk, and may be of greater value in the future. Improvements in commercial formulae offer an easier route. Further work is needed in neonatal nutrition in order to achieve the stated goal of an intra-uterine growth rate in very low birthweight infants (American Academy of Pediatrics 1977).

NEONATAL DEATH

In spite of the many improvements in neonatal medicine within the last three decades, death remains a frequent occurrence on a neonatal intensive care unit. Two major developments have taken place recently. The first involves the recognition of the emotional needs of parents and, very often, nursing and medical staff. The second encompasses the option of withdrawing extraordinary forms of treatment for babies whose survival could only be at the expense of serious handicap.

Grief and mourning are essential mechanisms in the acceptance of death. This applies to the loss of a newborn (Kennell et al 1970) or a stillborn baby (Lewis 1979) as much as to the loss of a more familiar relative. The death of one of a pair of twins involves particularly difficult emotional adjustments which are often underestimated (Bryan 1986). Rowe et al (1978) indicated that 60% of mothers were dissatisfied with the way their experience of perinatal death was managed. Staff on a neonatal unit may regard each death as an embarrassing failure and the emotional load can be considerable. Most neonatal units, following the pioneer work of Klaus and Kennell (1976), have evolved ways of managing bereavement in a sensitive and understanding manner. St George's Hospital, London (McIntosh and Eldridge 1984) sets a good example. Polaroid photographs help to provide permanent mementos of a dead baby. Parents are encouraged to fondle their dying or dead child in conditions of privacy. Funeral services are encouraged. The death of the child is discussed at staff meetings in order to ensure that the death is understood and that possible guilt reactions are resolved. The appointment of a bereavement officer in each maternity unit, who can assist with the formalities of registration and who is familiar with the technicalities of burial or cremation, was recommended by a recent working party (Royal College of Obstetricians and Gynaecologists 1985). Many paediatricians now interview parents a number of times after the death. An initial interview at which the death is announced is usually followed by another away from the bustle of the neonatal unit at which the autopsy findings may be discussed. A third meeting may take place after an interval to help resolve any new questions and to discuss the feelings of the parents.

Death as an acceptable form of management has recently been reviewed by Whitelaw (1986). Guidelines for the withholding or withdrawal of supportive care in very damaged babies have been sparse. Spina bifida, severe asphyxia and trisomy 18 are exceptions. However, the case of an eminent paediatrician who was charged with the murder of a rejected baby with Down's syndrome was an important lesson. Nevertheless, it seems ethically (if not legally) wrong to pursue intensive life support when there is little chance of meaningful later survival. As the accuracy of prediction of severe handicap improves with ultrasound, the option of death becomes more relevant. White-law explains how, as a result of a unanimous decision by the neonatal team, the possibility of discontinuation of treatment was put to the parents. Only 7% disagreed with the medical assessment and 47 babies died who would have been severely handicapped. Whitelaw's article adds support and a degree of legitimacy to decisions which paediatricians, in isolation, have long been obliged to make for their patients.

FUTURE STRATEGY

There are many questions of strategy which need answers, but two may be of general interest. First, where should the new technology be located? Should the burgeoning regional neonatal intensive care centres carry the load or is it reasonable for district general hospitals to look after their own sick babies? Second, and more fundamental, what is the limit of neonatal care in terms of birthweight and gestation? Is it right to strive for survival at ever decreasing gestational ages or will ethics, economy or even common sense call a halt?

For the first question the answer is not as clear as it might appear. There are many expressions of opinion from similar regional units and it would not be surprising to find a uniformity of view. From the standpoint of a district paediatrician, the author's view differs. It is clear that specialist units, drawing resources from central funds, have charted a path which others can follow. Transfer of high-risk babies to the agency with the most resources would appear to be logical. However, analyses can be biased by the selection of patients with socio-economic and other advantages. The variations in practice that change over a period of time are not always taken into account. Two recent controlled evaluations showed similar reductions in birthweight-specific mortality between areas which had, or did not have, regionalisation programs (Seigel et al 1985, McCormick et al 1985). Furthermore, central units may act as 'black holes' into which resources and staff are drawn, never to emerge again. This seems unlikely to improve overall effectiveness since expertise and confidence erodes at the periphery where most of the babies are born and die. In the UK there are lessons to be learned from the North. When babies had to be refused admission to the regional unit in Manchester, their mortality rate was high (Sims et al 1982). As a result, neonatal intensive care was developed in a district general hospital and has shown superb results. Blackburn's mortality figures, in a location of social disadvantage and without the assistance of regional funding, have now fallen below regional levels (Jivani 1986). However, great pressures are put upon those paediatricians in general hospitals who attempt to offer neonatal intensive care for their patients. When a regional centre offers adequate facilities, any death at the periphery can be seen as avoidable.

Perinatal death should, however, not be the sole criterion on which judgement is made. The personal cost for parents to visit distant central units can be alarming (Smith & Baum 1983). Subsequent problems of bonding (Klaus & Kennell 1982) are not surprising. Babies who have received intensive care are three times more likely than other babies to be re-admitted to hospital soon after discharge (Lewry & Wailoo 1985). Regional centres are usually unable to cope with these later admissions and are usually inappropriate because of distance. Admission to the familiar district hospital, where the baby was managed after birth, avoids the need for a sudden traumatic reaffiliation. Later management of babies who have passed through the local neonatal unit may be very satisfying for the team in a peripheral hospital, with consequent reduction in the stress experienced by the staff (Walker 1982). Few UK regions show the breadth of vision shown in the US and Canada (Hein 1980, Horwood et al 1982), where designated centres take responsibility for the regional figures for perinatal mortality as well as for the education of peripheral personnel and the upgrading of local facilities. Many UK peripheral hospitals still have staff and facilities which fall well below the minimum standards outlined by the British Paediatric Association (1983). Regional centres should help to ensure that their district hospitals are adequately staffed and equipped to cope with the demands of modern neonatal care. Efforts to increase the effectiveness of peripheral units by integrating them into programmes of audit should be a priority of the centre. Centrally funded, better-staffed regional units should assist in regional development instead of subtracting 'top-sliced' regional resources at the expense of the majority.

The second question is more difficult. Where should the line be drawn, if a line should be drawn at all, in the attempted salvage of smaller and smaller babies? Technology now makes possible extracorporeal membrane oxygenation (Bartlett et al 1985), and in theory this technique could be used for the smallest babies. But is it right, ethically or economically, to use this sort of technology to salvage the life of a 23-week baby of a 14-year-old mother who became pregnant by accident? The ethical question has recently been discussed by Bissenden (1986), who identifies the difficulty as not 'whether to provide such care but to justify not providing it'. It is easy and tempting to avoid the dilemma by enthusiastically attempting the maximum at all times. Campbell (1982) argues the value of a 'cut-off' weight below which intensive care would not normally be offered, suggesting 750 g. Mitchell (1985), in a gloomy article highlighting the contribution of a poor maternal social environment, suggests 700 g. It would seem proper for each unit to set out its own guidelines. Of course these should include the circumstances of the family as well as the condition, birthweight and gestational age of the baby. Consultation with families during the crisis immediately after birth is often difficult and not usually productive, but it is always essential. The burden is likely to remain that of the paediatrician.

The costs involved in neonatal intensive care have recently been evaluated in Liverpool (Sandhu et al 1986). Each survivor born at less than 1500 g cost about £5000 at 1984 levels. A similar Birmingham study (Newns et al 1984) indicated that survivors of less than 1000 g may cost twice as much as this figure. These analyses fail to indicate the magnitude of ongoing costs of management after discharge from hospital. The potential benefits to the nation from the future earnings of the survivors remain questionable. It seems very likely that the smaller the infant, the greater will be the economic loss (Boyle et al 1983). Although it could never be argued that cost alone should be a reason for withholding intensive care from very low birthweight babies, and since proper management of babies weighing 1000–1499 g is probably cost-effective (Dunn 1984), any attempt to follow priorities where resources are scarce would dictate restraint in attempts to save the smallest babies.

REFERENCES

Aiken G, Lenney W 1986 Calcium and phosphate content of intravenous feeding regimens for very low birthweight infants. Archives of Disease in Childhood 61: 495–501
Alberman E, Benson J, Kani W 1985 Disabilities in survivors of low birthweight. Archives of Disease in Childhood 60: 913–919
American Academy of Pediatrics (Committee on Nutrition) 1977 Nutritional needs of low-birth-weight infants. Pediatrics 60: 519–530
Baerts W, Meradji M 1985 Cranial ultrasound in preterm infants: long term follow up. Archives of Disease in Childhood 60: 702–705
Bartlett R H, Roloff D W, Cornell R G et al 1985 Extracorporeal circulation in neonatal respiratory failure: a prospective randomised study. Pediatrics 76: 479–487
Beverley D W, Chance G W, Inwood M J, Schaus M, O'Keefe B 1984 Intraventricular haemorrhage and haemostasis defects. Archives of Disease in Childhood 59: 444–448
Beverley D W, Pitts-Tucker T J, Congdon P J, Arthur R J, Tate G 1985 Prevention of intraventricular haemorrhage by fresh frozen plasma. Archives of Disease in Childhood 60: 710–713
Bissenden J G 1986 Ethical aspects of neonatal care. Archives of Disease in Childhood 61: 639–641
Black L, David R J, Brouillette R T, Hunt C E 1986 Effects of birthweight and ethnicity on incidence of sudden infant death syndrome. Journal of Pediatrics 108: 204–208
Boyle M H, Torrance G W, Sinclair J C, Horwood S P 1983 Economic evaluation of neonatal care of very low birthweight infants. New England Journal of Medicine 308: 1330–1337
British Paediatric Association 1983 Minimal standards of neonatal care. Archives of Disease in Childhood 58: 943–944
Bryan E 1986 The intrauterine hazards of twins. Archives of Disease in Childhood 61: 1044–1945
Campbell A G M 1982 Which infants should not receive intensive care? Archives of Disease in Childhood 57: 569–571
Chiswick M L, Johnson M, Woodhall C et al 1983 Protective effect of vitamin E (DL-alpha-tocopherol) against intraventricular haemorrhage in premature babies. British Medical Journal 287: 81–84
Collaborative Group on Antenatal Steroid Therapy 1981 Effect of antenatal dexamethasone administration on the prevention of respiratory distress syndrome. American Journal of Obstetrics and Gynecology 141: 276–286
Cooke R W I 1985 Neonatal cranial ultrasound and neurological development at follow up. Lancet ii: 494–495
Cooke R W I, Rolfe P, Howat P 1979 Apparent cerebral blood flow in newborns with respiratory disease. Developmental Medicine and Child Neurology 21: 154–160
Davies P A 1984 Follow up of low birthweight children. Archives of Disease in Childhood 59: 794–797
Donn S M, Goldstein G W, Roloff D W 1986 Prevention of intraventricular hemorrhage with Phenobarbital therapy: now what? Pediatrics 77: 779–780

Doyle L W, Kitchen W H, Ford G W, Rickards A L, Lissenden J V, Ryan M M 1986 Effects of antenatal steroid therapy on mortality and morbidity in very low birthweight infants. Journal of Pediatrics 108: 287–292

Drillien C M 1961 The incidence of mental and physical handicap in school age children of very low birth weight. Pediatrics 27: 452–464

Dunn P M 1984 Neonatal intensive care in the United Kingdom—problems and priorities. In: Neonatal intensive care a dilemma of resources and needs, Spastics Society, London, pp 7–12

Eilers B L, Desai N S, Wilson M A, Cunningham M D 1986 Classroom performance and social factors of children with birth weights of 1250 grams or less: follow up at 5 to 8 years of age. Pediatrics 77: 203–208

Evans N J, Rutter N 1986 Percutaneous respiration in the neonatal period. Journal of Pediatrics 108: 282–286

Field D, Milner A D, Hopkin I E 1985 Manipulation of ventilator settings to prevent active expiration against positive pressure ventilation. Archives of Disease in Childhood 60: 1036–1040

Georgieff M K, Hoffman J S, Periera G R et al 1985 Effect of neonatal calorie deprivation on head growth and 1-year developmental status in preterm infants. Journal of Pediatrics 107: 581–587

Gerard P, Bachy A, Battisti O et al 1985 Mortality in 504 infants weighing less than 1501 grams at birth and treated in four neonatal intensive care units of South-Belgium between 1976 and 1980. European Journal of Pediatrics 144: 219–224

Gill A, Yu V Y H, Bajuk B, Astbury J 1986 Postnatal growth in infants born before 30 weeks gestation. Archives of Disease in Childhood 61: 549–553

Greenough A, Roberton N R C 1985 Morbidity and survival in neonates ventilated for respiratory distress syndrome. British Medical Journal 290: 597–600

Greenough A, Wood S, Morley C J, Davies J A 1984 Pancuronium prevents pneumothoraces in ventilated premature infants who actively expire against positive pressure ventilation. Lancet i: 1–4

Greenough A, Morley C J, Pool J et al 1985 Are fast ventilation rates an effective alternative to paralysis? Pediatric Research 19: 1077 (abstract)

Hambleton G, Wigglesworth J S 1976 Origin of intraventricular haemorrhage in the preterm infant. Archives of Disease in Childhood 51: 651–659

Hein H 1980 Evaluation of a rural perinatal care system. Pediatrics 66: 540–546

Horwood S P, Boyle M H, Torrance G W, Sinclair J C 1982 Mortality and morbidity of 500–1499 gram birth weight infants live-born to residents of a defined geographic region before and after neonatal intensive care. Pediatrics 69: 613–620

Jivani S K M 1986 Evolution of neonatal intensive care in a district general hospital. Archives of Disease in Childhood 61: 148–152

Kennell J H, Slyter H, Klaus M H 1970 The mourning response of parents to the death of a newborn infant. New England Journal of Medicine 283: 344–349

Klaus M H, Kennell J H 1976 Caring for parents of an infant who dies. In: Maternal–infant bonding, Mosby, St Louis, pp 209–239

Klaus M H, Kennell J H 1982 Caring for the parents of premature or sick infants. In: Maternal–infant bonding, 2nd edn, Mosby, St Louis, pp 151–226

Kuban K K, Leviton A, Krishnamoorthy K S et al 1986 Neonatal intracranial hemorrhage and phenobarbital therapy. Pediatrics 77: 443–450

Kwong M S, Egan E A, Notter R H, Shapiro D L 1985 Double-blind clinical trial of calf lung surfactant extract for the prevention of hyaline membrane disease in extremely premature infants. Pediatrics 76: 585–592

Lesko S M, Mitchell A A, Epstein M F et al 1986 Heparin use as a risk factor for intraventricular haemorrhage in low-birth-weight infants. New England Journal of Medicine 314: 1156–1160

Levene M I, Starte D R 1981 A longitudinal study of post-haemorrhagic ventricular dilation in the newborn. Archives of Disease in Childhood 56: 905–910

Levene M I, Wigglesworth J S, Dubowitz V 1981 Cerebral structure and intraventricular haemorrhage in the neonate: a real time study. Archives of Disease in Childhood 56: 416–424

Levene M I, Wigglesworth J S, Dubowitz V 1983 Haemorrhagic ventricular leucomalacia in the neonate: a real time study. Pediatrics 71: 794–797

Lewis E 1979 Mourning by the family after a stillbirth or neonatal death. Archives of Disease in Childhood 54: 303–306

Lewry J, Wailoo M P 1985 Pattern of illness in babies discharged from a special care baby unit. Archives of Disease in Childhood 60: 1068–1081

Liggins G C, Howie R N 1972 A controlled trial of antepartum glucocorticoid treatment for the prevention of respiratory distress syndrome in premature infants. Pediatrics 50: 515–525

Lucas A, Gore S M, Cole T J et al 1984 Multicentre trial on feeding of low birthweight infants: effects of diet on early growth. Archives of Disease in Childhood 59: 722–730

Mactier H, Alroomi L G, Young D G, Raine P A M 1986 Central venous catheterisation in very low birthweight infants. Archives of Disease in Childhood 61: 449–453

Markestad T, Fitzharding P M 1981 Growth and development in children recovering from bronchopulmonary dysplasia. Journal of Pediatrics 98: 597–602

McCormick M, Shapiro S, Starfield B 1985 The regionalisation of perinatal services. Summary of the evaluation of a national demonstration program. Journal of the American Medical Association 253: 799–804

McIntosh N, Eldridge C 1984 Neonatal death—the neglected side of neonatal care. Archives of Disease in Childhood 59: 585–587

Mehta A, Wright B M, Callan K, Stacey T E 1986 Patient-triggered ventilation in the newborn. Lancet ii: 17–19

Ment L R, Duncan C C, Ehrenkrantz R A et al 1985 Randomised indomethacin trial for prevention of intraventricular haemorrhage in very low birth weight infants. Journal of Pediatrics 107: 937–943

Mitchell R G 1985 Objectives and outcome of perinatal care. Lancet ii: 931–933

Morgan M E I, Benson J W T, Cooke R W I 1981 Ethamsylate reduces the incidence of periventricular haemorrhage in very low birth weight babies. Lancet ii: 830–831

Morley C J 1983 Will exogenous surfactant treat respiratory distress syndrome? Archives of Disease in Childhood 58: 312–323

Morley C J, Bangham A D, Miller N, Davies J A 1981 Dry artificial lung surfactant and its effects on very premature babies. Lancet i: 64–68

Neligan G A, Kolvin I, Scott D M, Garside R F 1976 Born too soon or born too small. In: Clinics in developmental medicine No 61 (Spastics International Medical Publications), Heinemann, London

Nelson K B, Ellenberg J H 1986 Antecedents of cerebral palsy. Multivariate analysis of risks. New England Journal of Medicine 315: 81–86

Newns B, Drummond M F, Durbin G M, Culley P 1984 Cost and outcome in a regional intensive care unit. Archives of Disease in Childhood 59: 1064–1067

Nickel R E, Bennett F C, Lamson F N 1982 School performance of children with birthweight of 1000 g or less. Americal Journal of Diseases of Children 136: 105–110

Northway W H 1979 Observations on bronchopulmonary dysplasia. Journal of Pediatrics 95: 815–818

Northway W H, Rosan R C, Porter D Y 1967 Pulmonary disease following respirator therapy of hyaline membrane disease—bronchopulmonary dysplasia. New England Journal of Medicine 276: 357–368

Orgill A A, Astbury J, Bajuk B, Yu V Y H 1982 Early neurodevelopmental outcome of very low birthweight infants. Australian Paediatric Journal 18: 193–196

Pagani G, Rezzonico R, Marini A 1985 Trials of high frequency jet ventilation in preterm infants with severe respiratory disease. Acta Paediatricia Scandinavica 74: 681–686

Pape K E, Wigglesworth J S 1979 The clinico-pathological relationship and aetiological aspects of intraventricular haemorrhage. In: Haemorrhage, ischaemia and the perinatal brain, Heinemann, London

Pape K E, Cusick G, Houang M T W et al 1979 Ultrasound detection of brain damage in preterm infants. Lancet i: 1261–1264

Powell T G, Pharoah P O D, Cooke R W I 1986 Survival and morbidity in a geographically defined population of low birthweight infants. Lancet i: 539–543

Ross G, Lipper E G, Auld P A M 1985 Consistency and change in the development of premature infants weighing less than 1501 grams at birth. Pediatrics 76: 885–891

Rowe J, Clyman R, Green C, Mikkelsen C, Haight J, Ataide L 1978 Follow up of families who experienced a perinatal death. Pediatrics 62: 166–170

Royal College of Obstetricians and Gynaecologists 1985 Report of the RCOG Working Party on the Management of Perinatal deaths, Chameleon Press, London

Sandhu B, Stevenson R C, Cooke R W I, Pharoah P O D 1986 Cost of neonatal intensive care for very low birthweight infants. Lancet i: 600–603

Sauve R S, Singhal N 1985 Long term morbidity of infants with bronchopulmonary dysplasia. Pediatrics 76: 725–733

Schanler R A, Garza C, Nichols B L 1985a Fortified mother's milk for very low birth weight infants: results of growth and nutrient balance studies. Journal of Pediatrics 107: 767–774

Schanler R A, Garza C, Smith E O'B 1985b Fortified mother's milk for very low birth weight infants: results of macromineral balance studies. Journal of Pediatrics 107: 437–445

Seigel E, Gillings D, Campbell S, Guild P 1985 A controlled evaluation of rural regional perinatal care: impact on mortality and morbidity. American Journal of Public Health 55: 156–160

Shapiro D L, Notter R H, Morin F C et al 1985 Double-blind, randomised trial of calf lung surfactant extract administered at birth to very premature infants for prevention of respiratory distress syndrome. Pediatrics 76: 593–599

Sims D G, Wynn J, Chiswick M L 1982 Outcome for newborn babies declined admission to a regional neonatal intensive care unit. Archives of Disease in Childhood 57: 334–337

Sinha S K, Sims D G, Davies J M, Chiswick M L 1985 Relation between periventricular haemorhage and ischaemic brain lesions diagnosed by ultrasound in very pre-term infants. Lancet ii: 1154–1155

Smith M A, Baum J D 1983 Cost of visiting babies in special care baby units. Archives of Disease in Childhood 58: 56–59

Stahlman M T, Cheatham W, Gray M E 1979 The role of air dissection in bronchopulmonary dysplasia. Journal of Pediatrics 95: 878–882

Stewart A, Turcan D, Rawlings G et al 1978 Outcome of infants at high risk of major handicaps. Ciba Foundation Symposium 59: 151–164

Szymonowicz W, Yu V Y H, Walker A, Wilson F 1986 Reduction of periventricular haemorrhage in preterm infants. Archives of Disease in Childhood 61: 661–665

Tonz O, Schubiger G 1985 Feeding of very-low-birth-weight infants with breast-milk enriched with energy, nitrogen and minerals: FM85. Helvetica Paediatrica Acta 40: 235–247

Vohr B R, Coll C T G 1985 Neurodevelopmental and school performance of very low-birth-weight infants: a seven-year longitudinal study. Pediatrics 76: 345–350

Walker C H M 1982 Neonatal intensive care and stress. Archives of Disease in Childhood 57: 85–88

Werthammer J, Brown E R, Neff R K, Taeusch H W Jr 1982 Sudden infant death syndrome in infants with bronchopulmonary dysplasia. Pediatrics 68: 336–340

Whitelaw A 1986 Death as an option in neonatal intensive care. Lancet ii: 328–331

Wigglesworth J S, Pape K E 1978 An integrated model for haemorrhagic and ischaemic lesions in the human brain. Early Human Development 2: 179–199

Yu V Y H, James B, Hendry P, MacMahon R A 1979 Total parenteral nutrition in low birthweight infants: a controlled trial. Archives of Disease in Childhood 54: 653–661

Yu V Y H, Orgill A A, Lim S B, Bajuk B, Astbury J 1983 Growth and development of very low birth weight infants recovering from bronchopulmonary dysplasia. Archives of Disease in Childhood 58: 791–794

Yu V Y H, Watkins A, Bajuk B 1984 Neonatal and postneonatal mortality in very low birthweight infants. Archives of Disease in Childhood 59: 987–999

Yu V Y H, Wong P Y, Bajuk B, Szymonowicz W 1986a Pulmonary air leak in extremely low birthweight infants. Archives of Disease in Childhood 61: 239–241

Yu V Y H, Loke H L, Bajuk B, Szymonowicz W, Orgill A A, Astbury J 1986b Prognosis for infants born at 23 to 28 weeks gestation. British Medical Journal 293: 1200–1203

Very low birthweight babies

The outcome for infants born between 23 and 28 weeks' gestation has improved substantially over the last two decades (Kitchen et al 1985a, Philip et al 1981). The obstetrician, caring for a mother who appears likely to deliver before 29 weeks of gestation, requires accurate data on the infant's likelihood of survival and the risks of serious long-term morbidity. Such data have practical implications. The decision whether to transfer a mother for delivery in a tertiary centre, to monitor the fetus electronically, or to deliver by caesarean section for fetal indications can be influenced by the obstetrician's perception of the survival prospects. In one survey of those delivering babies in the State of Alabama, the estimates of fetal survival chances in a hypothetical situation were frequently erroneous in both directions, but most often survival chances were underestimated (Goldenberg et al 1982). Applying this misinformation to actual cases would have resulted in some potentially viable fetuses receiving less than optimal management and some mothers being subjected to caesarean section with negligible chances of a surviving child.

A knowledge of the risks of long-term morbidity is equally important when discussing with parents the treatment options. Ideally, these data should be available to the obstetrician for the region or for the centre where the delivery will take place. However, late mid-trimester live births are comparatively rare, comprising only 9.8 per 1000 live births in our tertiary centre (Kitchen et al 1985b). Results of follow-up of survivors are frequently not available. Reliance must be placed on published reports which are few in number, particularly since most studies of long-term outcome are related to birthweight categories rather than to gestational age.

There are reports of in-hospital mortality in relationship to gestational age (Dillon & Egan 1981, Herschel et al 1982, Verloove-Vanhorick et al 1986) but we are aware of only three studies (in the English literature) that also include the long-term outcome of infants born at less than 29 weeks' gestation. Milligan et al (1984) reported their experience in a tertiary centre in Toronto of intensive perinatal management of a cohort of preterm infants, which included 267 live births over 4 years between 23 and 28 weeks' gestation, with survivors followed for at least 6 months after discharge from hospital. The gestational age accepted was that noted by the obstetrician antenatally in over 99% of cases in their study. Yu et al (1986b), in their most recent publication, reported their experience of 356 live births in one of the three tertiary perinatal centres in Melbourne between 1977 and 1984, with most survivors followed to at least 2 years of age. In our most recent report (Kitchen et al 1985b) we detailed the outcome of 338 live births in another tertiary centre in Melbourne between 1977 and 1982. In both the Melbourne studies, the obstetricians' estimates of gestation were used exclusively. These three reports, supplemented with additional data from our own study, provide the basis for most of this chapter.

ACCURACY OF ASSIGNED GESTATIONAL AGE

Nobody is more aware of the difficulties in assessing the gestational age of the fetus than the obstetrician. Where a reliable menstrual history, regular menstrual cycles and early ultrasonic estimation of the size of the gestational sac or crown–rump length of the fetus are available, the gestation of the fetus is rarely in dispute (Robinson 1973). With less precise information, the obstetrician is in a dilemma; indeed, in our study we had to exclude 13 (4%) of infants judged on paediatric assessment to be of 24–28 weeks' gestation because the obstetrician was unable to estimate the gestational age of the fetus antenatally. Obstetricians may not realize the difficulties and inaccuracy of the paediatric assessment of gestational age in infants of border-line viability. The most commonly used scoring system (Dubowitz et al 1970, Dubowitz and Dubowitz 1977) cannot be accurately applied to a moribund infant or to one attached to the paraphernalia of modern neonatal intensive care. Even if a satisfactory paediatric assessment is technically feasible, it is now apparent that scoring systems are inaccurate in the extremely premature infant; under 33 weeks the Dubowitz system overestimates gestational age (Spinnato et al 1984), and Vogt et al (1981) reported that at early gestations the 95% confidence limits were ±5 weeks. We therefore chose, as did Yu et al (1986b), to accept the obstetrical dates as closest to the truth. Among the 338 infants in our study, there was not a single occasion when the paediatric assessment was less than that of the obstetrician; however, in 16 infants (4.7%) there was a strong presumption (based on paediatric assessment, birthweight far above the expected range) that the infant was between 3 and 8 weeks more mature than the obstetrical estimate. Dillon and Egan (1981) also noted that the paediatric estimate of gestation was frequently more advanced than the obstetrical assessment. If there is an obstetrical error, it is usually in the direction of underestimating gestational age or birthweight (Bowes et al 1979) and therefore underestimating survival prospects.

MORTALITY

In the context of mortality, we will confine discussion to live births occurring within tertiary centres. This is not to imply that events in a defined geographical region are unimportant; it is only by such data that the overall impact of perinatal intensive care can be judged (Sinclair et al 1981). Regional and community-based studies are difficult enough with a clearly defined parameter such as birthweight. Bearing in mind our earlier reservations regarding assessment of gestation, the pooling of unstandardized and non-validated data from numerous sources has serious problems; accurate regional mortality data for between 23 and 28 weeks' gestation do not exist, with the exception of the recent report of Verloove-Vanhorick et al (1986).

Survival data from tertiary centres also require close scrutiny. Because of the lack of data regarding all live births outside tertiary centres, outborn infants must be excluded from calculations. In our study 166 out of 338 (49%) of our live inborn babies died during their primary hospitalization, and the age at which they died is of interest: 20% (33 out of 166) of deaths occurred in the delivery room; by the end of the seventh day 85% (142 out of 166) had died; by 28 days 96% (160 out of 166) were dead; and the remaining 4% of deaths occurred between 5 and 24 weeks. This experience of late neonatal and infant deaths in hospital has been reported by others (Yu et al 1986b, Herschel et al 1982, Milligan et al 1984). The mortality risk does not cease when the extremely premature infant goes home; sudden infant death syndrome (SIDS) occurred in 6 of our study children and in 3 in the study of Yu et al (1986b). Post-hospital mortality is now well recognized in infants of very low birthweight or extreme prematurity (Hack et al 1980, Sells et al 1983).

Major malformations, incompatible with life, are prevalent in infants of borderline viability, occurring in 2% (6 out of 388) in our study, with similar figures from other studies (3.9% Yu et al 1986b, 5.2% Milligan et al 1984). Some variation in the prevalence of lethal malformations may be due to the inclusion or exclusion of those cases referred to tertiary centres specifically for termination late in the second trimester, lethal malformations having been diagnosed in utero. Our policy has been to exclude these particular cases since the obstetrician is in no doubt regarding the prognosis, but to include these malformations in booked patients and in those referred late for management of a pregnancy complication where the diagnosis of a major malformation had not been made before admission. Milligan et al (1984) noted that over half of the major malformations were unlikely to be diagnosed antenatally. These then are some of the pitfalls in the uncritical interpretation of mortality data.

What survival can we expect in late second-trimester and early third-trimester births? In Figure 11.1, the uncorrected mortality between 23 and 28 completed weeks of gestation are given from four studies with a sample size above 100; Yu et al (1986b) reported survival to 1 year, whereas the other studies considered survival to hospital discharge. The individual data have been pooled, but the range at each week is quite wide. In our study, survival at 23 and 24 weeks is poor in comparison with the other reports, probably because of our less aggressive approach to infants of these gestational ages.

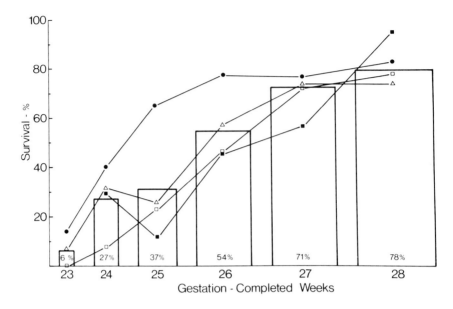

Fig. 11.1 In-hospital survival between 23 and 28 weeks' gestation. The histograms indicate the pooled survival rates, and the width of each histogram is proportional to the sample size. Survival rates from individual studies are included to illustrate the range ($\bullet$ = Milligan et al 1984, $n = 267$; $\triangle$ = Yu et al 1986b, $n = 356$; $\square$ = Kitchen et al 1985a, $n = 338$; $\blacksquare$ = Herschel et al 1982, $n = 136$)

OBSTETRICAL FACTORS AFFECTING SURVIVAL

Figure 11.1 indicates that increasing gestational age is an important factor in improving survival prospects—from 6% at 23 weeks' to 78% at 28 weeks' gestation. Additional obstetric factors associated with mortality observed in some or all studies are multiple births, pre-eclampsia or hypertension, breech presentation and failure to administer steroids antenatally to the mother (Dillon and Egan 1981, Herschel et al 1982, Kitchen et al 1985b, Yu et al 1986b). However, other risk factors cannot be evaluated without adjustment for gestational age differences. An idea of the relative statistical importance of some obstetric factors in association with improved survival in our study was: increasing gestation 9, no hypertension 3, singleton pregnancy 3, and antenatal steroid therapy 2.5 (Kitchen et al 1985b). Figure 11.2 illustrates survival in our study from 24 to 28 weeks' gestation and indicates that the use of antenatal steroids conferred a survival advantage above average of about two-thirds of a week of gestation, and multiple births had the equivalent of the loss of 1 week of gestation; other obstetric factors, including the presence of premature rupture of the membranes and breech presentation, were not statistically significant after adjustment for discrepancies in gestational age.

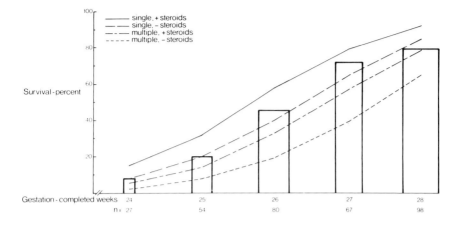

Fig. 11.2   In-hospital survival (%) of live-born infants at 24–28 weeks of gestation. The predicted survival for singleton and multiple pregnancies, with and without antenatal steroid therapy, is represented by lines; the actual survival is represented by histograms, with the width of each histogram being proportional to the sample size at each week of gestation (from Kitchen et al 1985b)

Caesarean section

The role of caesarean section for the delivery of extemely immature infants will only be settled by a randomized, controlled trial. Such are the practical difficulties, it is unlikely that these data will be obtained (Kitchen et al 1985b, Lumley et al 1985). We must rely on non-randomized data, adjusting for the fact that caesarean section is more likely to be used when prognosis for survival is a reasonable expectation; there is little evidence for the survival value of caesarean section in those studies where statistical adjustment has been made for confounding factors such as gestation (Herschel et al 1982, Barrett et al 1983, Worthington et al 1983, Olshan et al 1984, Kitchen et al 1985b). The tentative recommendation is that caesarean section should be considered on maternal grounds, such as severe pre-elcampsia, or when there is a fetal indication, such as fetal distress or malpresentation.

The question of the earliest gestation at which caesarean section is justified is a vexed one. Herschel et al (1982) performed caesarean section for fetal reasons at 26 weeks' gestation or more; Milligan et al (1984) are not specific on this point but regard 25 weeks as the time when the odds for a 'favourable result' are above 50%. Dillon and Egan (1981) noted that all four infants delivered by caesarean section at 24–25 weeks died, and this was our experience in six cases, with a survival following caesarean delivery of 73% (32 out of 44) between 26 and 28 weeks' gestation. All six infants delivered by caesarean section before 26 weeks in the State of Victoria in 1984 died (Consultative Council on Obstetric and Paediatric Mortality and Morbidity, 1986). At the present time, 26 weeks' gestation appears to be a practical lower limit, but in an individual situation where the fetus is 'irreplaceable', parents and obstetrician may decide on a lower gestation limit as a worthwhile risk.

Electronic fetal monitoring

This is an area of potential conflict between obstetrician and paediatrician. Many obstetricians are disinclined to use electronic fetal monitoring unless the fetus has reached a predetermined gestation—usually 26 weeks—when caesarean section would be seriously considered as an option for delivery if fetal distress develops. The technical problems involved in external monitoring of an extremely premature fetus during labour may be formidable, and the thin skull and delicate soft tissues at early gestations make internal monitoring potentially hazardous. Braithwaite et al (1986) reported that between 26 and 30 weeks a normal intrapartum cardiotocographical tracing was generally associated with a good outcome; an abnormal fetal heart tracing was predictive of 90% of the mortality, but half of those with an abnormal trace were free of mortality or morbidity. The paediatric viewpoint differs: because of the possibility of underestimation of gestation already referred to, monitoring at an earlier gestation is favoured. The presence or absence of fetal distress is an important part of the neonatal history. With evidence of prolonged intrapartum hypoxia, the paediatrician may well decide that the fetus that has been 'written off' in labour should not be vigorously resuscitated after birth; in the absence of this information, decision-making in the delivery room and intensive care unit is less rational.

Outcome in relation to weight for gestational age

In Figure 11.3, survival within each week of gestation (from 24 to 28 weeks) is given for weight groupings of 200 g for infants, in our own study; the tenth, fiftieth and ninetieth percentile lines are superimposed (Kitchen et al 1981). Two conclusions may be drawn from these data. Firstly, within each individual gestational age category, rising birthweight is associated with increasing survival. Secondly, the birthweights of some infants, *as judged on obstetric estimation*, are far above the ninetieth percentile, suggesting they were more mature; if so, this is a bonus for the obstetrician, who, as previously mentioned, sometimes tends antenatally to underestimate gestation and hence the survival chances. The enhanced survival of infants who are relatively large for gestational age may also reflect more vigorous paediatric treatment and fewer problems with the intricate techniques used in neonatal intensive care.

UTILIZATION OF NEONATAL INTENSIVE CARE RESOURCES

The obstetrician's initial reaction to this aspect may well be 'let the paediatrician worry about that'; however, if neonatal resources are in short supply, obstetrical decisions may be influenced by the lack of a ventilator bed. The

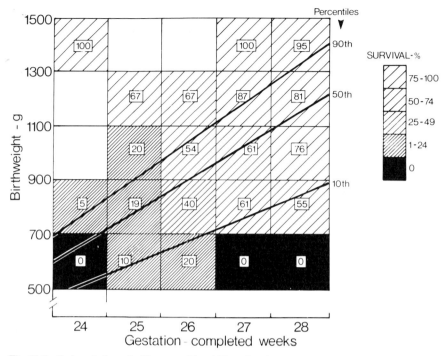

Fig. 11.3   In-hospital survival between 24 and 28 weeks of gestation in relation to birthweight in 200 g intervals after each week of gestation. The tenth, fiftieth and ninetieth percentile lines are superimposed.

distribution of some of these resources for infants from 24 to 28 weeks' gestation was investigated for the years 1982–1985 in our unit. Each week of gestation gained results in a reduction for the survivors of a mean of 8 days' ventilation, 9 days in the neonatal intensive care unit and 11 days in hospital, a compelling argument for obtaining the maximum time in utero at this gestation. To achieve a survivor at 28 weeks' gestation required less than half the neonatal resources as at 26 weeks.

LONG-TERM PROGNOSIS

The obstetrician, in discussing the antenatal and intrapartum treatment options, often finds that parents already have concerns extending beyond mere survival of their infant; the obstetrician needs information on the prevalence of long-term morbidity among survivors. An antenatal paediatric consultation should be helpful to obstetrician and parents; among other advantages, it gives the parents and paediatrician an opportunity to discuss at length and in an informed manner the treatment options—how vigorously to persist with resuscitation of a malformed infant or to continue ventilation in the presence of extensive cerebro-ventricular (intraventricular) haemorrhage, for example. The antenatal consultation makes any subsequent discussion of issues such as these just a little easier. Treatment decisions require input from well-informed parents and are not regarded merely as the prerogative of the professionals.

IMPAIRMENTS AND DISABILITIES

The World Health Organization (1980) recommends the use of the term 'impairment' to specify the diagnostic medical category of a sensory or neurological abnormality (e.g. cerebral palsy, blindness, deafness, developmental delay) and the use of the term 'disability' to indicate that the impairment causes restriction or lack of ability (e.g. severe motor disability in a child with spastic quadriplegia).

These criteria are used in the study of Yu et al (1986b) of predominantly 2-year-old children and in our study of 2-year-old children. Severe neurological impairment included children with one or more of the following: bilateral blindness, severe sensorineural deafness, cerebral palsy of any type or severity, or severe developmental delay (a mental developmental index on the Bayley Scales of Infant Development under 69, which is more than 2 SD below the test mean). The severe impairment rates for each individual week of gestation are tabulated for the individual studies of Yu et al (1986b) and Kitchen et al (1985b), and the data are then pooled (Table 11.1).

The overall rate of severe neurological impairment was disturbingly high at 16.8% (95% confidence intervals ±4.2%), substantially higher than the 2% we have found in 50 term children (Ford et al 1986). Because there are few survivors in some weeks of gestation, we have combined the data for 27–28 weeks' gestation and less than 27 weeks' gestation so as to obtain approximately equal numbers of severely impaired children in each category. The rate of severe neurological impairment for 27–28 weeks' gestation was 13.6% (±4.6%) and was significantly lower than the rate for 26 weeks' gestation or less of 24.4% (±8.9%) ($X^2 = 5.7, P < 0.05$).

Whereas the definition of impairment has a firm basis, the assessment of severe disability involves value judgement, not an easy task in 2-year-olds. Examples of children who would be defined as severely impaired but not severely disabled would be cerebral palsy with mild motor disability, and sensorineural deafness without developmental delay. The severe disability rates for the study of Yu et al are tabulated, together with our study children classified on the same criteria. The rate of severe neurological disability for 27–28 weeks' gestation was 8.0% (±3.6%), and again was significantly lower than the rate for 26 weeks' gestation or less of 17.8% (±7.9%) ($X^2 = 5.3$, $P < 0.05$).

The only other study giving long-term outcome in relation to gestational age was by Milligan et al (1984). The minimum age of follow-up was 6 months corrected age, and the outcome of survivors was described in terms of 'major developmental handicap' on criteria that cannot be pooled with the other

Table 11.1 Severe impairments and severe disability in relation to gestation at delivery. The majority of children were aged 2 years, corrected for the degree of prematurity

Gestation (completed weeks)	Severe impairment			Severe disability		
	Yu et al (1986b)	Kitchen et al (1985a)	Pooled data	Yu et al (1986b)	Kitchen et al (1985a)	Pooled data
23	50% (1/2)	—	50% (1/2)	50% (1/2)	—	50% (1/2)
24	15% (2/13)	0% (0/2)	13% (2/15)	8% (1/13)	0% (0/2)	7% (1/15)
25	45% (5/11)	0% (0/6)	29% (5/17)	27% (3/11)	0% (0/6)	18% (3/17)
26	26% (9/35)	24% (5/21)	25% (14/56)	20% (7/35)	19% (4/21)	20% (11/56)
27	14% (9/63)	14% (4/28)	14% (13/91)	10% (6/63)	11% (3/28)	10% (9/91)
28	15% (10/68)	11% (6/54)	13% (16/122)	7% (5/68)	6% (3/54)	7% (8/122)
Total	19% (36/192)	13.5% (15/111)	16.8% (51/303)	12% (23/192)	9% (10/111)	11% (33/303)

two studies. In particular, a mental developmental index below 80 was the criterion for 'mental retardation'; 21% (33 out of 159) had a major developmental handicap and their data showed no statistically significant relationship between handicap and gestational age.

LESSER IMPARIMENTS AND HEALTH PROBLEMS

The obstetrician should appreciate that the severe impairments found in surviving infants represent the more extreme end of the spectrum of long-term morbidity. In our study, in addition to the 13.5% of survivors with severe impairments, there were another 23% (26 out of 111) who had moderate developmental delay at 2 years; these children will require a longer period of follow-up to decide their outcome.

Although an extensive range of difficulties have been described for infants weighing under 1500 g and particularly for those weighing less than 1000 g, these data are not available in relation to gestational age (Desmond et al 1980, Ford et al 1985, Ford et al 1986, Hack et al 1981). The list, which is by no means exhaustive, includes lesser degrees of developmental delay, soft neurological signs, ocular morbidity other than bilateral blindness, iatrogenic sequelae of intensive care, poor physical growth, frequent rehospitalizations, behaviour disorders and school learning difficulties. These children may impose a continuing heavy burden on medical and educational resources and parents; psychiatric problems in one study were found in 25% of mothers of very low birthweight infants (Ryan et al 1985).

WHY ARE SOME SURVIVORS IMPAIRED?

This question can only be answered in general terms because the prediction from perinatal data of the outcome *for individuals* is usually not possible. Factors causing later impairments may operate before, during or after birth.

Some late mid-trimester births clearly represent part of the inevitable reproductive wastage associated with malformations or chromosomal defects. There is apprehension that less obvious developmental defects may also occur; for example, there is an increased prevalence of minor dysmorphic features in very low birthweight infants (Ford et al 1986). A substantial number of cases of cerebral palsy cannot be explained by intrapartum or postnatal events, raising the suspicion that they have a prenatal origin (Kitchen et al 1986).

It has long been an article of faith that adverse perinatal events may be responsible for continuum of reproductive wastage, from death at one extreme to survival with sequelae, the severity of which relates to the severity of perinatal insult (Lilienfeld & Parkhurst 1951). The close association of adverse perinatal events with perinatal death is still accepted, but the causal relationship of such insults to morbidity in survivors is being increasingly questioned (Hensleigh et al 1986, Shennan et al 1985). This should not be taken as licence for inadequate intrapartum care but rather as an indication that the main influence of obstetric care is to minimize death.

Some later morbidity in survivors is clearly related to neonatal events. Cerebro-ventricular haemorrhage that has extended into brain tissue is an example, although even in this extreme situation up to half of the survivors are free of major impairments (Kitchen et al 1985c). As techniques to assess structural and functional abnormalities of the brain improve, it is likely that a rather better correlation between neonatal morbidity and later impairment will be established (de Vries et al 1985).

PROSPECT FOR SUBSEQUENT PREGNANCIES

We are unaware of any published reports of the later reproductive performance of women who deliver in the late second trimester, i.e. in terms in gestational age. However, Kossman and Bard (1982) reviewed the outcome in 84 women aged less than 40 years and who had not had a tubal ligation, who sustained a neonatal death of a baby weighing less than 1000 g; 90% of the 40 mothers who subsequently became pregnant had a surviving child. Yu et al (1986a) found that of 103 mothers who delivered an infant weighing less than 1000 g at birth, 40% decided against subsequent pregnancy, a decision made significantly more often by older mothers and those where the index child had survived. Although there was a substantial pregnancy wastage over the next 3 years, 87% of mothers who became pregnant ultimately achieved at least one surviving child. In both studies, the mothers often conceived within a year, which may lead to later psychological problems as the result of the mothers' unresolved mourning experiences. These studies highlight some important maternal issues. Some mothers are reluctant to embark on another pregnancy for a variety of reasons that may include advancing maternal age and the negative experience of intensive care for a neonate. This experience is extremely stressful, whether it culminates either in death of the baby or an extremely protracted and anxious neonatal course before survival is assured; the survival of an impaired child may be a strong deterrent to attempting subsequent pregnancies. For those who become pregnant, the majority achieve a living child, although pregnancy losses and complications are frequent. Presumably pre-pregnancy counselling and a high standard of antenatal care are among the factors leading to a more favourable outcome in subsequent pregnancies. The obstetrician managing an individual mother may be able to make a more accurate estimate of future reproductive performance, the spectrum extending from 'an irreplaceable fetus' to a pregnancy complication that is unlikely to recur in the future.

OTHER CONSIDERATIONS

Increased survival has raised a number of ethical, moral and economic problems. The provision of intensive obstetrical and neonatal care is expensive, requiring substantial financial resources and highly trained personnel who may be in short supply; this has resulted in financial and economic evaluations of intensive care for very low birthweight infants (Boyle et al 1983, McCarthy et al 1979, Phibbs et al 1981, Pomerance et al 1978, Walker et al 1985). There continues to be apprehension about the long-term outcome of these infants who, until recently, would have been regarded as inevitable, perhaps even desirable, reproductive losses; we have no cut-off point below which the chances of intact survival are unacceptably low (Milligan et al 1984).

OPTIONS FOR THE OBSTETRICIAN

The obstetrician managing a pregnancy that is likely to terminate in the late second trimester is faced with important and difficult decisions. Ideally there will be up-to-date and reliable information on the prospects for both survival and intact survival from his or her own perinatal centre, rather than relying on data from other obstetrical services as reviewed in this chapter. With aggressive obstetric and paediatric management, surprisingly good survival rates can be achieved, but the rate of impairment is dauntingly high. In a slightly different context of genetic counselling, many parents faced with a 25% risk of an inherited neurological abnormality in their offspring would opt for termination of pregnancy; the overall risk for major neurological impairments of survivors under 27 weeks' gestation of 24.4% is close to this rate. If time permits, discussion with well-informed parents is an essential feature in planning whether managment will be aimed at achieving a survivor at all costs; sometimes the joint decision will be to let nature take its course.

REFERENCES

Barrett J M, Boehm F H, Vaughn W K 1983 The effect of type of delivery on neonatal outcome in singleton infants of birthweight of 1000 g or less. Journal of the American Medical Association 250: 625–629
Bowes W A, Halgrimson M, Simmons M A 1979 Results of the intensive perinatal management of very-low-birth-weight infants (501 to 1,500 grams). Journal of Reproductive Medicine 23: 245–250
Boyle M H, Torrance G W, Sinclair J C, Horwood S P 1983 Economic evaluation of neonatal intensive care of very-low-birth-weight infants. New England Journal of Medicine 308: 1330–1337
Braithwaite N D J, Milligan J E, Shennan A T 1986 Fetal heart rate monitoring and neonatal mortality in very preterm infants. American Journal of Obstetrics and Gynecology 154: 250–254
Consultative Council on Obstetric and Paediatric Mortality and Morbidity 1986 Annual Report for the Year 1984, Health Commission of Victoria, Melbourne
Desmond M M, Wilson G S, Alt E J, Fisher E S 1980 The very low birth weight infant after discharge from intensive care: anticipatory health care and developmental course. Current Problems in Pediatrics 10: 1–59
DeVries L S, Dubowitz L M S. Dubowitz L, Kaiser A, Whitelaw A, Wigglesworth J S 1985 Predictive value of cranial ultrasound in the newborn baby: a reappraisal. Lancet ii: 137–140
Dillon W P, Egan E A 1981 Aggressive obstetric management in late second-trimester deliveries. Obstetrics and Gynecology 58: 685–690
Dubowitz L M S, Dubowitz V 1977 Gestational age of the newborn, Addison-Wesley, Reading, Massachusetts
Dubowitz L M S, Dubowitz V, Goldberg C 1970 Clinical assessment of gestational age in the newborn infant. Journal of Pediatrics 77: 1–10

Ford G W, Rickards A L, Kitchen W H, Lissenden J V, Keith C G, Ryan M M 1985 Handicaps and health problems in 2 year old children of birth weight 500 to 1500 g. Australian Paediatric Journal 21: 15–22

Ford G W, Rickards A L, Kitchen W H, Lissenden J V, Ryan M M, Keith C G 1986 Very low birthweight and normal birthweight infants: a comparison of continuing morbidity. Medical Journal of Australia 145: 125–128

Goldenberg R L, Nelson K G, Dyer R L, Wayne J 1982 The variability of viability: the effect of physicians' perceptions of viability on the survival of very low-birth weight infants. American Journal of Obstetrics and Gynecology 143: 678–684

Hack M, Merkatz I R, Jones P K, Fanaroff A A 1980 Changing trends of neonatal and postneonatal deaths in very-low-birth-weight infants. American Journal of Obstetrics and Gynecology 137: 797–800

Hack M, DeMonterice D, Merkatz I R, Jones P, Fanaroff A A 1981 Rehospitalization of the very-low-birth-weight infant: a continuum of perinatal and environmental morbidity. American Journal of Diseases of Childhood 135: 263–266

Hensleigh P A, Fainstat T, Spencer R 1986 Perinatal events and cerebral palsy. American Journal of Obstetrics and Gynecology 154: 978–981

Herschel M, Kennedy J L, Kayne H L, Henry M, Cetrulo C L 1982 Survival of infants born at 24 to 28 weeks' gestation. Obstetrics and Gynecology 60: 154–158

Kitchen W H, Bajuk B, Lissenden J V, Yu V Y H 1981 Intrauterine growth charts from 24 to 29 weeks' gestation. Australian Paediatric Journal 17: 269–272

Kitchen W H, Rickards A L, Ford G W, Ryan M M, Lissenden J V 1985a Live-born infants of 24 to 28 weeks' gestation: survival and sequelae at two years of age. In: Porter R, O'Connor M (eds) Abortion: medical progress and social implications (Ciba Foundation Symposium 115), Pitman, London pp 122–135

Kitchen W H, Ford G W, Doyle L W et al 1985b Cesarean section or vaginal delivery at 24 to 28 weeks' gestation: comparison of survival and neonatal and two-year morbidity. Obstetrics and Gynecology 66: 1079–1087

Kitchen W H, Ford G W, Murton L J et al 1985c Mortality and 2 year outcome of infants of birthweight 500–1500 g: relationship with neonatal cerebral ultrasound data. Australian Paediatric Journal 21: 253–259

Kitchen W H, Doyle L W, Ford G W, Rickards A L, Lissenden J V, Ryan M M 1986 Cerebral palsy in very low birth weight infants surviving to 2 years with modern perinatal intensive care. American Journal of Perinatology 4: 29–35

Kossman J-C, Bard H 1982 Subsequent pregnancy following the loss of an early preterm newborn infant weighing less than 1000 grams. Obstetrics and Gynecology 60: 74–76

Lilienfeld A M, Parkhurst E 1951 A study of the association of factors of pregnancy and parturition with development of cerebral palsy. American Journal of Hygiene 53: 262–282

Lumley J, Lester A, Renou P, Wood C 1985 A failed RCT to determine the best method of delivery for very low birth weight infants. Controlled Clinical Trials 6: 120–127

McCarthy J T, Koops B L, Honeyfield P R, Butterfield L J 1979 Who pays the bill for neonatal intensive care? Journal of Pediatrics 95: 755–761

Milligan J E, Shennan A T, Hoskins E 1984 Perinatal intensive care: where and how to draw the line. American Journal of Obstetrics and Gynecology 148: 499–503

Olshan A F, Shy K K, Luthy D A, Hickock D, Weiss N S, Daling J R 1984 Cesarean birth and neonatal mortality in very low birth-weight infants. Obstetrics and Gynecology 64: 267–270

Phibbs C S, Williams R L, Phibbs R H 1981 Newborn risk factors and costs of neonatal intensive care. Pediatrics 68: 313–321

Philip A C S, Little G A, Polivy D R, Lucey J F 1981 Neonatal mortality risk for the eighties: the importance of birth weight gestational age groups. Pediatrics 68: 122–130

Pomerance J J, Ukrainski C T, Ukra T, Henderson D H, Nash A H, Meredith J L 1978 Cost of living for infants weighing 1,000 grams or less at birth. Pediatrics 61: 908–910

Robinson H P 1973 Sonar measurement of fetal crown–rump length as means of assessment maturity in first trimester of pregnancy. British Medical Journal 4: 28–31

Ryan M M, Rickards A L, Cook R, Kitchen W H, Lissenden J V 1985 Mental health of mothers of very low birthweight infants. In: Festschrift for Winston S. Rickards, Vital Instant Press, Melbourne, pp 142–149

Sells C J, Neff T E, Bennett F C, Robinson N M 1983 Mortality in infants discharged from a neonatal intensive care unit. American Journal of Diseases of Childhood 137: 44–47

Shennan A T, Milligan J E, Hoskins M 1985 Perinatal factors associated with death or handicap in very preterm infants. American Journal of Obstetrics and Gynecology 151: 231–238

Sinclair J C, Torrance G W, Boyle M H, Horwood S P, Saigal S, Sackett D I 1981 Evaluation of neonatal intensive care programs. New England Journal of Medicine 305: 489–494

Spinnato J A, Sibai B M, Shaver D C, Anderson G D 1984 Inaccuracy of Dubowitz gestational age in low birth weight infants. Obstetrics and Gynecology 63: 491–495

Verloove-Vanhorick S P, Verwey R A, Brand R, Gravenhorst J B, Keirse M J N C, Ruys J H 1986 Neonatal mortality risk in relation to gestational age and birthweight. Lancet i: 55–57

Vogt H, Haneberg B, Finne P H, Stensberg A 1981 Clinical assessment of gestational age in the newborn infant: an evaluation of two methods. Acta Paediatricia Scandanavica 70: 669–672

Walker D J, Vohr B R, Oh W 1985 Economic analysis of regionalized neonatal care for very low-birth-weight infants in the state of Rhode Island. Pediatrics 76: 69–74

World Health Organization 1980 International classification of impairments, disabilities and handicaps. A manual of classifications relating to the consequences of disease, Geneva

Worthington D, Davies L E, Grausz J P, Sobocinski K 1983 Factors influencing survival and morbidity with very low birth weight delivery. Obstetrics and Gynecology 62: 550–555

Yu V H Y, Davis N G, Mercado M F, Bajuk B, Astbury J 1986a Subsequent pregnancy following the birth of an extremely low birth-weight infant. Australian and New Zealand Journal of Obstetrics and Gynaecology 26: 115–119

Yu V Y H, Loke H L, Bajuk B, Szymonowicz W, Orgill A A, Astbury J 1986b Prognosis for infants born at 23 to 28 weeks gestation. British Medical Journal 293: 1200–1203

Failed forceps

INTRODUCTION

Failed forceps is an interesting topic which addresses both historic and present day concerns. The history of failed forceps traces the advances in operative obstetrics over a period of 300 years. During that time failed forceps has preoccupied the leaders of our profession: their first interest was the reduction in maternal mortality associated with the procedure, and more recently their efforts have been directed towards the reduction of fetal death and injury. Management of failed forceps remains a problem in our time. Failure of forceps deliveries has allowed the continued use of midforceps by providing a means of withdrawing safely from a situation that has been misjudged. Whether this last use should be a planned or unplanned procedure is now subject to re-examination.

Failed forceps has always been a controversial subject. Failure is, in this instance, obvious to all; to the onlooker it is seemingly apparent that the cause of the failure is the doctor. The public, and more recently the courts, have not been reluctant to express their disapproval of this event and to give their judgements.

HISTORY OF FAILED FORCEPS

Prior to 1950

It is ironic that the first description of forceps use is concerned with a description of a failure of forceps. All the controversy, misjudgement and tragic results that are associated with failed forceps are exemplified by Hugh Chamberlen's well-documented case of failed forceps (Taussig 1915). Obstetrical forceps had been a secret of the Huguenot family (the Chamberlens) for over 100 years. Forceps use had allowed successive generations of the family to gain ascendancy over their rivals, the midwives. The family had reached the highest appointments in the country and then, through a combination of events, its fortunes declined. Hugh, the great grandson of the original

Huguenot physician, in urgent need of funds, set out to sell the family's secret to the French in 1670. He boasted in a sales talk to Louis XIV that he (Chamberlen), through the use of his secret, could deliver any woman within 10 minutes. In the summer of that year and prior to the proposed sale, he was put to the test. His sensational failure was described in great detail and with some satisfaction by Mauriceau, the leader of French obstetrics of the day. The attempt took place in Paris's massive mediaeval hospital, the Hotel Dieu. By tradition, patients walked from the lying-in ward—the Salle Saint Joseph—to a room called the Chauffoy in which they were delivered. In this case it is hard to imagine that the walk took place, for Mauriceau had chosen for the demonstration a 'woman of small stature' who had been in labour for 8 days with a face presentation. For some 3 hours, Chamberlen, hidden beneath a sheet in order to better guard his secret, struggled in a vain attempt to deliver the infant. The child had died prior to the attempt; the mother was to do so shortly with a ruptured uterus. Louis XIV did not buy the Chamberlen family secret.

In 1752, William Smellie's book, *A Treatise on the Theory and Practice of Midwifery*, was published. This book was to set the standard for obstetrical care over the next 150 years. By the time Smellie's book was published, the description of forceps and the means of their use had become public knowledge, but the use of forceps was already surrounded with controversy. Smellie and his students were described by Mrs Nihell, a midwife and an outspoken critic of men-midwives, as 'wreaking havoc and spreading death and destruction' (Donegan 1978). Her diatribes became prophetic when failure of forceps occurred. Failure was managed by internal version or the use of crotchets (hooks) following craniotomy (Smellie 1752); the certain death of the infant and the almost certain death of the mother followed. Failure and its disastrous consequences affected not only the patient, but impugned the whole concept of the participation of the doctor in the delivery process. Smellie recognized that the major cause of failure was the attempt to deliver the infant when the station of the fetal head was high. To free himself, and his pupils, from the temptation of reaching high into the pelvis, he advocated the use of short-handled forceps only.

It is only a century ago, following the introduction of anaesthesia, asepsis and the realization of the need to suture the uterus after delivery, that caesarean section became an option in the management of failed forceps. Yet this was an option that could not be readily accepted. At that time the caesarean sections which were done were of the classical type, and the risk of postoperative peritonitis was prohibitively high. Eardley Holland (Holland 1921) pointed out that a classical caesarean section performed on a patient who was not in labour had a maternal mortality rate of 1.6%, but if the caesarean section was performed following failed forceps (in which case the uterus was invariably infected), the maternal mortality was 26%. A similar experience had been previously reported (Frank 1908) in Germany. Thus, at the beginning of the twentieth century the therapeutic options for the obstetrician were in effect limited to those described by Smellie in the middle of the eighteenth century.

In the early part of the century the public's unfavourable attention was attracted by the consequences of the improper use of forceps; in particular their failure was decried. Interest in the subject was said to have '. . . permeated every home in the land' (Hendry 1928). A public meeting with widespread lay and governmental representation was held at Westminster Central Hall in 1928 to debate the subject. The consensus of the meeting was expressed by Lady Selborne, who declared: 'there is danger in the doctor' (Hendry 1928). The profession responded with a detailed examination of the subject at the annual meeting of the British Medical Association of that same year. Along with other papers a large (523) collected series of failed forceps was presented (Miller 1928). In cases of failed forceps, maternal mortality was shown to be 10%, and fetal mortality 63%. The cause of failure was attributed to contracted pelvis (40% of cases), occipito-posterior position (31%) or premature application of forceps (29%). Caesarean section was performed in only 2% of cases of failure, and in those few instances one-quarter of the mothers died in the postoperative period. It was hoped that the incidence of failed forceps would decrease with improved medical education and better prenatal care. Little change in care was suggested for those patients in whom failure had occurred. An appeal for the public's understanding was made (Shaw 1928).

Change in the management of failed forceps, and with it the care of cephalopelvic disproportion or malpresentation, came only through the acceptance of the transverse lower uterine segment operation (Case et al 1971). The operation had been introduced to the English-speaking world by Munro Kerr and popularized by St George Wilson. There was quick realization that peritonitis and death did not occur with the same frequency following the lower segment operation as following the classical operation. Acceptance of the lower segment operation was such that within a few years it had for the most part replaced the classical operation. For the first time it became possible to accept the failure of forceps. It was no longer necessary to use high forceps or traction bars, to attempt internal version, and to perform a craniotomy. The consequence of these changes was an uninterrupted decline in maternal mortality over the ensuing years. By 1950, maternal mortality had reached 2% in cases of failed forceps, but fetal mortality remained high at 34% (Freeth 1950).

After 1950

Attention was now concentrated on the eradication of fetal death and injury that resulted from failed forceps. It was suggested by Douglas and Kaltreider (1953) that forceps should be abandoned as soon as unforeseen difficulties with delivery were encountered. Their paper was primarily concerned with a review of 2000 pelvimetry examinations and the subsequent labours of the patients. Three of the cases were delivered by caesarean section following attempts at forceps delivery. There is no suggestion in their paper that difficulty had been predicted, and no suggestion that the attempt had taken place in an operating room with all preparations made for a possible caesarean section. There is no reason to believe that the cases described were not in fact failures. The easy acceptance of failure was clearly stated:

> 'The regime very briefly consists of the correction of abnormalities of position when this can be done easily and of gentle traction with the forceps. If further progress is not obtained, the forceps are removed and the patient delivered abdominally.'

The only difference is that the name had changed from 'failure of forceps' to 'trial forceps', a change of name that was to allow failure to become acceptable with improved maternal and neonatal outcome. In this instance the truth of an old proverb was contradicted:

> To change the name, and not the letter,
> Is a change for the worse, and not for the better
>
> (Anonymous)

Within a few months of the publication of Douglas and Kaltreider's article, another authoritative paper brought the concept forward (Jeffcoate 1953). It was now suggested that, even in the face of predicted difficulty, careful attempts at forceps delivery could be made. Qualifications were also suggested: 'the possibility of failure should be voiced prior to the attempt, and the attempt should be made in the operating theatre with provisions for immediate caesarean section'; no further cases were described. The ambiguity over definition and intent persists to this day.

No meaningful series of trial forceps was to be published during the next 30 years. There are a number of possible explanations for this. Failed forceps occurred infrequently; lower segment caesarean section was resorted to after Barton's forceps on only 11 occasions amongst 625 midforceps deliveries (2%) in a total population of 20 394 (Parry-Jones 1972). This was not unusual; some years before Miller had reported only three cases of failed forceps among 6000 patients who had been examined antenatally (Miller 1927). The infrequency of failed forceps was presumably related to the well-developed clinical acumen of the obstetricians (the increasing frequency of the event relates perhaps to a loss of those same skills by present-day obstetricians). A second possibility is that failed forceps might have been less frequent in the past because obstetricians of that era may have delivered the infant with trauma which would now be considered unacceptable. Finally, obstetricians may have been reluctant to publish failures that did occur.

The results of this policy (of easy acceptance of failure) were first detailed by Cardozo et al (1983). The neonatal outcomes of 20 cases of failed forceps amongst 2708 consecutive deliveries were compared with neonatal results following spontaneous, non-rotational forceps, ventouse, Kielland's forceps and emergency caesarean section deliveries (caesarean sections in the first stage were included). The neonatal results of infants delivered by caesarean

Table 12.1   Outcome by method of delivery

| | Method of delivery | | | | |
	Spon-taneous	Low forceps	Mid-forceps	Caesarean section for failure to progress	Caesarean section for failed forceps
Number of cases	2760	2353	1276	82	53
Depression at birth (%)					
Moderate	2.0	1.7	4.0*	11.0*	11.3
Severe	0.3	0.3	0.3	2.4*	1.9
Encephalopathy (%)	0.1	0.1	0.4	2.4*	5.7*
Meconium aspiration (%)	0.4	0.3	0.4	2.4	3.8*
Fractures or palsies (%)	0.6	1.2*	5.1*	0	3.8*
Admission to neonatal intensive care unit (%)	7.9	8.7	13.8*	23.2*	24.5*

*$P < 0.05$ as compared with spontaneous deliveries. From Obstetrics and Gynecology, with permission.

section following failed trial of forceps or ventouse showed the infants' Apgar scores to be similar to those of infants delivered by emergency caesarean section; furthermore, in instances of failed trial of forceps, there was 'no evidence of severe birth trauma or neurological abnormality'. The study was further refined (Traub et al 1984): 20 cases of failed Kielland's forceps deliveries amongst 16 376 consecutive deliveries were compared with 101 caesarean sections performed in the second stage of labour and also with 132 successful uses of Kielland forceps. The 'neonatal outcome was no different' in the group of failed Kielland's deliveries from the other two groups. The neonatal result of spontaneous vaginal delivery or non-rotational forceps delivery was not described. The study did not distinguish between primigravidae and multigravidae as Cardozo et al's (1983) study had done. In neither study were compounding maternal or fetal variables such as antepartum haemorrhage, pre-eclampsia or prematurity removed from analysis. With these concerns in mind, Boyd et al (1986) addressed the subject. Their study included 81 cases of failed forceps amongst 22 247 consecutive deliveries. The study population was limited to primigravidae (10 501), in whom 98% of the failed forceps occurred. If compounding maternal or fetal factors were present which could independently cause asphyxia or trauma, the cases were removed. The final study population consisted of 53 cases of failed forceps among 6524 consecutive primigravid deliveries. Neonatal results of spontaneous delivery, low and midforceps delivery and caesarean section for failure to progress (in the second stage) and for failed forceps were then compared (Table 12.1).

As shown in Table 12.1, spontaneous delivery is clearly associated with fewer adverse neonatal outcomes than any operative delivery, including low forceps delivery. There was significant trauma associated with successful mid-forceps delivery: 67 out of 1276 infants delivered sustained some injury or were depressed at birth. The complications are not common: stated positively, 94% of the time midforceps deliveries result in the delivery of an undamaged infant. The trauma is rarely permanent; clavicular fractures and skull fractures heal readily, and facial and brachial palsies for the most part disappear. Eight infants out of 1276 midforceps deliveries showed abnormal cerebral signs, and one of these infants had convulsions and suffered permanent disability. It is often unappreciated that adverse outcomes cannot be eliminated by re-placing midforceps deliveries with caesarean section. Caesarean sections in the second stage for failure to progress have more adverse outcomes than successful midforceps deliveries (Table 12.1).

The neonatal ill-effects following failed forceps deliveries are similar to those that can be expected to follow caesarean section in the second stage for failure to progress. Failed forceps delivery is disadvantageous when com-pared with successful midforceps delivery; with these there are significantly increased numbers of neonates with moderate asphyxia, admission to neonatal intensive care unit, meconium aspiration and encephalopathy.

PRESENT-DAY MANAGEMENT

The present-day concern regarding midforceps use is not only with their failure but whether they should be used at all. It has been suggested that 'few if any midforceps operations can be justified' (Chez et al 1980). The neonatal outcomes on which such recommendations are based are found in a single 15-year-old study of 656 patients selected for abnormal labour patterns or clinically abnormal labour, which does not take modern practice into account (Friedman & Sachtleben 1971).

It is generally recognized that if the criteria for their use have been met, midforceps deliveries may be attempted. The prerequisites for midforceps delivery have been well described (Paintin 1982, Cardozo et al 1983, Kadar 1985). With such criteria forceps deliveries may be attempted but should be promptly discontinued if undue difficulty is encountered during the appli-cation of forceps, or with the attempted rotation of the vertex, or when more than moderate traction is found to be necessary. Data on discontinuation of forceps after failure and the resort to an unplanned caesarean section suggest that it is a safe procedure (Cardozo et al 1983, Traub et al 1984, Boyd et al 1986).

The principles of midforceps use up to this point are clear, but confusion arises on whether or not in cases 'where difficulty is anticipated or doubt about the feasibility of vaginal delivery exists . . .' proper management should consist of attempting the delivery in the operating room (Kadar 1985). It has been the author's contention that there were no data to support such an undertaking.

Until recent months there was no published series which took separate note of trial forceps deliveries that did succeed (in the sense that vaginal delivery occurred). Lowe (1987) has corrected this. His paper compares the neonatal outcome of primary second stage caesarean section with the neonatal outcome following unexpected failure of instrumentation and with that of trial forceps which did not succeed. He showed 'trials of instrumental delivery' to be safe as compared with unexpected failures or primary second stage caesarean section. Lowe (1987) did not, however, compare these results with those of midforceps deliveries in which no difficulty was anticipated and in which no difficulty occurred. Yet the cases in which a 'trial' is judged to be necessary are presumably more likely to be complicated by a higher station of the fetal head, more moulding and slower progress in the active phase of labour. It is reasonable to assume that the frequency of fetal asphyxia and trauma would have been higher than among those cases in which the accoucheur had no doubt that delivery would be uneventful, i.e. where the vertex was low in the pelvis, or where no moulding occurred. The author remains of the opinion that failure of forceps should be used as a safe means of withdrawing from a misjudged situation; it should not be used as a means of entering a situation fraught with potential difficulty.

The discussion of whether the attempt is to be a 'trial' or was a 'failure' is important not only with regard to the care of the patient, but also with regard to medico-legal considerations. In fact the courts have been reluctant to accept the term 'trial forceps' and have questioned it in the following terms: '. . . doubtful whether (the physician) was in fact undertaking a trial of forceps as opposed to an attempt at vaginal delivery which failed . . .' (Whitehouse vs Jordan and others 1981). The label 'trial' is often made after the fact; in no instance among the 81 cases described (Boyd et al 1986) was there documentation indicating the intent to undertake a 'trial', and in no case did the attempt take place in an operating theatre. The attending physician had judged vaginal delivery to be possible, and was unsuccessful in the attempt; all the cases were therefore called 'failed forceps' (Paintin 1982).

In an earlier era, failure of forceps most often occurred following attempts to deliver which were made away from the hospital. Failures now occur within the hospital setting and the occurrence is more than occasional (Myerscough 1982). The failure rate of midforceps deliveries has been variously reported as 4, 10, 15 or 20%; the difference may be explained by the frequency of midforceps use (Boyd et al 1986, Vacca et al 1983, Traub et al 1984, Cardozo et al 1983). The frequency of failure is sometimes expressed as a percentage of the primary caesarean section rate; this has been reported to be 1% (Quilligan & Zuspan 1982).

It has been recommended that caesarean section should be preferred to midforceps delivery when fetal distress is the indication for rapid delivery (Paintin 1982). In our experience, those cases of failed forceps where fetal distress was present appeared to have an unduly high number of adverse fetal outcomes (4 out of 17) compared with the incidence of adverse outcomes

Table 12.2   Role of fetal distress in affected infants (where fetal monitoring results were available)

	With fetal distress	Without fetal distress
Caesarean section for failed forceps	4 out of 17 (24%)	1 out of 33 (3%)
Caesarean section for failure to progress	0 out of 25 (0%)	4 out of 50 (8%)

when fetal distress did not precede failed forceps (Table 12.2). The diagnosis of fetal distress in these cases was based for the most part on the presence of an abnormal fetal heart tracing in the first and/or second stage, or the presence of meconium. The diagnosis of fetal distress must be considered to be imprecise, however, for it was not always confirmed by the determination of the fetal blood pH. Lowe (1987) excluded patients with suspected fetal distress in the second stage from his study group. The incidence of birth hypoxia among these infants was inordinately high.

Our data did not demonstrate a need for immediate caesarean section should forceps fail (Table 12.3). The mean period of time from failed forceps to

Table 12.3   Timing of failed forceps (i.e. the number of cases of failed forceps where the time of attempt and delivery were clearly specified—34 out of 53 cases)

	With fetal distress	Without fetal distress
Number of cases	9	25
Full dilatation to forceps application (min)	56	96
Forceps application to delivery (min)	33	51
Total second stage (min)	89	147

caesarean section was 46 minutes; in 10 cases the delay was over 60 minutes. In only one of these 10 cases was there any need for resuscitation. The findings suggest that delay did not affect the infant's condition in caesarean section for failed forceps. It may be that pre-existing fetal distress, which may prompt the attempted forceps delivery, is a more important concern.

MEDICO-LEGAL ASPECTS

'*Post hoc, ergo propter hoc*' is a phrase that refers to the fallacy of believing that there is always a cause and effect relationship between events which follow each other. Despite the illogicality, adverse fetal outcome following forceps delivery often results in the censure of the doctor. This is especially true following failed forceps. Doctors involved in these cases have had a major problem in mounting a viable legal defence. The problem is particularly acute should the infant suffer with long-term neurological defects. In spite of evidence confirming the importance of other factors in the determination of fetal outcome (Niswander et al 1984), such cases are assuming increasing importance in Canada and elsewhere.

REFERENCES

Anonymous 1802–71 In Chambers R (ed) Book of days, vol i, p 723
Boyd M E, Usher R H, McLean F H, Norman B E 1986 Failed forceps. Obstetrics and Gynecology 68: 779–783
Cardozo L D, Gibb M F, Studd J W W, Cooper D J 1983 Should we abandon Kielland's forceps? British Medical Journal 287: 315–317
Case B D, Corcoran R, Jeffcoate T N A, Randle G H 1971 Caesarean section and its place in modern obstetric practice 78: 203–214
Chez R A, Ekbladh L, Friedman E A, Hughey M J 1980 Mid-forceps delivery: is it an anachronism? Contemporary Obstetrics and Gynecology 15: 82–100
Donegan J B 1978 Art of midwifery: In: Women and men midwives, Greenwood Press, Westport, Connecticut, p 167
Douglas L H, Kaltreider D F 1953 Trial forceps. American Journal of Obstetrics and Gynecology 65: 889–896
Friedman E A, Sachtleben M R 1971 High risk labour. Journal of Reproductive Medicine 7: 28–32
Frank M 1908 Die geburtshilfliche therapie des engen Beckens. Muenchener Medizinische Wochenschrift 55: 363
Freeth H D 1950 The cause and management of failed forceps. British Medical Journal 2: 18–21
Hendry J 1928 Unsuccessful forceps cases. British Medical Journal 2: 185–188
Holland E 1921 The results of a collective investigation into Caesarean sections performed in Great Britain and Ireland from 1911 to 1920 inclusive. Journal of Obstetrics and Gynaecology of the British Empire 28: 358–446
Jeffcoate T N A 1953 The place of forceps in present-day obstetrics. British Medical Journal 2: 951–955
Kadar N 1985 The second stage. In: Studd J (ed) The management of labour, Blackwell, Oxford, pp 268–286
Lowe B 1987 Fear of failure: a place for the trial of instrumental delivery. British Journal of Obstetrics and Gynaecology 94: 60–66
Miller D 1927 The failed forceps case and its treatment. British Medical Journal 2: 685–687
Miller D 1928 Observations on unsuccessful forceps cases: causation, management and end-results. British Medical Journal 2: 183–185
Myerscough P R 1982 Operative obstetrics, Baillière Tindall, London, p 291
Niswander K, Henson B, Elbourne D et al 1984 Adverse outcome of pregnancy and the quality of obstetric care. Lancet 2: 827–831
Paintin D B 1982 Commentary: mid-cavity forceps delivery. British Journal of Obstetrics and Gynaecology 89: 495–496
Parry-Jones E 1972 Barton's forceps, Williams & Wilkins, Baltimore, pp 103–113
Quilligan E J, Zuspan F P 1982 Caesarean section. In: Douglas-Stromme operative obstetrics, 4th edn, Appleton-Century-Crofts, New York, p 603
Shaw W F 1928 Unsuccessful forceps cases. British Medical Journal 2: 188–190
Smellie W 1752 A treatise on the theory and practice of midwifery, D Wilson Printer, London, pp 296–306
Taussig F J 1915 Chamberlen and Mauriceau: an unsuccessful forceps application in the year 1670. Interstate Medical Journal 22: 59–62
Traub A I, Morrow R J, Ritchie J W K, Dornan K J 1984 A continuing use for Kielland's forceps? British Journal of Obstetrics and Gynaecology 91: 894–898
Vacca A, Grant A, Wyatt B, Chalmers I 1983 Portsmouth operative delivery trial: a comparison of vacuum extraction and forceps delivery. British Journal of Obstetrics and Gynaecology 90: 1107–1112
Whitehouse vs Jordan and others 1981 Weekly law reports (Parliament, House of Lords), p 262

The management of intra-uterine death

The death of a fetus at any stage of pregnancy is a tragic event. Whilst the onus is on the obstetrician to establish the diagnosis and investigate the cause, particular sensitivity is required in conducting the delivery and subsequent counselling of the parents. This chapter reviews all these aspects of management after 20 weeks' gestation. Changes have occurred in recent times which allow one a greater choice in accomplishing delivery of the fetus. Prostaglandins have revolutionised induction of labour remote from term, and a substantial quantity of literature has accumulated to guide one in their use. Some skills have been lost for better or for worse, notably many of the destructive operations which allowed vaginal delivery of the dead fetus. In replacement, the indications for abdominal delivery have become more clearly defined. Information continues to accrue on grief relating to stillbirth, although until recently one needed to look beyond the obstetric literature. All obstetricians should have a good working knowledge of this process and its aberrations, as they are in a primary position to help these unfortunate parents.

HISTORICAL CONSIDERATIONS

On 5 November, 1817, Princess Charlotte of Wales had laboured for 26 hours in the first stage and for 15 hours in the second stage when the uterine discharge became a dark green colour. It was then suspected that the child might be dead or be born in a state of suspended animation (Holland 1951). This suspicion was of interest because auscultation of the fetal heart was only described in the subsequent year. The delivery of a stillborn infant after 50 hours, followed by maternal death and the later suicide of Croft, the *accoucheur*, is a well-described tale.

Ramsbotham (1844) also wrote of the difficulties in establishing the diagnosis of intra-uterine death. He placed great reliance upon stethoscopic examination but acknowledged the common view that the diagnosis was essentially of academic interest, since it did not influence one's recourse to craniotomy where delivery was requisite.

A plethora of destructive procedures are described in the historical literature. Avoidance of abdominal delivery was all important and prompted Friedrich Benjamin Osiander (1759–1822) to write: 'It cannot be denied that of the women who undergo Caesarean section more than two-thirds die, and barely a third are saved. Caesarean section belongs to those operations of which the outcome is entirely uncertain. Before, then, undertaking this procedure, one should allow the patient to draw up her will and grant her time to prepare herself for death.' (McIntosh Marshall 1939)

ESTABLISHING THE DIAGNOSIS AND RELATING A CAUSE

The absence of fetal heart sounds remains the mainstay of clinical diagnosis, supported by lack of fetal movements and regression of uterine size. Auscultation of the fetal heart by Pinard stethoscope is dependent upon the experience of the operator, and reported lack of fetal movements may be unreliable. There are additional psychological benefits to the patient when ancillary aids are used to confirm the diagnosis, as well as the reassuring certainty of the diagnosis that ensues. The Doppler apparatus is a useful device where management depends upon an immediate diagnosis, for example after major placental abruption. When the membranes have ruptured, a fetal electrode may be used, but the pitfall of monitoring transmitted maternal cardiac activity must be acknowledged. Zlatnik (1986) suggested manoeuvres to overcome this error, such as maternal breath holding, which alters the maternal heart rate and should be reflected in the recorded trace. If this is not considered then Caesarean section for assumed fetal bradycardia may result.

Radiological confirmation of the diagnosis has become unpopular although no less valid. Overlapping of the fetal skull bones (Spalding's sign) or gas in the fetal circulatory system (Roberts' sign) are significant radiological findings (Russell 1973). Ultrasound diagnosis of death is recognised by an absent fetal heart pattern, skull collapse, a poorly visualised midline falx echo and retraction of brain tissue. Scheer & Nubar (1977) describe a zig-zag M-mode type pattern produced by the heart valves when the scanning arm is slowed while crossing the cardiac area, which is virtually always reproducible when the fetus is viable. The absence of this pattern, in association with an empty fetal bladder, a non-filled aorta and the signs already mentioned, allow a definitive diagnosis to be made. In addition, ultrasonography has the unspoken advantage of being an image with which the patient can more readily identify.

An attempt should always be made to determine the cause of the fetal death because this may dictate further management. The pendulum is swinging away from treatment as a matter of urgency, towards allowing parents time to consolidate their thoughts and prepare themselves for the subsequent delivery. There are situations, however, where advice should be given for delivery without delay. The presence of ruptured membranes with a retained dead fetus is a recipe for intra-uterine sepsis if this is not already present. A major placental abruption is associated with a risk of rapid onset coagulopathy.

In these circumstances, expeditious delivery is indicated in the interests of the mother.

PROBLEMS ASSOCIATED WITH THE RETAINED DEAD FETUS

Three potential problems are associated with retention of the dead fetus, these being infection, maternal distress and coagulopathy. Infection involving the dead fetus is a potential risk for which there is a paucity of support in the literature. Certainly, if the membranes remain intact, the risk of infection remains very low indeed. Additionally, there is no proof that the hasty induction of labour, and delivery within a short time, lessens the anguish for the parents. Indeed it may be that undue haste contributes to the trauma of the event rather than relieving it. Kellner et al (1984) allowed 69 patients with no medical indication for delivery a choice of immediate induction or awaiting the spontaneous onset of labour. Of these, 32 patients (46.4%) chose immediate induction and 37 (53.6%) chose to wait!

Coagulation system changes

In 1950, Weiner et al described the development of coagulation system changes in immunised Rh-negative women carrying a dead fetus. Death of the fetus rather than isoimmunisation was subsequently identified as the significant factor (Reid et al 1953, Pritchard & Ratnoff 1955). Coagulopathy only seems to occur after 16 weeks' gestation, and in general only when the dead fetus has been retained in utero for more than 4 weeks (Pritchard 1959, Pritchard 1973). Although a slow decline of the plasma fibrinogen level is the usual feature, Goldstein & Reid (1963) have reported abrupt changes over the course of a few days. There may also be elevation of fibrin degradation products (FDP) and a fall in the platelet count, while the prothrombin and partial thromboplastin time may become prolonged. Fibrinogen usually falls at a rate of approximately 50 mg/dl per week, and is unlikely to be associated with an increased bleeding tendency until its level has fallen below 100 mg/dl.

The coagulopathy is considered to result from fibrinogen consumption following the release of thromboplastin from the retained products of conception (Pritchard 1973). Jimenez & Pritchard (1968) described a case where anti-fibrinolytic agents failed to reverse an established coagulopathy but infusion of heparin caused the concentration of fibrinogen to rise. Fibrinolysis may contribute to the bleeding diathesis as a secondary event. Pfeffer (1966) described the successful treatment of a patient with ε-aminocaproic acid, although the balance of evidence indicates primary fibrinogen consumption as the cause. From a practical point of view one should therefore measure the fibrinogen level rather than relying upon FDP as an indirect measure of disseminated intravascular coagulation (Romero et al 1985).

This particular complication of the retained dead fetus therefore dictates a necessity to empty the uterus, but only after 4 weeks in most instances. Spontaneous abortion or labour will occur in 80% of women within 2 weeks, and only 10% remain undelivered for more than 3 weeks (Zlatnik 1986). Interestingly, Townsend & Shelton (1964) found evidence of delayed spontaneous labour when the fetal death was due to Rh-isoimmunisation, 50% of mothers remaining undelivered after 5 weeks. In addition, Ursell (1972) found the onset of coagulopathy to occur before 4 weeks in five patients with fetal death due to Rh-isoimmunisation. Deaths due to this cause therefore appear to be an exception to the '4-week' rule, and it would be of interest to determine whether deaths due to non-immunological hydrops are also an exception. Nevertheless, these examples demonstrate that when a conservative approach to management is chosen, fibrinogen levels, FDP and platelets should be measured on a weekly basis, and intervention is indicated after a maximum interval of 4 weeks.

What of the patient presenting with an established coagulopathy? If the patient is not in labour, the use of heparin to arrest consumption of coagulation factors and allow time for spontaneous recovery is well described (Kent & Goldstein 1976, Pritchard et al 1985, Romero et al 1985). Maintenance of the partial thromboplastin time at 2.5 times the control level until the fibrinogen concentration rises above 200 mg/dl is the aim. Heparin may then be stopped and labour induced safely after 6 hours (Romero et al 1985). The use of heparin has also been described by Skelly et al (1982) for the successful treatment of coagulopathy developing after the death of one fetus at 22 weeks in a triplet pregnancy. Treatment was continued until 35 weeks when a second infant died and the third was delivered liveborn. A further case involving the death of one twin at 27 weeks was described by Hainline & Nagey (1982). Fibrinogen, FDP and platelet counts did not deviate from normal levels during monitoring until induction of labour at 39 weeks, illustrating that coagulopathy is by no means invariable in this circumstance. If the patient presents with coagulopathy in labour or there is active haemorrhage, heparin is contraindicated. Treatment should then be directed towards replacement of deficient factors using fresh blood, cryoprecipitate or fresh frozen plasma. The urgency of replacement therapy must be balanced against the requirement to empty the uterus, as only then will the consumption of the coagulation factors be arrested. In our opinion there is insufficient evidence to recommend the use of anti-fibrinolysins in this situation.

ACCOMPLISHING DELIVERY OF THE FETUS

Conduct of the established labour

Caesarean section for fetal reasons after disappearance of the heart sounds is rarely indicated. The exception is perhaps where death of the fetus occurs during preparation for an otherwise indicated Caesarean section. The paediatric staff need to be assured that the infant for potential resuscitation is within

10 minutes of death. This procedure must never become a means of demonstration to the mother that everything possible was done in the interests of her child.

Vaginal delivery should be the aim unless there are specific indications for abdominal delivery, as will shortly be discussed (see below). Analgesia should be offered liberally, including epidural analgesia, after demonstration of an intact coagulation cascade. Sedation should be available upon request but not unduly promoted.

The induction of labour

The therapeutic options available are hypertonic solutions administered intra-amniotically, oxytocin or prostaglandins, which may be given by various routes. The use of hypertonic solutions in the presence of a dead fetus has become obsolete and is mentioned only for completeness.

Intra-amniotic saline administration has been described by Csapo (1966), Goplerud & White (1968), and Rozenman et al (1980). Most patients are delivered within 24 hours, but coagulopathy similar to that seen in association with placental abruption may occur (Pritchard 1973), and maternal deaths have been recorded (Wagatsuma 1965, Cameron & Dayan 1966). Hypertonic glucose has also been used successfully for the induction of labour by Lewis et al (1969), but it is associated with unacceptable infectious morbidity (Peel 1962, MacDonald et al 1965). The use of hypertonic urea has also been described by Greenhalf & Diggory (1971), but it confers no particular advantage.

The obstetric literature is replete with advice about induction of labour in the presence of fetal death. After appraisal of the evidence, one could be pardoned for confusion. We do believe, however, that certain principles may be listed as follows:

1. Any agent which increases uterine tone has the potential capacity to rupture the uterus.
2. The myometrium is sensitive to prostaglandin at any gestation, but there is evidence that sensitivity increases with advancing gestation (Schulman et al 1979).
3. It does not matter which prostaglandin is administered or which route is used, as there will always be a dose–effect relationship. Nevertheless, some analogues and some methods of administration are associated with a lower incidence of side-effects.
4. The myometrium is relatively insensitive to oxytocin remote from term, although sensitivity usually increases with advancing gestation.
5. Cervical 'ripeness' or 'favourability', as defined by the Bishop score, reflects oxytocin sensitivity.
6. The simultaneous administration of prostaglandin and oxytocin is most commonly associated with iatrogenic damage to the uterus and cervix.

The logical principles of management then follow:

1. Oxytocin should be used for the induction of labour when the cervix is 'favourable' (Bishops score >4), which generally equates to an advanced gestation (>35 weeks).
2. The prostaglandin chosen should be one which is available, familiar to the obstetrician concerned and authorised for use by local regulations. These factors are more relevant than any purported superiority of one to another.
3. When prostaglandin is used the initial dose should be adjusted according to the gestation and further doses should be administered according to the uterine response.
4. One should always beware of the simultaneous administration of prostaglandin and oxytocin.

Table 13.1 demonstrates the multiple routes of administration and types of prostaglandin which may be used. We believe that the preferred route is by extra-amniotic infusion, as this allows both the dose and the rate of administration to be controlled while delivering the prostaglandin to the site of response. With limited systemic absorption, all side-effects are minimised. A 12 or 14 French gauge Foley catheter is passed through the cervix using a bivalve speculum and a single-toothed vulsellum if necessary. The balloon is inflated with 20–40 ml of normal saline, and an infusion pump is used to instil prostaglandin, after considering the catheter dead space (approximately 3 ml). In Manchester we have used prostaglandin E_2 (PGE$_2$) in a concentration of 100 µg/ml, commencing the infusion at 0.5 (or 1.0) ml/h and increasing it hourly by 0.5 (or 1.0) ml increments to a maximum of 3.0 ml/h. The infusion dose and rate is titrated against uterine response and the whole protocol is very simple. Uterine response is monitored clinically, although others have described tocodynamometric monitoring (Miller et al 1972) or intra-uterine pressure monitoring (Embrey et al 1974). Oxytocin for augmentation is indicated if the catheter is passed spontaneously or the patient remains undelivered for 24 hours, but *only* after the prostaglandin administration has ceased and uterine activity has abated. The risk of uterine or cervical trauma is increased when the synergistic effect of combined prostaglandin and oxytocin is inflicted on the uterus, especially at advanced gestations or in multiparous patients (Schulman et al 1979, Lauersen et al 1980, Kent et al 1984). We agree with the current view of Lawson (1986, personal communication) that combined prostaglandin and oxytocin is a dangerous method of emptying the uterus in the presence of fetal death.

Vaginal PGE$_2$ has been popular in North America used as a 20 mg pessary inserted at 2–8 hourly intervals. Some authors recommend a reduction of the dose to 5–10 mg beyond 28 weeks to avoid uterine hypertonicity (Bailey et al 1975, Zlatnik 1986). Schulman et al (1979) described an elaborate oxytocin challenge test with measurement of intra-uterine pressure to determine the initial dose of prostaglandin to be administered. They also described the use of a contraceptive diaphragm to confine the drug to the paracervical

Table 13.1 The use of prostaglandin for the induction of labour with intra-uterine fetal death

Author	Method	Patients (number)	Success (%)	Dose (mg)	Interval (hours)
Antsaklis et al (1979)	IA PGF$_{2\alpha}$	30	100.0	40.0	5.3
Antsaklis et al (1984)	IM 15-Me PGF$_{2\alpha}$	52[a]	100.0	0.8	7.3
Bailey et al (1975)	VAG PGE$_2$	20	100.0[b]	32.0	8.7
Embrey et al (1974)	EA PGE$_2$	12[c]	100.0	0.8	7.6[d]
Gruber & Baumgarten (1980)	IV PGE$_2$ IV Sulprostone	10 10	90.0[e] 100.0[f]	3.3 0.9	8.1 8.8
Karim et al (1982)	IM 15-ME PGF$_{2\alpha}$	282	97.2	0.9	10.5
Kent et al (1984)	VAG PGE$_2$	46	95.7[g]	NS	8.7
Kent & Goldstein (1976)	VAG PGE$_2$	19	94.7[h]	48.2	7.9[i]
Lauersen et al (1980)	VAG PGE$_2$	80	97.5[j]	NS	8.9[k]
Miller et al (1972)	EA PGE$_2$	60[l]	100.0[m]	2.5	15.75[n]
Phelan & Cepalo (1978)	VAG PGE$_2$	25	100.0	56.0	7.0
Saarikoski et al (1980)	IV Sulprostone	12	100.0	1.1	13.0
Scher et al (1980)	EA PGE$_2$ VAG PGE$_2$	26 23	100.0[o] 91.3[q]	1.8 45.2	8.6[p] 9.2[p]
Schwartz & Brenner (1980)	IA PGF$_{2\alpha}$	3	100.0	47.3	28.3
Southern et al (1978)	VAG PGE$_2$	709	96.9[r]	60.4	10.7

IA = intra-amniotic, EA = extra-amniotic, IM = intramuscular, IV = intravenous, VAG = vaginal, NS = not stated
[a] One patient with an extra-uterine pregnancy is excluded from further consideration.
[b] 10% of patients required evacuation of retained products of conception (ERPC).
[c] PGF$_{2\alpha}$ was used in one patient.
[d] Two patients were given oxytocin after passing the extra-amniotic catheter.
[e] 30% of patients required ERPC, and one was undelivered at 24 hours.
[f] 30% of patients required ERPC.
[g] One patient required hysterectomy after sustaining a cervical laceration during delivery. Oxytocin was used for augmentation in this case.
[h] 26.3% of patients required ERPC.
[i] Four patients required augmentation with oxytocin after spontaneous rupture of the membranes.
[j] 50% of patients required ERPC.
[k] Concomitant oxytocin was used in 38 out of 80 (47.5%) patients.
[l] PGF$_{a\alpha}$ was used in eight patients.
[m] 52% of patients required ERPC.
[n] Oxytocin was used in 10 out of 60 (16.7%) patients remaining undelivered after 24 hours.
[o] 3.8% of patients required ERPC.
[p] Oxytocin was used for augmentation in some patients.
[q] 23.8% of patients required ERPC.
[r] 13% of patients required ERPC.

area in an attempt to reduce side-effects. Scher et al (1980) assessed side-effects when they compared extra-amniotic PGE$_2$ given to 26 patients and vaginal PGE$_2$ given to 23 patients. There was no significant difference in the success rate of delivery or the induction–delivery interval, but a greater incidence of side-effects was noted when the vaginal route was used (Table 13.2). The dose required for vaginal administration was 25 times that for extra-amniotic administration, suggesting that prostaglandin administered vaginally is system ically absorbed before acting upon the uterus, thus accounting for the higher incidence of side-effects. The occurrence of prostaglandin-induced pyrexia when the vaginal route is used is also of note, and this rarely occurs when extra-amniotic prostaglandin is used. It can be quite dramatic and simulate endotoxic shock (Phelan et al 1978). Nevertheless, many authors attest to the efficacy of vaginally administered prostaglandin in achieving delivery (Bailey et al 1975, Kent & Goldstein 1976, Phelan & Cepalo 1978, Southern et al 1978, Lauersen et al 1980, Kent et al 1984).

Table 13.2   Side-effects of prostaglandin therapy: extra-amniotic vs vaginal administration (adapted from Scher et al 1980)

Signs	Group I (extra-amniotic administration)	Group II (vaginal administration)
Temperature >100°C	0	10 out of 23 (43.5%)*
Tachycardia	0	3 out of 23 (13.0%)
Gastrointestinal symptoms	4 out of 26 (15.4%)	13 out of 23 (56.5%)*
Vomiting	2 out of 26 (7.7%)	9 out of 23 (39.1%)
Diarrhoea	2 out of 26 (7.7%)	6 out of 23 (26.1%)

* Significant ($P<0.005$).

Antsaklis et al (1979) described the use of intra-amniotic $PGF_{2\alpha}$ administered as a single dose. Their 100% success rate with a mean induction–delivery interval of 5.3 hours looks impressive, but one patient from their series of 30 sustained a cervical laceration, and this may reflect a lack of control over the uterine response when this method is used. Schwartz & Brenner (1980) surmounted this problem by the use of an intra-amniotic catheter passed transabdominally, through which fractional doses of $PGF_{2\alpha}$ were administered. The risk with this method concerns the possible development of an intraperitoneal liquor leak when high intra-uterine pressures are generated.

Intravenous administration of the classical prostaglandins caused too many gastrointestinal side-effects to be clinically useful (Toppozada 1986), but the availability of newer analogues has again popularised this route of administration in some centres. The intravenous administration of 16-phenoxy prostaglandin E_2 methyl sulfonylamide (Sulprostone) has been described by Gruber & Baumgarten (1980) and Saarikoski et al (1980) with satisfactory results. The intramuscular administration of another analogue, 2a-2b-dihomo-15(S)-15-methylprostaglandin $F_{2\alpha}$ methyl ester (15-Me-$PGF_{2\alpha}$), was described by Karim et al (1982) in a large multicentre trial conducted in Singapore, Indonesia and Malaysia. 15-Me-$PGF_{2\alpha}$ was used in a dose of 0.5 mg intramuscularly 8-hourly to effect delivery in 97.2% of patients with a mean induction–delivery interval of 10.5 hours. Similar results were reported in a later study by Antsaklis et al (1984). This method of administration may be particularly useful for those patients with ruptured membranes who are resistant to the use of oxytocin.

Oxytocin per se may be used for the induction of labour near term when the cervix is 'favourable'. In spite of well-intentioned use, either alone or following prostaglandin, one may still encounter a degree of uterine resistance. When fetal death is present, high concentrations of syntocinon up to 200 iu/1 can be used, although the principle of commencing with low doses and increasing according to uterine response still applies. The dose of oxytocin should be altered by increasing the concentration rather than by increasing the infusion rate, as the anti-diuretic effect of oxytocin at high doses is significant, especially when used with large volumes of aqueous dextrose. Water intoxication in this circumstance was first reported by Liggins (1962). Whalley & Pritchard (1963) produced experimental evidence to suggest that oxytocin infused at a rate of 50 milliunits per minute inhibited urine flow by more than 90% when given to women with either prolonged retention of a dead fetus or an incomplete abortion. The clinical syndrome has been described by Morgan et al (1977), Pedlow (1970) and Eggers & Fliegner (1979). Drowsiness, confusion and vomiting is followed by fitting and coma. Hyponatraemia in the range of 125 mmol/1 or lower is usual, and this may occur with a positive fluid balance of as little as 4 litres in 24 hours. Recovery is usual although cerebral function may remain abnormal for some weeks. Fluid balance and electrolyte status must therefore be carefully monitored whenever high doses of oxytocin are used, and the infusion medium should contain electrolytes.

When oxytocin is used alone, there is debate over whether the membranes should be ruptured or left intact. Both Ursell (1972) and Rozenman et al (1980) provide evidence to suggest that the induction–delivery interval is shortened without significant increase in the incidence of infection, when amniotomy is performed. Ursell used prophylactic antibiotics in some patients, being guided by the presence of potential pathogens on high vaginal swabs taken before the induction of labour. We would recommend this measure as a routine procedure.

When one is faced with protracted failure of the uterus to respond to either oxytocin or prostaglandin, consideration should be given to the presence of an extra-uterine pregnancy. Orr et al (1979) presented four cases of failure to respond to prostaglandin where this diagnosis was eventually made. A further case was reported by Antsaklis et al (1984) and another by Cohn & Goldenberg (1976), where the pregnancy was located in an unattached uterine horn.

The place of Caesarean section and fetal destruction

With reference to Caesarean section for delivery of the dead fetus, McIntosh Marshall wrote in 1939: 'I have no qualms of conscience in this matter. Actually I do not perform Caesarean section in order to save foetal life.

It is only a happy coincidence that this line of treatment does so often lead to such a result.' Table 13.3 shows what we believe, in present times, are indications for Caesarean section in the presence of a dead fetus. These are based upon similar concerns for maternal safety as expressed by McIntosh Marshall in 1939. We acknowledge that each case needs individual consideration, and management will often depend upon the experience of the operator. There is of course a paucity of controlled studies comparing destructive procedures with Caesarean section. Golgoi (1971) considered the management of 158 grossly infected patients in late labour, in most of whom labour was obstructed. 107 patients underwent Caesarean section with a maternal mortality rate of 12.1%. This compared with a mortality rate of 2.7% for those undergoing fetal craniotomy or decapitation, and the single maternal death in this latter group was associated with pre-existing anaemic cardiac failure. The two groups, however, were not comparable as Caesarean section was generally chosen when the lower uterine segment was on the verge of rupture, and hence these patients were generally in a more advanced stage of obstructed labour.

Table 13.3 Indications for Caesarean section in the presence of a dead fetus

Absolute indications
Known placenta praevia of a major degree
Severe cephalo-pelvic disproportion, where the fetal head remains high in the maternal pelvis or where crushing the base of the fetal skull would be necessary to achieve delivery
Previous classical Caesarean section
Two (or more) previous Caesarean sections
Incipient uterine rupture—most commonly in the presence of a neglected obstructed labour
In the presence of uterine rupture

Relative indications
In the presence of one previous Caesarean section. Other factors need consideration such as degrees of disproportion and the extent of fetal maceration
With a transverse lie or shoulder presentation near term, in advanced labour with ruptured membranes. The alternative is decapitation, but this is rarely used in modern obstetric practice
Where there is a fetal tumour or abdominal distension which would otherwise require evisceration—operator experience is relevant

While Caesarean section will often be in the best interests of the mother, there are occasions when destructive procedures can be used to expedite delivery. Perhaps the most common procedure is craniotomy, as eruditely described by Lawson (1982) and Myerscough (1982). Here, a Simpson's perforator can be used to inflict a cruciate incision in the cranium, after which the intracranial contents are disrupted. Traction on the cranial bones with the aid of multiple clamps is associated with expulsion of the contents and a reduction in the diameter of the presenting part. Both authors warn against crushing of the cranium and especially against crushing of the base of the skull, as they frequently cause maternal trauma. Craniotomy is contraindicated when the obstructed head remains high in the pelvis as a result of inlet contracture, but may be performed in the case of face presentation when an approach is made through the palate or the orbit. It may also be effective in reducing the size of the aftercoming head in breech presentation by subcutaneous tunnelling along the posterior fetal neck and perforation of the occiput. Kampf et al (1979) described the use of a trocar and cannula designed for intercostal thoracic drainage (Argyle No 28) for perforation of the fetal cranium and suction evacuation of its contents.

When the lie is transverse and the membranes are intact, version under deep general anaesthesia is preferred. With an impacted transverse lie or shoulder presentation and the liquor drained away, uterine rupture is a grave risk if version is attempted. Decapitation or delivery by Caesarean section are therefore the alternatives and the experience of the operator may well be the deciding factor in modern obstetrics. Again, Lawson (1982) and Myers-cough (1982) described the technique of decapitation using the Blond-Heidler saw for those who are interested.

A further destructive procedure of use is that of cleidotomy, where one or both clavicles are divided by the use of heavy straight scissors to achieve delivery in the presence of shoulder dystocia. Identification of the ventral from the dorsal aspect of the fetus is important to prevent the spines of the scapulae from being divided in error.

INVESTIGATION INTO THE CAUSE OF FETAL DEATH

Attempts should be made to establish the cause of death of the fetus, with a view to prevention or treatment in a subsequent pregnancy. Information from the mother, the fetus and the placenta should be considered simultaneously. It is surprising how little attention has been paid in the past to placental pathology when attempts to categorise the cause of death are made. Rayburn et al (1985) highlighted this where they found that histological placental examination was the sole contributor in explaining the cause of death in 11% of cases when 89 stillborn placentae were examined.

We cannot stress too strongly that the responsibility for documentation of events surrounding an intra-uterine death, and co-ordination of the investigations which should follow, rests solely with the obstetrician under whose care the baby is delivered. A protocol designed to fulfil the requirements and the resources of any particular hospital will assist in this matter and prevent the omission of important investigations on the assumption that 'somebody else will do it'. In the development of a protocol, the guidelines given below may be useful.

Photographic documentation

This may be of great value when immediate consultation regarding dysmorphism is not available, but should only supplement a detailed description of any abnormalities present.

Radiology

It has been advocated that radiographs be taken in any case of stillbirth (Mueller et al 1983, Zlatnik 1986) and we would agree. They are obviously mandatory in the presence of external malformation or dwarfism.

Cytogenetics

We agree with the indications suggested by Mueller et al (1983) for the attempted karyotyping of the stillborn infant. These are shown in Table 13.4. Bauld et al (1974) found a 10.2% chromosomal abnormality rate in

Table 13.4   Indications for attempted karyotyping of the stillborn infant (adapted from Mueller et al 1983)

Indications
Where obvious fetal anomalies are present
In the presence of intra-uterine growth retardation without other obvious cause
Where there is a family history of abnormal children or an obstetric history of recurrent pregnancy losses
In the presence of non-immunological hydrops fetalis
Where the Potter phenotype is apparent

their Edinburgh study of 61 perinatal deaths with severe congenital malformations. When 29 primary CNS abnormalities were excluded, the incidence rose to 18.8%. Blood may be used for lymphocyte culture where the fetus has been dead for less than 8 hours, but fibroblast culture using a variety of tissues is more likely to be successful. Skin, gonad and retina have all been used and should be forwarded to the laboratory in a sterile container without additives. The fetus which has been dead in utero for up to 48 hours, or delivered and refrigerated at 4°C for longer periods of time, may yield useful specimens. Machin (1974) described the successful culture of placental amnion from macerated stillbirths in some cases.

Autopsy examination

This is of vital importance in determining the presence or absence of congenital malformations, in establishing the actual cause of death where possible, and in evaluating the extent of intra-uterine stress which has preceded the fetal death. Evidence of chronic stress may manifest itself by growth retardation and thymic involution and act as a pointer to potentially recurrent obstetric events. Manchester & Shikes (1980) have produced an excellent review on the interpretation of perinatal autopsies which we recommend to interested readers.

When requesting permission for autopsy, the obstetrician should give the parents guidelines on what information may be expected from the examination. They should also be told what arrangements will be made to discuss the findings. The obstetrician also has responsibility to relay all the appropriate clinical information to the pathologist so that the autopsy can be 'tailored' to suit the circumstance.

Maternal investigations

Many maternal tests may be applicable to particular clinical situations and will not be discussed here. There are two tests, however, that should be considered after any intra-uterine death. These are the Kleihauer-Betke acid elution test for the detection of fetal red blood cells in the maternal circulation, and the measurement of lupus anticoagulant. Laube & Schauberger (1982) found 4 out of 29 (13.8%) otherwise unexplained stillbirths to have evidence of fetomaternal transfusion ranging in amount from 30 to 66% of the circulating fetal blood volume. Lubbe et al (1984) described the obstetric implications of lupus anticoagulant, a circulating immunoglobulin which may be present in patients both with and without systemic lupus erythematosus. These patients are prone to both early and late fetal loss, although suppression of this immunoglogulin with high-dose steroids may allow subsequent successful pregnancies.

PUERPERAL CARE AND BEREAVEMENT SUPPPORT

Stress to the parents can be reduced if medical and nursing staff are familiar with local regulations relating to the registration of a stillborn infant. All too often this familiarity is lacking and an opportunity to assist these patients in a simple and practical way is missed. Care should also be taken to ensure that the appropriate certificates are correctly completed, as rejection may occur when these are presented to a local government office. Forrest et al (1981) have outlined the registration procedures and options for disposal of the infant which are applicable in the UK. Again, familiarity with local options will be of immense benefit to the parents, and will serve as a platform upon which further bereavement counselling and support can be built.

It is beyond the scope of this chapter to consider bereavement counselling in depth. A review of this subject was recently published in the 'Progress' series (Giles 1985). In addition, Kirkley-Best & Kellner (1981) have constructed a useful annotated bibliography to acquaint obstetricians with the literature pertaining to grief at stillbirth. There are, however, some aspects of bereavement management that can only benefit from highlighting, and can be summarised in the sentiments of Bourne (1977) who stated: 'The danger lies not in the grief and distress [that follows stillbirth], the danger is in bypassing it'. One should appreciate that the grief response following stillbirth is severe and similar to that following the loss of an adult family member (Kellner et al 1984). A stage of shock and disbelief upon learning of the death is typically followed by yearning for the lost infant, personal disorientation, then slow reorganisation of lifestyle as resolution of grief proceeds. This process may take a considerable time, although the majority of patients will have resolved their grief within 12 months (Furlong & Hobbins 1983). Acceptance of the infant as a real person facilitates the inevitable grief process. To this end, the obstetrician should, as much as possible, attempt to manage the labour and delivery like normal. Seeing, holding and naming the baby may be beneficial for many parents, although it should not become a new rigid orthodoxy. The importance of photographs and other momentos are recognised as important in this process (Kellner et al 1981, Beckey et al 1985). A requirement for privacy should be respected, both at the time of delivery and in subsequent management on the ward. However, not all patients will wish to return to a non-obstetric ward and should be offered choice where possible; some may prefer a return to where the staff are familiar, as they will after all be exposed to other peoples' babies in everyday life a short time later. Above all else, the mother should not feel ostracised, regular visits by the medical and nursing staff being particularly important in this respect. Answers to questions and grievances should be honest and comprehensive, although explanations may need to be repeated several times.

After delivery, lactation suppression should be considered, and we have found bromocriptine effective for this purpose. Before leaving the hospital, contraception should also be discussed. Additionally, the obstetrician should ensure that parents have access to continuing supportive care either by direct contact with the obstetric team or through the general practitioner. Local self-help organisations are usually available and their value is illustrated by one medical practitioner's personal account of experience with stillbirth (Oglethorpe 1983). A scheduled 6-week appointment is a convenient time to review results and assess the parents' ability to cope with their tragedy. Plans for future pregnancies are often discussed at this visit, although parents should be dissuaded from embarking upon another pregnancy until grieving for the lost infant has waned.

The obstetrician need not assume the role of psychiatrist in the management of these patients, but should be sufficiently familiar with the grief reaction to recognise its aberrations. Some patients will then derive immense benefit from collaboration and consultation with others in the field of bereavement support.

REFERENCES

Antsaklis A, Diakomanolis E, Karayannopoulos C, Aravantinos D, Kaskarelis D 1979 Induction of abortion by intra-amniotic administration of prostaglandin $F2_{2\alpha}$ in patients with intrauterine fetal death and missed abortion. International Surgery 64: 41–43
Antsaklis A, Politis J, Diacomanolis E, Aravantinos D, Kaskarelis D 1984 The use of 15-methylated derivative of prostaglandin $F_{2\alpha}$ for the therapeutic termination of pregnancy and management of late fetal death. International Surgery 69: 63–68

Bailey C D H, Newman C, Ellinas S P, Anderson G G 1975 Use of prostaglandin E₂ vaginal suppositories in intrauterine fetal death and missed abortion. Obstetrics and Gynecology 45: 110–113

Bauld R, Sutherland G R, Bain A D 1974 Chromosome studies in investigation of stillbirths and neonatal deaths. Archives of Disease in Childhood 49: 782–788

Beckey R D, Price R A, Orkerson M, Walker Riley K 1985 Development of a perinatal grief checklist. Journal of Obstetric, Gynecologic and Neonatal Nursing (Philadelphia) 14(3): 194–199

Bourne S 1977 Stillbirth, grief and medical education. British Medical Journal 1: 1157

Cameron J M, Dayan A D 1966 Association of brain damage with therapeutic abortion induced by amniotic-fluid replacement; report of two cases. British Medical Journal 1: 1010–1013

Cohn F L, Goldenberg R L 1976 Term pregnancy in an unattached uterine horn. Obstetrics and Gynecology 48: 234–236

Csapo I A 1966 The termination of pregnancy by the intra-amniotic injection of hypertonic saline. In: Greenhill J P (ed) Year book of obstetrics and gynecology (1966–1967 Year Book Series), Year Book Medical, Chicago, p 126–163

Eggers T R, Fliegner J R 1979 Water intoxication and syntocinon infusion. Australian and New Zealand Journal of Obstetrics and Gynaecology 19: 59–60

Embrey M P, Calder A A, Hillier K 1974 Extra-amniotic prostaglandins in the management of intrauterine death, anencephaly and hydatidiform mole. Journal of Obstetrics and Gynaecology of the British Commonwealth 81: 47–51

Forrest G C, Claridge R S, Baum J D 1981 Practical management of perinatal death. British Medical Journal 282: 31–32

Furlong R M, Hobbins J C 1983 Grief in the perinatal period. Obstetrics and Gynecology 61: 497–500

Giles P F H 1985 The psychological response to stillbirth and neonatal death. In: Studd J (ed) Progress in obstetrics and gynaecology, vol 5, Churchill Livingstone, Edinburgh, pp 134–145

Goldstein D P, Reid D E 1963 Circulating fibrinolytic activity—a precursor of hypofibrinogenaemia following fetal death in utero. Obstetrics and Gynecology 22: 174–180

Golgoi M P 1971 Maternal mortality from Caesarean Section in infected cases. Journal of Obstetrics and Gynaecology of the British Empire 78: 373–376

Goplerud C P, White C A 1968 Delivering the dead fetus. Postgraduate Medicine 43(4): 167–171

Greenhalf J O, Diggory P L C 1971 Induction of therapeutic abortion by intra-amniotic injection of urea. British Medical Journal 1: 28–29

Gruber W S, Baumgarten K 1980 Intravenous prostaglandin E₂ and 16-phenoxy prostaglandin E₂ methyl sulfonylamide for induction of fetal death in utero. American Journal of Obstetrics and Gynecology 137: 8–14

Hainline S W, Nagey D A 1982 Prospective obstetric management of a twin pregnancy complicated by death of one twin. North Carolina Medical Journal 43: 708–709

Holland E 1951 The Princess Charlotte of Wales: a triple obstetric tragedy. Journal of Obstetrics and Gynaecology of the British Empire 58: 905–919

Jiminez J M, Pritchard J A 1968 Pathogenesis and treatment of coagulation defects resulting from fetal death. Obstetrics and Gynecology 32: 449–459

Kampf D, Jaschevatzsky O E, Georhiou P, Andermon S, Grunstein S 1979 A technique for management of obstructed labour with fetal death. Australian and New Zealand Journal of Obstetrics and Gynaecology 19: 32–35

Karim S M M, Ratnam S S, Hatabarat H et al 1982 Termination of pregnancy in cases of intrauterine fetal death, missed abortion, molar and anencephalic pregnancy with intramuscular administration of 2a 2b dihomo 15(S) 15 methyl PGF₂α methyl ester—a multicentre study. Annals of the Academy of Medicine 11: 508–512

Kellner K R, Kirkley-Best E, Chesborough S, Donnelly W H, Green M 1981 Perinatal mortality counselling program for families who experience a stillbirth. Death Education 5: 29–35

Kellner K R, Donnelly W H, Gould S D 1984 Parental behavior after perinatal death: lack of predictive demographic and obstetric variables. Obstetrics and Gynecology 63: 809–814

Kent D R, Goldstein A I 1976 Prostaglandin E₂ induction of labour for fetal demise. Obstetrics and Gynecology 48: 475–478

Kent D R, Goldstein A I, Linzey E M 1984 Safety and efficacy of vaginal prostaglandin E₂ suppositories in the management of third trimester fetal demise. Journal of Reproductive Medicine 29: 101–102

Kirkley-Best E, Kellner K R 1981 Grief at stillbirth: an annotated bibliography. Birth and the Family Journal 8: 91–99

Laube D W, Schauberger C W 1982 Fetomaternal bleeding as a cause for 'unexplained' fetal death. Obstetrics and Gynecology 60: 649–651

Lauersen N H, Cederqvist L L, Wilson K H 1980 Management of intra-uterine death with prostaglandin E₂ vaginal suppositories. American Journal of Obstetrics and Gynecology 137: 753–757

Lawson J 1982 Delivery of the dead or malformed fetus. Clinics in Obstetrics and Gynecology 9(3): 745–756

Lewis R V, Smith J W G, Speller D C E 1969 Penicillin prophylaxis during termination of pregnancy by intra-amniotic glucose. Journal of Obstetrics and Gynaecology of the British Commonwealth 76: 1008–1012

Liggins C C 1962 Treatment of missed abortion by high dosage Syntocinon intravenous infusion. Journal of Obstetrics and Gynaecology of the British Commonwealth 69: 277–281

Lubbe W F, Butler W S, Liggins G C 1984 The lupus-anticoagulant: clinical and obstetric implications. New Zealand Medical Journal 97: 398–402

MacDonald D, O'Driscoll M K, Geoghegan F J 1965 Intra-amniotic dextrose—a maternal death. Journal of Obstetrics and Gynaecology of the British Commonwealth 72: 452–455

Machin G A 1974 Chromosome abnormality and perinatal death. Lancet i: 549–551

McIntosh Marshall C 1939 Caesarean section—lower segment operation, John Wright, Bristol

Manchester D K, Shikes R H 1980 The perinatal autopsy: special considerations. Clinical Obstetrics and Gynecology 23(4): 1125–1134

Miller A W F, Calder A A, MacNaughton M C 1972 Termination of pregnancy by continuous intrauterine infusion of prostaglandins. Lancet ii: 5–7

Morgan D B, Kirwan K W, Hancock K W, Robinson D, Ahmad S 1977 Water intoxication and oxytocin infusion. British Journal of Obstetrics and Gynaecology 84: 6–12

Mueller R F, Sybert V P, Johnson J, Brown Z A, Chen W 1983 Evaluation of a protocol for post-mortem examination of stillbirths. New England Journal of Medicine 309: 586–590

Myerscough P R 1982 Munro Kerr's operative obstetrics, 10th edn, Baillière Tindall, London, pp 330–336

Oglethorpe R J L 1983 Stillbirth: a personal experience. British Medical Journal 287: 1197–1198

Orr J W, Huddleston J F, Goldenberg R L, Knox G E, Davis R O 1979 Association of extrauterine fetal death with failure of prostaglandin E₂ suppositories. Obstetrics and Gynecology (suppl) 53: 56S–58S

Pedlow P R B 1970 Syntocinon induced convulsions. Journal of Obstetrics and Gynaecology of the British Commonwealth 77: 1113–1114

Peel J 1962 Inducing labour by intra-amniotic injection. British Medical Journal 2: 1397–1398

Pfeffer R I 1966 Hypofibrinogenemia in the dead fetus syndrome treated with aminocaproic acid. American Journal of Obstetrics and Gynecology 95: 1095–1098

Phelan J P, Cepalo R C 1978 A better approach to fetal demise—PGE₂ suppository. Contemporary Obstetrics and Gynecology 11: 93–95

Phelan J P, Meguiar R V, Matey D, Newman C 1978 Dramatic pyrexia and cardiovascular response to intravaginal prostaglandin E₂. American Journal of Obstetrics and Gynecology 132: 28–32

Pritchard J A 1959 Fetal death in utero. Obstetrics and Gynecology 14: 573–580

Pritchard J A 1973 Haematological problems associated with delivery, placental abruption, retained dead fetus, and amniotic fluid embolism. Clinics in Haematology, 2(3): 563–586

Pritchard J A, Ratnoff O D 1955 Studies of fibrinogen and other haemostatic factors in women with intrauterine death and delayed delivery. Surgery, Gynecology and Obstetrics 101: 467–477

Pritchard J A, MacDonald P C, Gant N F 1985 Williams' obstetrics, 17th edn, Appleton-Century-Crofts, New York, pp 412–415

Ramsbotham F H 1844 The principles and practice of obstetric medicine and surgery in reference to the process of parturition, 2nd edn, Churchill, London

Rayburn W, Sander C, Barr M, Rygiel R 1985 The stillborn fetus: placental histologic examination in determining a cause. Obstetrics and Gynecology 65: 637–641

Reid D E, Weiner A E, Roby C C, Diamond L K 1953 Maternal afibrinogenaemia associated with long standing intrauterine fetal death. American Journal of Obstetrics and Gynecology 66: 500–506

Romero R, Copel J A, Hobbins J C 1985 Intrauterine fetal demise and hemostatic failure: the fetal death syndrome. In: Pitkin R M, Scott J R, Weiner C P (eds) Clinical Obstetrics and Gynecology, vol 28, no 1, Harper and Row, Hagerstown, pp 24–31

Rozenman D, Kessler I, Lancet M 1980 Third trimester induction of labour with fetal death in utero. Surgery, Obstetrics and Gynecology 151: 497–499

Russell J G B 1973 Radiology in obstetric and antenatal paediatrics, Butterworth, London, pp 119–136

Saarikoski S, Selander K, Pystynen P 1980 Induction of labour with Sulprostone after foetal death and in hydatidiform mole. Prostaglandins 20: 481–485

Scheer K, Nubar J C 1977 Rapid conclusive diagnosis of intra-uterine fetal death. American Journal of Obstetrics and Gynecology 128: 907–908

Scher J, Jeng D, Moshipur J, Kerenyi T D 1980 A comparison between vaginal prostaglandin E_2 suppositories and intrauterine extra-amniotic prostaglandins in the management of fetal death in utero. American Journal of Obstetrics and Gynecology 137: 769–772

Schulman H, Saldana L, Lin C C, Randolph G 1979 Mechanism of failed labour after fetal death and its management with prostaglandin E_2. American Journal of Obstetrics and Gynecology 133: 742–748

Schwartz M L, Brenner W E 1980 Termination of pregnancy complicated by anencephaly with intra-amniotic prostaglandin $F_{2\alpha}$. American Journal of Obstetrics and Gynecology 136: 203–204

Skelly H, Marivate M, Norman R, Kenoyer G, Martin R 1982 Consumptive coagulopathy following fetal death in a triplet pregnancy. American Journal of Obstetrics and Gynecology 142: 595–596

Southern E M, Gutknecht G D, Mohberg N R, Edelman D A 1978 Vaginal prostaglandin E_2 in the management of fetal intrauterine death. British Journal of Obstetrics and Gynaecology 85: 437–441

Toppozada M K 1986 Prostaglandin in mid-trimester abortion. Prostaglandin Perspectives 2: 1–3

Townsend L, Shelton J G 1964 Intra-uterine death due to foetal crythroblastosis. Australian and New Zealand Journal of Obstetrics and Gynaecology 4: 85–89

Ursell W 1972 Induction of labour following fetal death. Journal of Obstetrics and Gynaecology of the British Commonwealth 79: 260–264

Wagatsuma T 1965 Intra-amniotic injection of saline for therapeutic abortion. American Journal of Obstetrics and Gynecology 93: 743–745

Weiner A E, Reid D E, Roby C C, Diamond L K 1950 Coagulation defects with intrauterine death from Rh isosensitization. American Journal of Obstetrics and Gynecology 60: 1015–1021

Whalley P J, Pritchard J A 1963 Oxytocin and water intoxication. Journal of the American Medical Association 186: 601–603

Zlatnik F J 1986 Management of fetal death. In: Pitkin R M, Scott J R, Cruickshank D P (eds) Clinical Obstetrics and Gynecology, vol 29, no 2, Harper and Row, Hagerstown, pp 220–229

The sex ratio, and ways of manipulating it

One of the first things most people want to know about a new born baby is its sex.

The primary sex ratio—the ratio of boys to girls at birth—is similar throughout the world at about 1.06 boys to 1.0 girls. It is often quoted as the number of males born divided by the number of females, with the quotient sometimes multiplied by 1000 to give a more manageable number. The alternative term of 'masculinity' is rarely used nowadays. The size of the ratio (which humans share with many other animal species) is not constant, and there have been many reports of pronounced variations, particularly in relatively small areas and often over relatively short times (Lyster 1970, Walby et al 1981a, b). Some variations, such as those reported from Third World countries, rarely occur when statistics are collected carefully (Rehan 1982).

The sex ratio is not constant. It approaches unity in the early reproductive years, and from then the higher mortality rates that males have had from conception leads to an excess of females. The primary determinant of sex is the chromosome complement of the fertilizing spermatozoon, and there is no reason to suspect that the ratio between X- and Y-carrying spermatozoa is other than unity. Tricomi et al in 1960, using sex chromatin typing of early human embryos collected following spontaneous abortions, showed that male embryos were aborted preferentially, with only 93 out of 242 specimens being female. This work was continued by looking at embryos collected following early surgical termination of pregnancy; Serr and Ismajovich (1963) found that of 125 fetuses 78 were male, giving a male:female ratio of 165.9:100 between the fifth and eighth week (menstrual age) of pregnancy.

Male sexual differentiation is associated with the presence of the male specific antigen (H-Y), the presence of which directs the gonads to form testes. There are reports of animal and human males without it. Male mice without the H-Y antigen have spermatogenic failure (Burgoyne et al 1986). Inseminating mice with semen that has been treated with H-Y antiserum does not seem to affect the sex ratio of the progeny (Bennett and Boyse 1973). In animals, but not humans, the banded krait minor satellite DNA sequences are associated with male sexual differentiation (Kiel-Metzger et al 1985).

There are many factors that may influence the sex ratio at birth. Some mammals manipulate sex ratio when the environment changes (Austad & Sunquist 1986); there is no evidence that humans share this ability. Other factors include race, other genetic factors (but this factor is less important when data are carefully collected), socioeconomic status, the season of the year [in England and Wales relatively more females are born in late autumn and winter (Macfarlane & Mugford 1984), although this does not seem to be the case for Hungary (Czeizel 1980)], ABO and Rh blood groups of mother and child, the sex of siblings and the pH of male blood serum (McWhirter, 1956). There is no theory that unifies all observations, but much literature includes reports on environmental toxins decreasing the proportion of boys born, and changes in dietary minerals, especially calcium and magnesium, affecting the sex ratio.

More boys than girls are born as fathers age; this is well recognized. Szilard (1960) suggested that this was the result of ageing on the testes, particularly random chromosomal damage leading to death of those cells without an X-chromosome, but survival of those losing only a Y-chromosome. This leads to a relative deficit of Y-chromosome containing spermatozoal stem cells. Szilard predicted that there should be a 2% reduction in the numbers of boys born for every 12-year increment in paternal age. This seems to be the case in the USA. There is also a decrease in the probability of the birth of male children as birth order increases; this too is a small effect. There is a marked increase in the proportion of sons born to women over the age of 45 (Hytten 1982).

In most societies there is an increase in the proportion of sons born during and shortly after war. This has been attributed to some inbuilt urge to repopulate, although it would seem more sensible to increase the proportion of females. James (1986b) suggested that the altered sex ratio was due to the increased frequency of intercourse that soldiers who have limited time away from military duties, or who are returning home after service away, have. This in turn leads to a greater probability of conception in the earlier part of the cycle, which may make male births more likely. This is discussed later. This phenomenon may also explain the relatively higher proportion of boys born amongst babies conceived in the first few weeeks of marriage in those couples who were not living together before they were married.

In 1967, Kirby et al suggested that if there were more male than female embryos present in early pregnancy, then either fertilization produced more male than female embryos, or female embryos implanted less successfully than male ones. Since most laboratories report no difference in the numbers of male and female embryos formed following either in vivo or in vitro fertilization, it would seem that the failure of implantation theory is the more likely. There is a rich literature on the immunological events surrounding implantation, e.g. zygotes antigenically dissimilar from the mother have been said to be favoured at implantation, and male embryos differ in the Y-linked antigens they carry, so Kirby et al felt that male embryos should be slightly favoured. This is true in inbred populations, where the relative difference imported by the Y-linked antigens is more noticeable. In consanguineous marriages, and some inbred animal species, more males than females are born. Immunological dissimilarity may also explain the higher sex ratio (55.7% male) of infants of mothers with the AB blood group compared with those from all other blood groups combined (51.9% male). Infants of blood group O are more likely to be male.

THE SEX RATIO IN DISEASE

Alterations in the sex ratio sometimes follow illness in a parent. This may be due to a reduction in births of one sex (usually male, because male embryos are more vulnerable throughout pregnancy), or it may reflect a real alteration in the type of spermatozoa or embryo formed, or there may be no obvious cause. Among the diseases studied are multiple sclerosis (excess of sons born to women with the disease, Alperovitch & Feingold 1981), non-Hodgkin's lymphoma (excess of daughters born to parents with the disease, Olsson & Brandt 1982), infectious hepatitis (female births increase, Robertson & Sheard 1973), schizophrenia (excess of daughters, Lane 1969), maternal smoking (excess of daughters, Fraumeni & Lundin 1964), excessive maternal alcohol consumption (excess of females born with the fetal alcohol syndrome, Qazi & Masakawa 1976) and even pregnancies occurring after treatment of endometriosis (excess of males, Barbieri et al 1982). Perhaps linked with this is the observation that female fetuses are more likely to produce severe hyperemesis in the mother than male fetuses (Pickard et al 1982). There is no factor explaining or linking these observations except that most have a female birth relative excess.

When environmental pollution leads to an increase in the proportion of female births, this seems to be mediated by a reduction in the number of boys born, whilst the numbers of girls born remains constant. This suggests that if a toxic factor is involved in a disease process, it acts on the sex ratio by depressing male rather than female births.

James (1986a) suggested that the reason for the differing anatomical levels of neural tube defects in male and female infants was because of the effect of an environmental teratogen acting at the same maternal time in pregnancy, affecting fetuses that had been conceived at differing stages in the menstrual cycle. He hypothesised that if male infants were preferentially conceived in the early part of the cycle, they would be developmentally more advanced at a point where an external teratogen produced failure to close the neural tube.

Some authors have reported an apparent excess of female births after the use of clomiphene. This may relate to maternal gonadotrophin levels (for a review of which see James 1986b), or may relate to an effect of clomiphene on cervical mucus. Rohde et al (1973) suggested that Y-bearing spermatozoa were the first to enter cervical mucus, but they studied mucus from healthy ovulating women, none of whom were undergoing induction of ovulation. The equivalent experiment using mucus from women taking clomiphene has not been performed. Not all authors (e.g. Cholst et al 1981) agree that there is a link between induction of ovulation and alterations in the sex ratio.

THE SEX RATIO FOLLOWING ENVIRONMENTAL STRESS

Environmental stresses can sometimes alter the sex ratio in a predictable direction. Among the most detailed studies have been those of Lyster, who has documented sex ratio in several parts of Australia following changes, presumably of mineral content, in the water supply (Lyster 1970, 1974, 1977b) and following environmental pollution (Lyster 1974, 1977a). In those parts of Australia dependent on rainfall for part of their drinking water, especially those areas that depend on dams fed by rainfall, there are marked changes in sex ratio following heavy storms. The most interesting feature is that the alteration in water supply precedes a reduction in male births by 320 days. Stormy weather may stir up sediments in river and dam beds, so changing the mineral content (particularly magnesium and calcium levels) and hardness of water; this remains uproven, but it is of interest that Stolkowski and Lorrain (1980) claim to be able to manipulate the sex ratio by altering the diet, particularly its mineral composition. The Japanese Sex Selection Society (whose members have a monopoly over the use of these preparations) use drugs rich in calcium, and this is believed by them to ensure the birth of a boy (Kasai et al 1982).

Other environmental pollutants include arsenic (excess of male births, Lyster 1977b), general industrial pollution near an iron and steel complex (excess of females, Lyster 1977a), and the London smog of 1952 (excess of females, Lyster 1974). Much of the data from these studies relate to small numbers of births collected over relatively short periods of time, and sometimes from an incomplete data-base (e.g. in the study of births after the London smog one hospital refused access to its records, while the delivery records for several others could not be located).

Other stresses that have been reported to alter the sex ratio include the effect on men of flying high-performance military aircraft (excess of daughters born, Snyder 1961), commercial underwater diving for abalone (excess of females, Lyster 1982), and giving anaesthetics (excess of females fathered by male anaesthetists, Wyatt & Murray Wilson 1973). The latter effect may be related to anaesthetic agents (Fink et al 1967).

These variations have been the subject of much speculation by those searching for the philosopher's stone that will let sex selection become a practical possibility. No coherent pattern has emerged, although many studies seem to suggest that those stresses that increase the relative proportion of female births do so by decreasing the expected number of male births, and thus reducing the number of babies born. If male fetuses are more vulnerable throughout pregnancy, then perhaps those stresses produce their effect by decreasing the implantation rate of male embryos, or increasing their spontaneous abortion rate. It would also seem that such methods are potentially unsafe.

REASONS FOR SELECTING THE SEX OF A CHILD

Throughout recorded history couples have wanted to predict, or select, the sex of their children. This is particularly so for their first-born, whom most couples want to be a boy. This is usually for social reasons, often linked with inheritance, but in agrarian societies male infants are prized for their usefulness on the farm, and in others because they bring wealth to the family when they marry. In some parts of the world girls are expected to transfer their duty of care of the aged from their parents to their parents-in-law on marriage, so an elderly couple with only daughters and no social security system is disadvantaged. Girls are usually wanted only when families already have one or more boys, or when a sex-linked genetic disorder is present.

At a simple level sex selection is already widely practised, even in the West; more couples stop having children after a boy than after a girl.

THE EFFECT OF SEX-SELECTION PROCEDURES ON POPULATION GROWTH

Many demographers feel the world, and particularly the Third World, is overpopulated. If reliable, safe and simple sex-selection procedures were available, population growth will be slowed if couples could have a child of each sex. Since most couples seem to want more boys than girls, and want to start families with a boy, this will lead to a reduction in the breeding pool of women. This has been reviewed by Clark (1985), Markle & Nam (1982) and Rinehart (1975).

HISTORICAL BACKGROUND

Before the arrival of accurate antenatal diagnosis, attempts at sex selection were the only method of preventing sex-linked diseases. There is a long history to this: the Talmudic writings from the second century state that a boy whose two older brothers had died of bleeding following circumcision could not be circumcised, and the same was true if two of his mother's sisters had had male children die in similar circumstances (Rosner 1984). An Old Testament quote that may refer to sex selection is discussed later.

POTENTIAL METHODS OF ANTENATAL SEX-SELECTION

In theory, there have always been five possible approaches to selection of the sex of children: selective abortion or infanticide, timing of insemination or intercourse, manipulation of semen to select either the X- or the Y-bearing spermatozoa, the use of vaginal chemicals, condoms or diaphragms that destroy or incapacitate either X- or Y-bearing spermatozoa, or the immunization of women against Y-bearing spermatozoa (immunization against the X-chromosome would not be feasible).

In some societies abortion or infanticide is used to ensure a child of the wanted sex. Several thousand such abortions have been reported (Lancet 1983), which also describe the use of advertising hoardings in Amritsar identifying clinics where antenatal sex selection procedures are carried out. Of 7800 requests for amniocentesis in one large Bombay hospital, 94% were from couples wanting to avoid the birth of a daughter. Kumar (1985) reports that in China an estimated 250 000 baby girls were killed between 1979 and 1984. Clark (1985) reports that in some parts of China the male:female ratio of young children is 5:1, with selective abortion and infanticide of girls accounting for the bulk of the change. Feil et al (1984) studied college students, and found that more men than women approved of abortion for sex selection.

FOLKLORE METHODS OF SEX PRESELECTION

References to sex preselection are as old as the oldest medical writings. A Chinese manuscript of 4400 years ago discusses the subject, and an Egyptian papyrus of 2200 BC observed that a pregnant woman with a face of a greenish cast was certain to bear a son (Gordon 1958). Both Aristotle and the Talmud said that placing the marital bed in a north–south direction increased the likelihood of a son.

Leviticus 12:2 has been interpreted, by those who have read the original Hebrew rather than the King James version (translated from the Greek that was derived from the Hebrew), to imply that for women who 'emitted semen' first the resulting child would be male (Rosner 1979). This emission of semen has been interpreted as meaning either that the women reached orgasm before her partner, or that intercourse occurred after ovulation.

Mittwoch (1985) gives a detailed account of erroneous theories of sex determination, and her review is well worth reading. Anaxagoras (?500–425 BC) was the first of many to 'think right'; he felt that if couples had intercourse with the man lying on his right side, and if women lay on their right side afterwards, then fertilization would occur following fusion of humours from the right testis and the right side of the woman, and such an infant would undoubtedly be male. He was also the first to suggest that tying off the left testicle would ensure male children. This belief persisted well into the eighteenth century, when French noblemen were persuaded to submit to hemi-castration to produce male heirs (Glass 1977). Aristotle pointed out that men with only one testis could father children of either sex, but this did not interfere with the acceptability of the theory. Aristotle believed that it was the mother's imagination that influenced the sex of the child. One underlying feature of all of these theories is the constancy of the right side in producing males; the right side of the body was considered superior, as were males. This was expanded into beliefs such as making sure that the right foot was the first to touch the floor on leaving bed. An Alexandrian manuscript of the first century AD states that if a bull dismounts a cow from the right side, the calf will be male, whilst if it dismounts from the left the calf will be female.

DIFFERENCES IN THE TIMING OF INTERCOURSE

Empedocles was the first philosopher to link the timing of intercourse with the subsequent sex of the infant. Unfortunately, he believed that ovulation occurred during menstruation. Aristotle disagreed with him, pointing out that his theory could not explain twins of different sex. Many others since have studied the relationship between the timing of intercourse and the sex of subsequent offspring. This has been done utilising three groups of women: those who practise *niddah*—the ritual of sexual abstinence for the duration of menstruation and the next 7 days, those who have conceived following failures of the periodic abstinence method of contraception, and those who have been attending infertility clinics and have either conceived following artificial insemination or induction of ovulation. None of these three groups is necessarily representative of the rest of the population.

The evidence is that intercourse close to ovulation leads to a preponderance of female births, but Shettles suggests that the reverse is the case. Women who conceive following artificial insemination have infants with a sex ratio that mirrors those who conceive following intercourse.

Susan Harlap (1979) studied a population of 3658 infants born in Jerusalem. Jewish women were asked if they practised niddah. If they did, she predicted the closeness of the conception to ovulation using menstrual calendar data. Male infants comprised 53.3% of births conceived 2 days before presumed ovulation, 49.3% of those on the day of presumed ovulation, and 65.5% of those conceived 2 days after presumed ovulation. These data contradict much of our current knowledge about the longevity and fertilizing ability of oocytes, but do fit with other studies. Shettles (1976) says that among the Jewish population of tsarist Russia, the sex ratio was at least 150 boys to 100 girls at birth.

Other studies include those of Guerrero (1974, 1975). He studied women who conceived following failures of the rhythm method of contraception, and those who had been attending infertility clinics, the majority of whom had had artificial insemination. For women who conceived after intercourse there was a U-shaped distribution of the sex ratio, with the highest proportion of boys born when single acts of intercourse had occurred well before, or well after, the day of the temperature rise. There were naturally very few births in the right-hand arm of the U; the time after the temperature has risen has been shown by many to be a time of relative infertility.

Perhaps the most surprising feature of Guerrero's data was that sex ratios following insemination were a mirror-image of those following intercourse; male infants were much more likely following insemination on the day of the temperature shift, and less likely on the days before and after the shift. There is no explanation for this unless his argument is accepted—that there is a difference between insemination into the cervix and intercourse mediated by the differing pH of the two environments.

David et al (1980), in a well-controlled study looking at the results of single inseminations in 1188 women, failed to detect any differences in sex ratio. Another point against there being a significant effect mediated through timed insemination is the fact that most cattle in the West are conceived following timed insemination and artificial induction of ovulation; an effect on sex ratios would be of enormous commercial benefit, and has not yet been reported.

Mortimer and Richardson (1982) reported that artificial insemination, especially with cryopreserved semen, reduced the proportion of boys born, particularly when frozen semen was used. Mason and Smith (1985), reporting 3000 pregnancies fathered with donor semen, reported no differences in the sex ratio between infants born after the use of fresh or frozen semen, but did find that the combination of ovulation induction and artificial insemination increased the proportion of female births. Sampson et al (1983) reported similar results from a smaller group.

Revelle (1974), reviewing Guerrero's data, pointed out that a couple could double their chances of conceiving a male by restricting intercourse to the early part of the cycle, and abstaining for about 4 or 5 days before the rise in body temperature that indicates ovulation, although unfortunately they might have to wait 5 years or more for a live birth. Perez et al (1985) reported that the rhythm method could be utilized to increase the proportion of boys born to 0.58; France et al (1984), timing ovulation accurately by using a rapid assay for luteinizing hormone in early morning urine, were unable to alter the sex ratio significantly. Shiono et al (1982) reported that pregnancies resulting from failure of the rhythm method of family planning were more likely to produce males, but again the change (56.7% male) was small.

James (1986b) has explained these observations by hypothesising that there is a hormonal control of the sex ratio. Testosterone and oestradiol may have some importance, but the major hormonal control is mediated through gonadotrophins. He points out that in induction of ovulation, when the levels of gonadotrophins are artificially raised, the sex ratio is lowered, and the probability of this being a chance effect is <0.000001. When artificial insemination is coupled with the use of clomiphene, there is a similar reduction in the sex ratio. Twin pregnancies, which are often associated with raised levels of gonadotrophins, are also commonly associated with a decrease in the sex ratio. He also points out that since levels of gonadotrophins are higher in the early part of the cycle, pregnancies are more likely to produce males if conceptions occur then, and this fits with the data of Guerrero (1974,

1975) and Harlap (1979) as well as with the observations mentioned earlier about the sex ratio in children of newly married couples and in war time (both of which are said to be associated with a higher coital frequency and thus a higher likelihood of conception in the earlier part of the cycle).

Shettles has propounded his own theory of sex preselection. His views on the relationship between the timing of intercourse and ovulation are the reverse of all those reported by other authors; this does not seem to affect his success rates, which are quoted as 86.7%, based on 'a little over 3000 letters and innumerable phone calls, domestic and foreign' (Shettles 1978). The method for preselecting sex has been summarised by Vear (1977) and Daniell (1983). Prospective trials (Williamson et al 1978, Simcock 1985, France et al 1984) have not been successful.

Selection of a female fetus

1. A douche of 15–20 ml white vinegar in 500 ml of cooled boiled water is used 10–15 minutes before coitus.
2. Frequent coitus is performed in the 7–10 days before ovulation.
3. The last coitus should be at least 24 hours, and preferably more, before ovulation is expected to occur, and abstinence should then be practised for at least a week.
4. Intercourse should be face-to-face, and the ejaculate should be deposited low in the vagina, preferably just inside the introitus.
5. Intercourse should cease with ejaculation.
6. Female orgasm should not occur.

Selection of a male fetus

1. A douche of 5 g of baking soda in 500 ml of cooled boiled water is used before intercourse.
2. Abstinence should be practised from the end of menstruation until after ovulation has occurred.
3. Vaginal penetration should be from the rear, so that ejaculation will occur high in the vaginal vault, and preferably against the cervix. The man should have deep penetration at the moment of ejaculation.
4. Intercourse should cease with ejaculation.
5. Female orgasm should occur just before ejaculation.
6. The procedure should be repeated two or three times in the next 24–48 hours.

Using these techniques Vear achieved a success rate of 10 correct predictions out of 10 pregnancies, but it took 7 years to obtain those 10 couples from a practice delivering between 100 and 120 births annually. The couples are all carefully counselled beforehand, and 'it should be impressed on both parties that the procedure is a scientific exercise and not an emotional or erotic skirmish, and the chance of success is only of the order of 85%' Vear (1977).

For most people timing of intercourse or insemination is not a suitable method for sex preselection. There are dangers: there may be links between fertilization of ageing gametes and Down's syndrome (German 1968, Mulcahy 1978).

SEPARATION OF X- AND Y-BEARING SPERMATOZOA

Most modern literature on sex preselection suggests trying to separate X- and Y-carrying spermatozoa, and then inseminating artificially the resulting preparation. Unfortunately, insemination and the use of clomiphene to either induce ovulation or regulate cycles may introduce its own bias; this was found in the study of Beernink and Ericsson (1982).

The selection of spermatozoa for fertilization either in vivo or in vitro to produce infants of the desired sex depends on the differences that are said to exist between X- and Y-bearing spermatozoa. There are many such differences postulated; none are reliable. There are few differences between the two different types of spermatozoa. Shettles (1960a, b, c) found some, but Van Duijn (1960) pointed out that the differences were artefacts, and he and others (Bishop 1960, Rothschild 1960) have pointed out that much of the relevant scientific data are missing from his publications.

There are theoretical reasons for doubting the presence of characteristics that may differentiate between haploid cells on the basis of their genetic components. Most people believe that haploid cells do not express their genes.

DIFFERENCES BETWEEN X- AND Y-CARRYING SPERMATOZOA

The biggest single drawback in the literature of this field is that it comprises many papers that have concentrated on separating X-bearing from Y-bearing spermatozoa and many papers that have tried such methods in small numbers of couples (often reporting as results those still pregnant). There is doubt about the accuracy of many tests for Y-bearing spermatozoa. Gledhill (1983) points out that 5.6% of spermatozoa seem to have two Y chromosomes, as judged by the use of mepacrine (quinacrine) fluorescence (Barlow & Vosa 1970), which, if the test is accurate, gives an unacceptably high rate of non-disjunction. In-situ hybridization may be a good, rapid, simple test (Burns et al 1985), but is not yet widely available.

Perhaps one difference between the two types of spermatozoa that may be relevant is that spermatozoa carrying an X chromosome have, on average, 3.5% more DNA than those carrying a Y chromosome. DNA is dense and comprises most of the mass of a spermatozoon, so there should be a small, but significant, difference in the average mass between the two types of spermatozoa; the difference in specific gravity is only at the third or fourth decimal place (Harvey 1946).

It is a truth universally acknowledged that Y-bearing spermatozoa swim faster than those possessing an X chromosome. Unfortunately, there are few data to substantiate this belief.

PRACTICAL METHODS FOR SEPARATING DIFFERENT TYPES OF SPERMATOZOA

Many methods of separating X- from Y-bearing spermatozoa have been suggested. Most only enrich the Y-bearing fraction, some will separate X- from Y-bearing spermatozoa, but none has yet been validated in a carefully controlled trial using relatively large numbers.

Albumin column layering and sedimentation, in which the progressively motile spermatozoa, of which the majority are said to be Y-bearing, swim into the albumin layer (Ericsson et al 1973, Dmowski et al 1979). This is perhaps the most widely used technique, and has now been licensed by Ericsson. The technique does not work for everybody: Ross et al (1975) pointed out that this technique decreased the number of spermatozoa to about 1–5% of the original sample, and they failed to observe an alteration in the proportion of spermatozoa carrying a Y-chromosome. Evans et al (1975) similarly failed to achieve a significant separation, and emphasised that staining for the Y-body was perhaps the most important aspect of the procedure.

Among the other methods reported have been:

> Counter streaming centrifugation (Lindahl 1958)
> Albumin gradient centrifugation (Shilling & Thromaehlen 1977)
> Ficoll-sodium metrizoate density gradient centrifugation (Shastry et al 1977, Hedge et al 1977)
> Sephadex gel filtration (Corson et al 1983, Steeno et al 1975)
> Millipore filtration (Adimoelja et al 1977, Broer et al 1978)
> Electrophoretic separation (Shishito et al 1975)
> Density gradient ultracentrifugation on a discontinuous sucrose gradient (Rohde et al 1975)
> Convection counter streaming galvanization (Bhattacharya et al 1977, Daniell et al 1982)
> Percoll density gradient centrifugation (Kaneko et al 1983)

Most of these methods have some promise for the future; none has yet been validated on a significant scale.

ETHICS AND SOCIAL IMPLICATIONS OF ANTENATAL SEX SELECTION

This has been discussed in more detail elsewhere (e.g. Clark 1985, Fletcher 1983, Kumar 1985). It has become customary to criticise many aspects of the application of new technology to medicine, and particularly to the control of human reproduction. Swinbanks (1986) demonstrates that one factor might be a rush for publicity. He describes the problems that occurred when Japanese researchers were being monitored by a broadcasting company; the journalists recognised a good story, and so arranged premature publication that almost led to the closure of a research programme.

There are not many people prepared to argue that selective abortion is beneficial, except perhaps in the overall framework of reducing excess births in an overcrowded world. Even many who believe that abortion is a 'woman's right to choose' find abortion for sex selection unpleasant.

Sex selection through separating spermatozoa is perhaps different, but like so many potential changes in medicine there has been no opportunity for controlled research. Clark (1986) makes the interesting point that if a method for sex selection becomes widely available then women of low income and low social status will not use it (principally because they cannot afford it), while women of high income and social status will. Since parental influence is one of the most important determinants of one's eventual place in society, such a technique will eventually increase the numbers of men in positions of power and influence.

Other writers (reviewed by Clark 1985) have pointed out that a society with an increase in the numbers of men (assuming that more people want males selected rather than females) will have an increase in rape, child molestation and violence against women and children. Much of this is based on the analysis of societies with a large imbalance of men, usually following mass immigration. These are usually frontier societies, such as the American West in the last century, and there is no reason to assume that they would be representative of any other society, particularly one that planned a sex imbalance.

There are no methods of sex preselection that are likely to make much difference in the forseeable future. Perhaps before such a method does become available, society, and the medical profession in particular, should debate their attitudes to it.

REFERENCES

Adimoelja A, Hariadi R, Amitaba I G B, Adisetya P, Soeharno 1977 The separation of X- and Y-spermatozoa with regard to the possible clinical application by means of artificial insemination. Andrologia 9: 289–292
Alperovitch A, Feingold N 1981 Sex ratio in offspring of patients with multiple sclerosis. New England Journal of Medicine 305: 1157
Austad S N, Sunquist M E 1986 Sex-ratio manipulation in the common opossum. Nature 324: 58–60
Barbieri R L, Evans S, Kistner R W 1982 Danazol in the treatment of endometriosis: analysis of 100 cases with a 4-year follow-up. Fertility and Sterility 37: 737–746
Barlow P, Vosa C G 1970 The Y chromosome in human spermatozoa. Nature 226: 961–962
Beernink F J, Ericsson R J 1982 Male sex preselection through sperm isolation. Fertility and Sterility 38: 493–495
Bennett D, Boyse E A 1973 Sex ratio in progeny of mice inseminated with sperm treated with H-Y antiserum. Nature 246: 308–309
Bhattacharya B C, Shome P, Gunther A H 1977 Successful separation of X and Y spermatozoa in human and bull semen. International Journal of Fertility 22: 30

Bishop D W 1960 X and Y spermatozoa. Nature 187: 255–256

Broer K H, Dauber U, Kaiser R, Schumacher G F B 1978 The failure to separate human X- and Y- spermatozoa by the millipore filtration technique. Journal of Reproductive Medicine 20: 67

Burgoyne P S, Levy E R, Mclaren A 1986 Spermatogenic failure in male mice lacking H-Y antigen. Nature 320: 170–172

Burns J, Chan V T W, Jonasson J A, Fleming K A, Taylor S, McGee J O'D 1985 Sensitive system for visualising biotinylated DNA probes hybridised in situ: rapid sex determination of intact cells. Journal of Clinical Pathology 38: 1085–1092

Cholst I, Jewelewicz R, Dyrenfurth I, Vande Wiele L 1981 Gonadotrophin and the human secondary sex ratio. British Medical Journal 283: 1264–1265

Clark L R 1985 Sex preselection: the advent of the made-to-order child. The Pharos 48: 2–7

Corson S L, Batzer F R, Schlaff S 1983 Preconceptual female gender selection. Fertility and Sterility 40: 384–385

Czeizel A 1980 Time of fertilisation and sex of infants. Lancet ii: 199

Daniell J F 1983 Sex-selection procedures. Journal of Reproductive Medicine 28: 235–237

Daniell J F, Herbert C M, Repp J, Torbit C A, Wentz A C 1982 Initial evaluation of a convection counter streaming galvanization technique of sex separation of human spermatozoa. Fertility and Sterility 38: 233–237

David G, Czyglik F, Mayaux M J, Martin-Boyce A, Schwartz D 1980 Artificial insemination with frozen sperm: protocol, method of analysis and results for 1188 women. British Journal of Obstetrics and Gynaecology 87: 1022–1028

Dmowski W P, Gaynor L, Rao R, Lawrence M, Scommegna A 1979 Use of albumin gradients for X and Y sperm separation and clinical experience with male sex preselection. Fertility and Sterility 31: 52–57

Ericsson R J, Langevin C N, Nishino M 1973 Isolation of fractions rich in human Y sperm. Nature 246: 421–424

Evans J M, Douglas T A, Renton J P 1975 An attempt to separate fractions rich in human Y sperm. Nature 253: 352–354

Feil R N, Largey G P, Miller M 1984 Attitudes towards abortion as a means of sex selection. Journal of Psychology 116: 269–272

Fink B R, Shepard T H, Blandau R J 1967 Teratogenic activity of nitrous oxide. Nature 214: 146–148

Fletcher J C 1983 Is sex selection ethical? Research Ethics 128: 333–348

France J T, Graham F M, Gosling L, Hair P I 1984 A prospective study of the preselection of the sex of offspring by timing intercourse relative to ovulation. Fertility and Sterility 41: 894–900

Fraumeni J F, Lundin F E 1964 Smoking and pregnancy. Lancet i: 173

German J 1968 Mongolism, delayed fertilization and human sexual behaviour. Nature 217: 516–518

Glass R H 1977 Sex preselection. Obstetrics and Gynecology 49: 122–126

Gledhill B L 1983 Control of mammalian sex ratio by sexing sperm. Fertility and Sterility 40: 572–574

Gordon M J 1958 The contol of sex. Scientific American 199: 87–94

Guerrero R 1974 Association of the type and time of insemination within the menstrual cycle with the human sex ratio at birth. New England Journal of Medicine 291: 1056–1059

Guerrero R 1975 Type and time of insemination within the menstrual cycle and the human sex ratio at birth. Studies in Family Planning 6: 367–371

Harlap S 1979 Gender of infants conceived on different days of the menstrual cycle. New England Journal of Medicine 300: 1445–1448

Harvey E N 1946 Can the sex of mammalian offspring be controlled? Journal of Heredity 37: 71–73

Hegde U C, Shastry P R, Rao S S 1977 A simple and reproducible method for separating Y-bearing spermatozoa from human semen. Indian Journal of Medical Research 65: 738–740

Hytten F E 1982 Boys and girls. British Journal of Obstetrics and Gynaecology 89: 97–99

James W H 1986a Neural tube defects and sex ratio. Lancet ii: 573–574

James W H 1986b Hormonal control of the sex ratio. Journal of Theoretical Biology 118: 427–441

Kaneko S, Yamaguchi J, Kobayashi T, Iizuka R 1983 Separation of human X- and Y- bearing sperm using Percoll density gradient centrifugation. Fertility and Sterility 40: 661–665

Kasai K, Nakayama S, Shik S S, Yoshida Y 1982 Sex selection and recurrence of anencephaly. International Journal of Biological Research and Pregnancy 3: 21–24

Kiel-Metzger K, Warren G, Wilson G N, Erickson R P 1985 Evidence that the human Y chromosome does not contain clustered DNA sequences (BKM) associated with heterogametic sex determination in other vertebrates. New England Journal of Medicine 313: 242–245

Kirby D R S, McWhirter K G, Teitelbaum M S, Darlington C D 1967 A possible immunological influence on sex ratio. Lancet ii: 139–140

Kumar D 1985 Should one be free to choose the sex of one's child? Journal of Applied Philosophy 2: 197–204

Lancet correspondent 1983 Misuse of amniocentesis. Lancet i: 812–813

Lane E A 1969 The sex ratio of children born to schizophrenics and a theory of stress. Psychological Record 19: 579–584

Lindahl P E 1958 Separation of bull spermatozoa carrying X- and Y- chromosomes by counter-streaming centrifugation. Nature 181: 784

Lyster W R 1970 Sex ratio in the Australian Capital Territory. Human Biology 42: 670–678

Lyster W R 1974 Altered sex ratio after the London smog of 1952 and the Brisbane flood of 1965. British Journal of Obstetrics and Gynaecology 81: 626–631

Lyster W R 1977a Sex ratio of human births in a contaminated area. Medical Journal of Australia 1: 829–830

Lyster W R 1977b Arsenic and sex ratio in man. Medical Journal of Australia 2: 442

Lyster W R 1982 Altered sex ratio in children of divers. Lancet ii: 152

Macfarlane A, Mugford M 1984 Birth counts. Statistics of pregnancy and childbirth, HMSO, London

Markle G E, Nam C B 1982 Sex predetermination: its impact on fertility. Social Biology 29: 168–179

Mason B A, Smith S 1985 Artificial insemination by donor. British Medical Journal 291: 974

McWhirter K G 1956 Control of sex ratio in mammals. Nature 178: 870–871

Mittwoch U 1985 Erroneous theories of sex determination. Journal of Medical Genetics 22: 164–170

Mortimer D, Richardson D W 1982 Sex ratio of births resulting from artificial insemination. British Journal of Obstetrics and Gynaecology 89: 132–135

Mulcahy M T 1978 Down syndrome and parental coital rate. Lancet ii: 895

Olsson H, Brandt L 1982 Sex ratio in offspring of patients with non-Hodgkin lymphoma. New England Journal of Medicine 306: 367–368

Perez A, Eger R, Domenichini V, Kambic R, Gray R H 1985 Sex ratio associated with natural family planning. Fertility and Sterility 43: 152–153

Pickard B M, Mutch L, Elbourne D, Oakley A, Dauncey M, Samphier M 1982 Impact of sex ratio on onset and management of labour. British Medical Journal 285: 889

Qazi Q H, Masakawa A 1976 Altered sex ratio in fetal alcohol syndrome. Lancet ii: 42

Rehan N-H 1982 Sex ratio of live-born Hausa infants. British Journal of Obstetrics and Gynaecology 89: 136–141

Revelle R 1974 On rhythm and sex ratio. New England Journal of Medicine 291: 1083

Rohde W, Porstmann T, Prehn S, Dörner G 1975 Gravitational pattern of the Y-bearing human spermatozoa in density gradient centrifugation. Journal of Reproductive Fertility 42: 587–591

Rinehart W 1975 Sex preselection. Not yet practical. Population Reports (Series 1) 2: I-21–I-32

Robertson J S, Sheard A V 1973 Altered sex ratio after an outbreak of hepatitis. Lancet i: 532–534

Rohde W, Porstmann T, Dörner G 1973 Migration of Y-bearing human spermatozoa in cervical mucus. Journal of Reproductive Fertility 33: 167–169

Rosner F 1979 The biblical and Talmudic secret for choosing one's baby's sex. Israel Journal of Medical Sciences 15: 784–787

Rosner F 1984 Ancient descriptions of hemophilia and preconception gender selection. Journal of the American Medical Association 252: 900

Ross A, Robinson J A, Evans H J 1975 Failure to confirm separation of X- and Y-bearing human sperm using BSA gradients. Nature 253: 354–355

Rothschild 1960 X and Y Spermatozoa. Nature 187: 253–254

Sampson J H, Alexander N J, Fulgham D L, Burry K A 1983 Gender after artificial induction of ovulation and artificial insemination. Fertility and Sterility 40: 481–484

Serr D M, Ismajovich B 1963 Determination of the primary sex ratio from human abortions. American Journal of Obstetrics and Gynecology 87: 63–65

Shastry P R, Hegde U C, Rao S S 1977 Use of Ficoll-sodium metrizoate density gradient to separate human X- and Y-bearing spermatozoa. Nature 269: 58–60

Shettles L B 1960a X and Y spermatozoa. Nature 187: 254–255

Shettles L B 1960b Nuclear morphology of human spermatozoa. Nature 186: 648–649

Shettles L B 1960c Nuclear structures of human spermatozoa. Nature 188: 918–919

Shettles L B 1976 Sex selection. American Journal of Obstetrics and Gynecology 124: 441–442

Shettles L 1978 Sex preselection. Obstetrics and Gynecology 51: 513

Shilling E, Thormahlen D 1977 Enrichment of human X and Y spermatozoa by density gradient centrifugation. Andrologia 9: 106

Shiono P H, Harlap S, Ramcharan S 1982 Sex of offspring of women using oral contraceptives, rhythm, and other methods of birth control around the time of conception. Fertility and Sterility 37: 367–372

Shishito S, Shirai M, Sasaki K 1975 Galvanic separation of X- and Y- bearing human spermatozoa. International Journal of Fertility 20: 13

Simcock B W 1985 Sons and daughters—a sex preselection study. Medical Journal of Australia 142: 541–542

Snyder R G 1961 The sex ratio of offspring of pilots of high performance military aircraft. Human Biology 33: 1–10

Steeno O, Adimoejla A, Steeno J 1975 Separation of X and Y bearing human spermatozoa with the Sephadex gel-filtration method. Andrologia 7: 95

Stolkowski J, Lorrain J 1980 Preconceptional selection of fetal sex. International Journal of Gynaecology and Obstetrics 18: 440–443

Swinbanks D 1986 Gender selection sparks row. Nature 321: 720

Szilard L 1960 Dependence of the sex ratio at birth on the age of the father. Nature 186: 649–650

Tricomi V, Serr D, Solish G 1960 The ratio of male to female embryos as determined by the sex chromatin. American Journal of Obstetrics and Gynecology 79: 504–509

Van Duijn C Jun 1960 Nuclear structure of human spermatozoa. Nature 188: 916–918

Vear C S 1977 Preselective sex determination. Medical Journal of Australia 2: 700–702

Walby A L, Merrett J D, Dean G, Kirke P 1981a Unusual sex ratio in Ireland in 1978. Lancet ii: 760

Walby A L, Merrett J D, Dean G, Kirke P 1981b Sex ratio of births in Ireland in 1978. Ulster Medical Journal 50: 83–87

Williamson N E, Lean T H, Vengadasalam D 1978 Evaluation of an unsuccessful sex preselection clinic in Singapore. Journal of Biosocial Science 10: 375–388

Wyatt R, Murray Wilson A 1973 Children of anaesthetists. British Medical Journal 1: 675

Gamete intrafallopian transfer (GIFT)

INTRODUCTION

The birth of the first baby conceived through in vitro fertilisation (IVF) (Steptoe & Edwards 1978) heralded a new era in reproductive medicine, opening new awareness into the further understanding of the human reproductive process as well as initiating new ideas into the area of assisted reproduction. In a move to simplify the technique of IVF, Craft et al (1982) carried out the placement of oocytes and sperms into the uterine cavity. Though there were some pregnancies, this technique was abandoned due to the low overall success rate. Buster et al (1983) then introduced a technique called ovum donation which involved the flushing out of pre-implantation embryos from donor women and the transfer of these embryos to recipient uteri. The initial success of this technique was encouraging but unfortunately it did not find wide application presumably because of the technical difficulties involved and the scarcity of a pool of donors. In 1984, Asch et al reported the first pregnancy following translaparoscopic gamete intrafallopian transfer (GIFT), followed by the subsequent delivery of twins (Asch et al 1985a). The introduction of GIFT into the armamentarium of the reproductive endocrinologist was another major contribution to the further understanding of the reproductive process and a benefit to infertile couples desiring a pregnancy. This chapter provides a summary of what is known so far in this exciting technique.

CONCEPT OF GIFT

During a conception cycle, following a timely midcycle luteinising hormone (LH) surge, ovulation occurs and the oocyte enters the fallopian tube. Following coitus, sperm that are deposited in the vagina will ascend into the cervical canal, uterus and fallopian tubes where they meet the egg in the ampullary portion of the tube. Fertilisation occurs and the embryo undergoes a series of cell divisions as it makes its way down the fallopian tube where it reaches the uterine cavity 5 to 7 days later, followed by implantation.

In couples with unexplained infertility it is assumed that one or more aspects of this process may be defective or absent, hence contributing to infertility. Therefore, if normal physiology is simulated by placing egg(s) and sperm into the ampulla of the fallopian tube, would this not contribute to initiating a pregnancy? It was with this concept in mind that the technique of GIFT was conceived as a therapeutic alternative. Basically, the GIFT technique involves the placing of both gametes into the ampullary section of the fallopian tube, and therefore provides an alternative to IVF in patients with normal tubes.

STEPS IN A GIFT PROGRAMME

The treatment cycle in a GIFT programme would involve the following steps:

1. *Induction of multiple follicular development.* Experience with the IVF technique has shown that the pregnancy rate increases with the number of embryos replaced. Similarly in a GIFT programme, in order to increase the chances of pregnancy, it is thought that placing a few oocytes is better than placing one. Therefore, patients undergoing GIFT are preferably stimulated with preparations such as clomiphene, human menopausal gonadotrophin (hMG) or these in combination. Recently the use of gonadotrophin releasing hormone (GnRH) analogues in combination with hMG have been described.

2. *Monitoring of follicular development.* Monitoring of follicular development induced by the agents mentioned above usually includes serial ovarian ultrasonography and daily serum oestradiol measurement. Further doses of hMG are usually titrated to those parameters.

3. *Timing of human chorionic gonadotrophin (hCG).* hCG is usually given 24–30 hours after the last dose of hMG to stimulate an LH surge.

4. *Oocyte recovery.* Oocytes are recovered 34–36 hours after the hCG injection either by laparoscopy, mini-laparotomy or by ultrasound guidance.

5. *Semen preparation.* Semen preparation is carried out 2–2½ hours before oocyte recovery by a semen wash and swim-up technique using antibiotics in the culture medium (Wong et al 1986a).

6. *Oocyte identification and grading.* The oocytes recovered are then identified and graded and kept in short culture while awaiting oocyte recovery to be completed.

7. *Gamete loading and GIFT.* After oocyte recovery is complete, the eggs are selected and loaded into a catheter together with the sperm preparation. The catheter is then introduced into the fibrial ostium and the gametes expelled into the ampullary region of the fallopian tube.

8. *Luteal phase support.* The role of this is debatable and most centres do not use it. However, we routinely use intramuscular administration of progesterone in oil 25 mg daily in the luteal phase.

9. *Confirmation of pregnancy.* β-hCG is estimated 14 days after GIFT and two positive hCGs are required to confirm a pregnancy. Most centres now confirm pregnancy with an ultrasound scan 4–6 weeks after GIFT.

NON-HUMAN PRIMATE STUDIES

The technique of GIFT is very new and undoubtedly several modifications are inevitable as we gain further understanding of the procedure. In order to achieve this Wong et al (unpublished data) have developed an experimental model using the rhesus monkey (*Macaca mulatta*).

Their study consisted of 20 normal cycling adult female rhesus monkeys (group 1). These monkeys received hMG for the induction of multiple follicular development and were monitored by daily serum oestradiol measurement and laparoscopy; 36 hours after hCG administration, at laparotomy, oocytes were aspirated.

Three hours before surgery, semen was collected by electroejaculation into TALP/HEPES medium with bovine serum albumin. It was capacitated by the addition of caffeine and dibutryl CAMP.

Oocytes recovered were assessed and then transferred to the semen preparation. Two oocytes and 10 15 μl of semen preparation (containing 100 000–150 000 sperm) were drawn into a $3\frac{1}{2}$ inch Tomcat $3\frac{1}{2}$ French catheter for transfer into the ampulla of each fallopian tube via the fimbria.

Group 2 in this study consisted of five normal cycling adult female rhesus monkeys. They were not stimulated with hMG and acted as synchronised recipients based on laparoscopic assessment. They underwent GIFT and received the excess oocytes obtained from animals in group 1.

Six animals from group 1 did not respond to hMG stimulation and were dropped from the study. Pregnancy was confirmed in six animals (31.5%), five in group 1 and one in group 2. The outcome of pregnancy is summarised in Table 15.1.

Table 15.1 Outcome of pregnancy in rhesus monkeys undergoing GIFT

Animal	Type	Outcome of pregnancy
4	R	Miscarriage
5	D	Miscarriage
6	D	Twin miscarriages at 73 days post-GIFT
8	D	Term delivery
11	D	Miscarriage
12	D	Miscarriage

D = Donor (group 1); R = Recipient (group 2).

According to the authors, this was the first report of the technique of GIFT in non-human primates though successful IVF of non-human primate oocytes in the squirrel monkeys (Gould et al 1973, Kuehl & Dukelow 1982), baboon (Gould 1979), cynomolgus monkey (Kreitman et al 1982), rhesus monkey (Bavister et al 1983) and Chimpanzee (Gould 1983) has been attained.

The births of a baboon, a rhesus monkey and a cynomolgus monkey (Clayton & Kuehl 1984, Bavister et al 1984, Balmaceda et al 1984) conceived after IVF and embryo transfer have been reported in the literature. The overall pregnancy rate of 31.5% (6 out of 19) achieved in this group of monkeys was encouraging and was comparable with that obtained in the human (Asch et al 1986a). The incidence of early pregnancy loss—66.7% (4/6)—was high, however.

CLINICAL STUDIES

Since the first descriptions of the GIFT technique (Asch et al 1984, 1985a), numerous reports have appeared in the literature confirming its usefulness in the treatment of some types of infertility (Asch et al 1985b, 1986a,b, Madden et al 1986, Corson et al 1986, Confino et al 1986, Guastella et al 1985, 1986, Lim-Howe et al 1987, Molloy et al 1987, Wong et al 1986b, 1987a).

Pregnancy rates of 21–40% have been reported; these are equivalent to the results of most IVF units, if not better.

INTERNATIONAL MULTICENTRE STUDY

Since the technique of GIFT is new, its efficacy in the treatment of various causes of infertility requires proper evaluation. This can only be satisfactorily carried out if the number of patients analysed is sufficiently large. To this end, an international multicentre study was initiated in late 1985 to investigate the use of a common GIFT protocol in 10 centres worldwide. The centres involved are:

1. University of California at Irvine, USA (R H Asch and J P Balmaceda),
2. University of Palermo, (E Cittadini),
3. Clinic of Gynaecology, Rosario, Argentina (P Figuero-Casas),
4. University of Vancouver, (V Gomel),
5. University of Zurich, (M K Hohl),
6. Royal Women Hospital, Melbourne, (I Johnston),
7. Monash University, Melbourne, (J Leeton),
8. University of Paris Vasco, Bilbao, (F J Rodrigues-Escudero),
9. University of Munich, (U Noss),
10. National University of Singapore, (P C Wong).

800 couples with an average duration of infertility of 7.8 years (± 3.1 years SEM) were treated with a single attempt of GIFT.

The primary diagnoses of the 800 couples were unexplained infertility (499 cases—62%), endometriosis (91 cases—11%), male factor (84 cases—10%), previous failed artificial insemination with donor semen (65 cases—8%), periadnexial adhesions (32 cases—4%), cervical or immunological factor (3 cases), and premature overian failure (2 cases).

Eighty per cent of the procedures were performed through the laparoscope and 20% via a mini-laparotomy incision. A total of 3843 oocytes were collected (average 4.8 per patient) and 3014 oocytes were transferred (average 3.8 per patient).

Of the 800 cases of GIFT, there were 275 pregnancies; a pregnancy rate of 34.4%. There were 66 miscarriages (24%), 8 ectopic pregnancies (2.9%) and 69 multiple pregnancies (25%) (Table 15.2).

Table 15.2 Results of the international multicentre study of 800 couples undergoing GIFT

Results	Number of patients	%
Number of procedures	800	100.0
Clinical pregnancies	272	34.4
Delivered or ongoing >12 weeks	201	73.1
Miscarriages	66	24.0
Ectopic pregnancies	8	2.9
Multiple pregnancies	69	25.0

INDICATIONS FOR GIFT

Initially GIFT was conceived as a therapeutic option for patients with *unexplained infertility* (Asch et al 1984). The indications were later expanded to include that of *male factor* (i.e. low sperm count and/or low sperm motility) (Asch et al 1985a).

The use of GIFT in patients with *endometriosis* has been explored. Other indications for GIFT include *periadnexal adhesions* and *cervical factor*. Table 3. summarises the relative success rates of GIFT for various aetiologies.

Table 15.3 Relative success rates of GIFT for various aetiologies

Results by etiology	Cases	Number of clinical pregnancies (%)
Unexplained infertility	499	175 (35)
Endometriosis	91	35 (38)
Male factor	84	15 (18)
Failed AID	65	35 (54)
Periadnexal adhesions	32	9 (28)
Cervical factor	27	4 (15)
Premature ovarian failure	2	2 (100)
Total	800	275 (34.4)

Recently GIFT has also been applied to couples in whom *artificial insemination with donor semen* (AID) has failed as well as to oocyte donation in women with premature ovarian failure.

Over a 12-month period, 48 infertile couples with a duration of infertility of 9.5 ± 0.4 years (mean $\pm$ SEM) were recruited in the GIFT programme. The husbands were either azoospermic or severely oligospermic and had previously failed from 9 to 24 cycles of AID (13.5 ± 0.6) cycles (mean $\pm$ SEM), following spontaneous ovulation and also when ovulation was induced with clomiphene and hMG.

During the treatment cycle, multiple follicular development was achieved with either a protocol of clomiphene and hMG (Asch et al 1986b) or with pure FSH (follicle stimulating hormone, Metrodin) 300 iu intramuscularly on days 3 and 4 of the menstrual cycle and hMG (Pergonal) 150 iu intramuscularly from day 5 onwards until two or more follicles reached 16 mm in diameter on ultrasound scan and serum oestradiol levels reached 300 pg/μl per follicle.

Donors were selected among medical students according to the American Fertility Society (1986) guidelines. The semen samples obtained 2½ hours prior to the procedure were processed by the wash and swim-up technique as described by Wong et al (1986a). Oocyte recovery, identification, transfer of gametes, luteal phase support and monitoring were carried out as described previously (Asch et al 1986b).

All 48 couples were treated with one cycle of GIFT each; 27 couples conceived (56%). Eight patients (29%), however, miscarried during the first trimester while no ectopic pregnancies occurred. Four sets of twins and one set of triplets were confirmed, a multiple pregnancy rate of 18%.

The high success rate in these patients with failed AID may suggest that perhaps in these women there may be a defect in:

1. sperm transport to the site of fertilisation,
2. oocyte expulsion at time of ovulation, or
3. oocyte pick-up by the fallopian tube.

Hopefully further experience will shed more light on this area of reproduction.

We have explorted the use of oocyte donation in a GIFT programme for patients with *premature ovarian failure* (POF).

POF occurs in 1–3% of the general population (Coulam et al 1986), and until recently there was no satisfactory treatment. In 1984, Lutjen et al reported the first case of IVF with donated eggs and subsequent successful embryo transfer (ET) in a 25-year-old woman with POF. More recently Navot et al (1986) reported two successful pregnancies in eight patients in whom IVF–ET was performed using donated oocytes.

Asch et al (1987c) recently reported the first series of GIFT performed in eight patients with POF using donated oocytes. The recipients were between 24 and 36 years of age. They received β-oestradiol orally and progesterone in oil intramuscularly as previously described (Asch et al 1987a,b). Oocytes were obtained from GIFT patients whose eggs were not used for the transfer. From the eight patients who underwent the procedure, there were six clinical pregnancies, a pregnancy rate of 75%.

ABORTION AND ECTOPIC PREGNANCY

The overall rate of abortion in patients who conceive after GIFT is not excessive. Various authors have reported incidences of 11–25% (Nemiro &

McGoughey 1986, Guastella et al 1986, Molloy et al 1986, Asch et al 1986b, Wong et al 1987a). The data from the multicentre study showed an abortion rate of 24% (see Table 15.2).

The risk of ectopic pregnancy has been quoted to vary from 0% to 7% (Asch et al 1986b, Guastella et al 1986, Molloy et al 1986, Nemiro & McGoughey 1986, Wong et al 1987a). The corresponding data from the multicentre study showed an ectopic pregnancy rate of only 2.9% (see Table 15.2). This figure is not excessive when compared with the figure of 5% quoted for IVF pregnancies (Australian IVF Collaborative Group 1985).

MULTIPLE PREGNANCY

The transfer of several oocytes (normally up to four) in most centres increases the chances of pregnancy but also risks an increase in the incidence of multiple pregnancy. Multiple pregnancy rates of 21–55% have been reported by various authors (Asch et al 1986b, Guastella et al 1986, Molloy et al 1986, Nemiro & McGoughey 1986, Wong et al 1987a). The multicentre study showed a multiple pregnancy incidence of 25%.

Wong et al (1987a) showed that when four, three and two oocytes were transferred, the respective pregnancy rates were 33.9%, 30.8% and 14.3% (Table 15.4). There was more than a two-fold rise in the pregnancy rate

Table 15.4   Pregnancy and multiple pregnancy rates by the number of oocytes transferred

No. of oocytes transferred	No. of cycles	No. of conceptions (%)	No. of multiple pregnancies (%)
1	1	0 (0)	0 (0)
2	7	1 (14.3)	0 (0)
3	13	4 (30.8)	1 (25)
4	59	20 (33.9)	5 (25)

when four oocytes were transferred when compared with three oocytes. On the other hand, the multiple pregnancy rate remained at 25% when three or four oocytes were transferred. Hence, the transfer of four oocytes increased the chances of pregnancy without increasing the chances of multiple pregnancy. The authors feel therefore that four is the optimum number of oocytes to transfer.

THE CORRELATION OF IVF AND GIFT

Wong et al (1987a) compared the outcome of IVF of the excess oocytes with the outcome of GIFT. In 48 patients who underwent GIFT, there were six or more oocytes recovered from each patient. Four were used for GIFT and the remaining two used for IVF. The ability of excess oocytes to be fertilised in vitro did not correlate with the final outcome of GIFT (Table 15.5). It was argued that perhaps this was because the better quality oocytes had been

Table 15.5 Correlation of IVF of excess oocytes with success of GIFT

IVF of excess oocytes	Pregnant with GIFT	Not pregnant with GIFT
No fertilisation	5	13
Fertilisation	12	18
Total	17	31

pre-selected for GIFT, leaving the lower quality oocytes for IVF. Matson et al (1987) also drew the same conclusion. Larger numbers of patient cycles, using equal quality oocytes, need to be compared before the real correlation is known. This study is currently being undertaken.

COMBINED IVF AND GIFT

Figuero-Casas (personal communication, 1986) treated 10 patients with GIFT combined with IVF and ET, i.e. excess oocytes after GIFT were inseminated with the husband's sperm and the resultant embryos transferred to the uterine cavity in the same cycle. Of the 10 cases, there were six pregnancies. Two patients miscarried (33%) and in one case there was a tubal pregnancy in conjunction with an intrauterine gestation. All four patients have delivered. This is certainly an alternative approach in centres without facilities for embryo freezing or where such freezing procedures are not allowed, the only problem being that when a pregnancy ensues it is not known if it was from the IVF–ET or the GIFT procedure.

CRYOPRESERVATION OF EXCESS EMBRYOS

Although the fertilisation of excess oocytes after GIFT did not predict the outcome of the procedure (Wong et al 1987a), the embryos so derived could be frozen and thawed for subsequent transfer in a later cycle. Wong et al (1987b) recently showed that in 11 patients who received thawed embryos after a failed GIFT, there were two pregnancies (18.2%). This procedure therefore helps to increase the overall pregnancy rate in women undergoing GIFT.

THE FUTURE OF GIFT

One of the problems that GIFT has to address is the risk of multiple pregnancy. At the moment it appears that 3–4 is the optimum number of eggs to be transferred. However, if the technique could be refined further, perhaps a better selection of eggs may enable a comparable pregnancy rate with the transfer of a smaller number of eggs. In fact, Asch (1986) showed that none of his patients who had received grade 3 or less oocytes conceived. Perhaps the optimum may be to transfer 2–3 good grade oocytes.

In the near future, further simplification of the technique could inevitably be made. The trend is towards an outpatient procedure and perhaps ultrasound-directed oocyte recovery and hysteroscopic or ultrasound-guided cannulation of the fallopian tube (Jansen & Anderson 1987) via the cornual end for gamete transfer may be the convenient method of the future.

There have been two successful reports so far (Blackledge et al 1986, Devroey et al 1986) on the transfer of embryos into the fallopian tube using GIFT technique. A combination of all these techniques could be the answer in the future, i.e. ultrasound-guided oocyte recovery, in vitro fertilisation and tubal embryo transfer using ultrasound-guided fallopian tube cannulation techniques.

CONCLUSION

In the four years since GIFT was announced it has found application in many centres around the world. Though it started as a treatment for unexplained infertility, its usefulness is now known for patients with endometriosis, and male factor, cervical factor and immunological causes of infertility. More recent applications have been in patients in whom repeated AID attempts have failed and also in women with premature ovarian failure.

In the near future, further simplification of the technique may enable the procedure to be carried out entirely on an outpatient basis with further refinement to increase the overall pregnancy rate without increasing the risk of multiple pregnancy.

REFERENCES

The American Fertility Society 1986 New guidelines for the use of semen donor insemination. Fertility and Sterility 4 (suppl 2): 939–1103
Asch R H, 1986 Gamete intra-fallopian transfer (GIFT). Presented at the XI World Congress on Fertility and Sterility. Singapore, Oct 26–31
Asch R H, Ellsworth L R, Balmacdea J P, Wong P C 1984 Pregnancy following translaparoscopic gamete intrafallopian transfer (GIFT). Lancet ii: 1034–1035
Asch R H, Ellsworth L R, Balmaceda J P, Wong P C 1985a Birth following gamete intrafallopian transfer. Lancet ii: 163
Asch R H, Balmaceda J P, Ellsworth L R, Wong P C 1985b Gamete intra-fallopian transfer (GIFT): a new treatment for infertility. International Journal of Fertility 30: 41–45
Asch R H, Balmaceda J P, Ellsworth L R, Wong P C 1986a Preliminary experiences with GIFT (gamete intrafallopian transfer). Fertility and Sterility 45: 366–371
Asch R H, Balmaceda J P, Wong P C et al 1986b Gamete intrafallopian transfer (GIFT): use of minilaparotomy and an individualized regimen of induction of follicular development. Acta Europaea Fertilitatis and Sterility 17: 187–193
Asch R H, Balmaceda J P, Ord T et al 1987a Oocyte donation and gamete intrafallopian transfer is treatment for premature ovarian failure (letter). Lancet i: 687
Asch R H, Balmaceda J P, Ord T, Borrero C, Rodriguez-Rigau L J, Rojas E J 1987b Gamete intrafallopian transfer (GIFT) and oocyte donation—a novel treatment for infertility in premature ovarian failure. Case report. Gynecologic Endocrinology 1: 99–105
Asch R H, Balmaceda J P, Borrero C, Rojas E J 1987c Oocyte donation and GIFT in premature ovarian failure. Fertility and Sterility (in press)
Australian IVF Collaborative Group 1985 High incidence of pre-term birth and early losses in pregnancy after in-vitro fertilisation. British Medical Journal 291: 1160

Balmaceda J P, Pool T B, Arana J B, Heitman T S, Asch R H 1984 Successful in vitro
fertilisation and embryo transfer in cynomolgus monkeys. Fertility and Sterility 42: 791–795
Bavister B D, Boatman D E, Liebfried L, Loose M, Vernon M W 1983 Fertilization and
cleavage of rhesus monkey oocyte in vitro. Biology of Reproduction 28: 983–999
Bavister B D, Boatman D E, Collins K, Kierschke D J, Eisele S G 1984 Birth of rhesus monkey
infant after IVF and non-surgical embryo transfer. Proceedings of the National Academy
of Sciences of the United States of America 81; 2218–2222
Blackledge D G, Matson P L, Wilcox D L et al 1986 Pronuclear stage transfer and modified
gamete intra-fallopian transfer techniques for oligospermia cases. Medical Journal of Australia
145: 300
Buster J E, Bustillo M, Thorneycroft I H et al 1983 Nonsurgical transfer of in vivo fertilised
donated ova to five intertile women: Report of two pregnancies. Lancet i: 816–817
Clayton O, Kuehl T J 1984 The first successful in vitro fertilization and embryo transfer in
a non-human primate. Theriogenology 21: 228
Confino E, Friberg J, Gleicher N 1986 A new stirrable catheter for gamete intrafallopian tube
transfer (GIFT) Communications-in-brief. Fertility and Sterility 46: 1147–1149
Corson S L, Batzer F, Eisenberg et al 1986 Early experience with the GIFT procedure. Journal
of Reproductive Medicine 31: 219–223
Craft I, Djahanbakhch O, McLeod F et al 1982 Human pregnancy following oocyte and sperm
transfer to the uterus. Lancet i: 1031–1033
Coulam C B, Adamson S C, Annegers J U F 1986 Incidence of premature ovarian failure.
Obstetric Gynecology 67: 604–606
Devroey P, Braeckmans P, Smitz J et al (1986) Pregnancy after translaparoscopic zygote
intrafallopian transfer in a patient with sperm antibodies. Lancet i: 1329
Gould K G 1979 Fertilization in vitro of non-human primate ova: present status and rationale
for further development of the technique. In: Report of the Ethics Advisory Board, Appendix:
HEW Support of Research Involving Human In Vitro Fertilization and Embryo Transfer.
Washington D C, US government Printing Office, No 14, p 1
Gould K G 1983 Ovum recovery an in vitro fertilization in the Chimpanzee. Fertility and
Sterility 40: 378–383
Gould K G, Cline E M, Williams W L 1973 Observation on the induction of ovulation and
fertilization in vitro in the squirrel monkey (Saimiri sciureus). Fertility and Sterility 24: 260–
268
Guastella G, Comparetto A G, Gullo D 1985 Gamete intra-fallopian transfer (GIFT): a new
technique for the treatment of unexplained infertility. Acta Europaea Fertilitatis 16: 311–316
Guastella G, Comparetto A G, Palermo R, Cefalu E, Ciriminna R, Cittadini E 1986 Gamete
intrafallopian transfer in the treatment of infertility: the first series at the University of
Palermo. Fertility and Sterility 46: 417–423
Jansen R P, Anderson J C 1987 Catheterisation of the fallopian tubes from the vagina. Lancet
ii: 309–310
Kreitmann O, Lynch A, Nixon W E, Hodgen G D 1982 Ovum collection, induced luteal
dysfunction, in vitro fertilization, embryo development and low tubal ovum transfer in
primates. In: Hafez E S E, Semm K (eds) In vitro fertilization and embryo transfer. MTP
Press, Lancaster, p 303
Kuehl T J, Dukelow W R 1982 Time relations of squirrel monkey (Saimiri sciureus) sperm
capacitation and ovum maturation in an in vitro fertilization system. Journal of Reproduction
and Fertility 64: 135–137
Lim-Howe D, Studd J, Dooley M 1987 Gamete intra-fallopian transfer (GIFT). British Journal
of Hospital Medicine March: 241–244
Lutjen P, Trounson A, Leeton J, Findlay J, Wood C, Renon P 1984 The establishment and
maintenance of pregnancy using in vitro fertilisation and embryo donation in a patient with
primary ovarian failure. Nature 307: 174–175
Madden J D, Bookout D M, Siverstein E H et al 1986 GIFT-pregnancy by translaparoscopic
gamete intrafallopian transfer. Dallas Medical Journal 72: 15–17
Matson P L, Yovich J M, Bootsma B D, Spittle J W, Yovich J L 1987 The in vitro fertilisation
of supernumerary oocytes in a gamete intrafallopian transfer program. Fertility and Sterility
47: 802–806
Molloy D, Speirs A, du Plessis Y, McBain J, Johnston I 1987 A laparoscopic approach to
a program of gamete intra-fallopian transfer. Fertility and Sterility 47: 289–294
Navot D, Laufer N, Kopolovic J et al 1986 Artificially induced endometrial cycles and

establishment of pregnancy in the absence of ovaries. New England Journal of Medicine 314: 806–811

Nemiro J S, McGoughey R W 1986 An alternative to in vitro fertilisation embryo transfer: The successful transfer of human oocytes and spermatozoa to the distal oviduct. Fertility and Sterility 46: 644–652

Steptoe P C, Edwards R G 1978 Birth after reimplantation of a human embryo. Lancet ii: 366

Wong P C, Balmaceda J P, Blanco J D, Gibbs R S, Asch R H 1986a Sperm washing and swim-up technique using antibiotics removes microbes from human semen. Fertility and Sterility 45: 97–100

Wong P C, Ng S C, Edirisinghe W R, Ratnam S S 1986b Pregnancy following gamete intra-fallopian transfer (GIFT) Case report. Singapore Journal of Obstetrics and Gynaecology 17: 59–61

Wong P C, Ng S C, Hamilton M P R, Anandakumar C, Wong Y C, Ratnam S S 1987a Gamete intra-fallopian transfer—the Singapore experience. In: Teoh E S, Ratnam S S, Ng S C (eds) In vitro fertilization and other alternative methods of conception. Parthenon, Carnforth (in press)

Wong P C, Bongso A, Ng S C, Chan C L K, Ratnam S S 1987b Cryopreservation of embryos derived from in vitro fertilization (IVF) of excess oocytes increase pregnancy rate in a gamete intrafallopian transfer (GIFT) programme (submitted for publication)

New developments in contraception

It is now 25 years since the contraceptive revolution of the 1960s, when the Pill was introduced and the population explosion became a subject of popular concern. In the 1980s there has been a tendency towards contraceptive complacency, and developments in the technology of family planning have not been widely publicised. Nevertheless, factors such as 'Pill scares' and the Government's efforts to encourage the use of condoms could alter patterns of contraceptive use in the near future. This chapter will therefore briefly review recent developments in established methods, and discuss in more detail new methods, some of which are not yet ready for widespread use.

COMBINED ORAL CONTRACEPTIVE PILLS

Side-effects

The combined oral contraceptive pill (COC) remains the most popular form of contraception for young women, with about three million users in Britain and 60 million throughout the world (Wellings & Mills 1984, Shearman 1986). Recent developments have centred on concern about possible side-effects.

Cardiovascular disease

In 1970 a link between COCs and venous thromboembolism was attributed to the oestrogen content of the COC, and in 1980 evidence appeared that the progestogen content might be important in determining the risk of arterial disease (Kay 1980, Vessey 1980). Current COC formulations therefore employ the lowest effective dose of both oestrogen and progestogen (Fotherby 1985). Before the switch to low-dose COCs, the excess mortality attributable to COCs was around 20 per 100 000 users per year (Dalen & Hickler 1981); the majority of deaths, which were mainly due to cerebrovascular accidents and myocardial infarction, occurred in women over the age of 35 years, or in women who smoked or were hypertensive. Nowadays, therefore, women who smoke are not prescribed COCs after the age of 35 years (Sartwell & Stolley 1982, Drug and Therapeutics Bulletin 1986), though in the normotensive slim woman who has never smoked, COCs can be continued after

35, and possibly after 40 years, provided that the blood pressure is checked frequently (Bowen-Simpkins 1984). The suggestion that the excess risks in many of the epidemiological studies could be explained by bias (Realini & Goldzieher 1985) is controversial, but there is general agreement nowadays that the use of low-dose COCs in healthy young women is associated with little or no increase in the absolute risk of stroke (Longstreth & Swanson 1984, Vessey et al 1984).

Malignant disease

Of more concern recently has been the possibility that COCs may influence a woman's risk of developing cancer later in life (Drife & Guillebaud 1986, Khoo 1986). Several studies have demonstrated that COC-users have a reduced risk of cancer of the endometrium and the ovary; the risk is approximately halved after 1 year of use and the reduction in risk persists for at least 10 years after stopping COCs. An adverse effect on the incidence of cervical neoplasia has been suggested but has been difficult to prove because unprotected sexual intercourse is itself a risk factor for the condition (Vessey et al 1983). Nevertheless, regular cervical smears are essential for oral contraceptive users.

Breast cancer

Because breast cancer is the commonest lethal cancer in women, the question of a possible link with COC use is very important. The use of COCs after the first full-term pregnancy is not associated with any change in the risk of breast cancer, but there is some concern about COC use before first pregnancy, when the response of breast tissue to steroids may be different from that later in life (Drife 1986, Leading Article 1986). Some studies suggest an association between early COC use and breast cancer (Pike et al 1983, Meirik et al 1986), while others do not (Cancer and Steroid Hormone Study of the Centers for Disease Control 1986, Paul et al 1986). The reasons for this epidemiological uncertainty may include several factors: a long latent period between tumour initiation and clinical breast cancer, changes in prescribing patterns over the last 20 years, and possibly bias (including recall bias) in the studies themselves (McPherson & Drife 1986). At present it is still impossible to say with certainty that COC use early in life does not alter the risk of subsequent breast cancer, but there is no reason to alter our prescribing habits or to advise women to stop COC use after a certain number of years.

New progestogens

In an effort to find a formulation with minimum metabolic side-effects, several synthetic progestogens have been tested in humans and some have reached

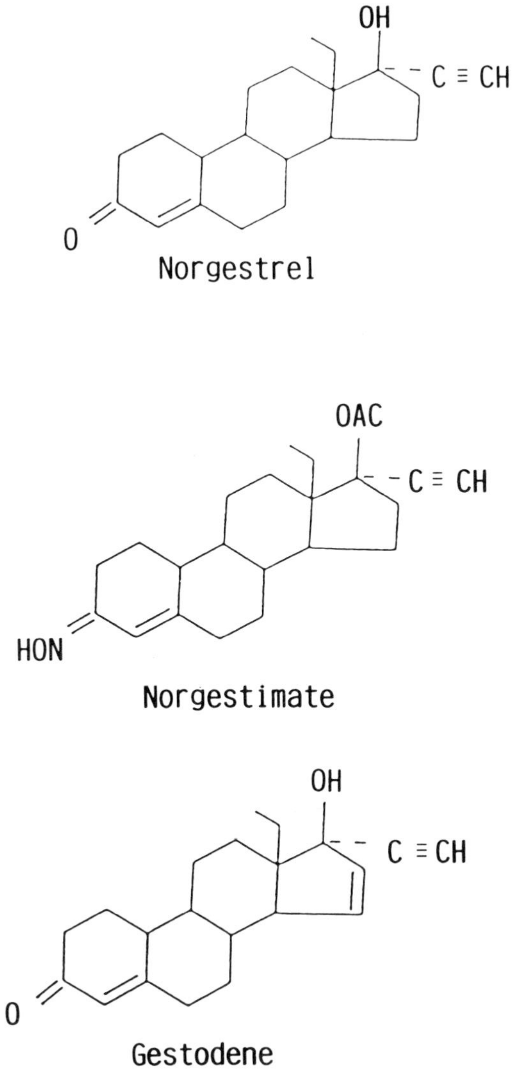

Fig. 16.1   Structural formulae of two new progestogens—norgestimate and Gestoden— compared with the formula of norgestrel

the stage of being introduced for clinical use. Gestodene (Fig. 16.1) is more potent than levonorgestrel (Fotherby 1984), and a combined formulation containing 30 µg ethinyloestradiol and 75 µg gestodene (Femodene) was introduced in the UK in 1987. Norgestimate (Fig. 16.1) has been thought to be a pro-drug (Fotherby 1984), but this has been disputed; a combination of 250 µg norgestimate and 35 µg ethinyloestradiol (Cilest) may be introduced in the UK. Initial clinical experience with gestodene suggests that cycle control is good and the incidence of side-effects is low (Loudon et al 1988), but it will be several years before the long-term risks and benefits of the new progestogens can be fully assessed.

Medico-legal aspects of COC prescribing

After a well-publicised legal action over the prescribing of COCs to minors without their parents' knowledge, in 1985 the House of Lords gave judgement which included guidelines to doctors faced with a request for COCs from a girl aged under 16 years (Dyer 1985). The doctor should try to persuade her to agree to her parents being told, but if she refuses the doctor may prescribe COCs provided that he/she is satisfied that:

1. the girl will understand his/her advice,
2. he/she cannot persuade the girl to tell her parents,
3. the girl will probably begin or continue having intercourse with or without contraception,
4. without contraception the girl's physical or mental health will suffer,
5. the girl's best interests require the doctor to give contraceptive advice or treatment without her parents' consent.

In 1986, the General Medical Council advised that if the doctor is not satisfied that the child can understand the issues involved, he/she may disclose the information to her parents, bearing in mind 'the patient's best medical interests and the trust which the patient places in the doctor' (Anonymous 1986). This advice was criticised by the British Medical Association (Havard 1986), who feared that it may prevent young girls from seeking advice from their doctors.

PROGESTOGEN-ONLY CONTRACEPTION

The progestogen-only pill is as effective as the intra-uterine contraceptive device (Loudon 1985, McEwan 1985), and may be particularly suitable for the older woman. However, it may cause irregular vaginal bleeding and has to be taken very regularly, with a leeway of only 3 hours on either side of a fixed time each day (Bowen-Simpkins 1984). There is therefore continuing interest in other methods of delivering progestogens to the body.

Injectables

Two injectable progestogens are currently licensed in Britain: medroxy-progesterone acetate (Depo-Provera, usually given every 12 weeks) and nor-ethisterone enanthate (Noristerat, given every 8 weeks). Only Depo-Provera is licensed for long-term use. They are extremely effective, with failure rates of less than 1%, and are as safe as any other drug on the market (McEwan 1985, Elder 1984). Their only significant disadvantage is irregular bleeding.

Nevertheless, because of public concern and fears that in the past patients have not been properly counselled before receiving these drugs, the Minister of Health has advised that doctors should prescribe Depo-Provera for long-term use only in special instances when other contraceptive methods have been proved unsuitable.

New delivery systems

Slow-release systems have several advantages over daily administration of a progestogen (Fotherby 1984, Elstein & Nuttall 1985). Daily administration involves regular fluctuations of blood levels, with the theoretical possibility of overdosage at some times of the day and the more immediate threat of underdosage—and reduced efficacy—at other times. Pills may be forgotten, and if they are not taken at the same time each day the method may fail. With slow-release systems, however, a single administration of a hormone can last for several weeks or months, a constant blood level can be achieved, problems with gastrointestinal absorption can be eliminated, and initial metabolism in the liver (the so-called 'first pass' effect) can be avoided. The advantages are of marginal importance in European countries, but may be vital in developing countries where there may be poorer facilities for distributing drugs regularly.

Subdermal implants

Twenty years ago, Croxatto and Segal suggested that subdermal capsules of Silastic could be used as a basis for long-term steroidal contraception (Segal 1983). Research and development was carried out by the Population Council through its International Committee for Contraception Research, first in Santiago, Chile, using the progestogen chlormadinone acetate, and then in India and Brazil, using megestrol acetate. Subsequently, implants containing norethisterone were tested, but this progestogen was too weak to be effective. Levonorgestrel proved to be more successful, and trials of levonorgestrel-containing implants have been carried out in over a dozen countries, though not in the UK. These implants—'Norplant'—are the only implantable contraceptive currently available.

'Norplant' consists of six capsules, each containing 36 mg of levonorgestrel and having a diameter of 2.4 mm and a length of 3.4 cm (Fig. 16.2). The capsules release levonorgestrel at a rate of 80 μg per day during the first 6–18 months of use, and thereafter a release rate of 30 μg per day is maintained for at least 5 years. The capsules are inserted subdermally into the palmar aspect of the upper arm or forearm using a specially designed trocar which is introduced through a 2 mm incision (WHO 1985). Sutures are not required. Removal is usually easy, though difficulty can be encountered if the insertion has been too deep. Another system—'Norplant 2'—which consists of two slightly longer rods, is also being tested.

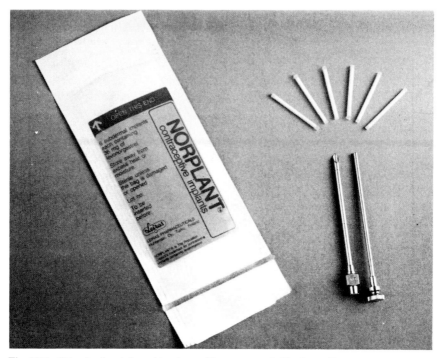

Fig. 16.2 'Norplant': subdermal implants of levonorgestrel. The figure illustrates a sterile package, a set of six implants and a trocar for insertion (from Leiras Pharmaceuticals, Turku, Finland, with permission)

Phase III trials of Norplant have been in progress for over 5 years in several centres, and the total clinical experience exceeds 50 000 woman months of use. Ovulation is suppressed in at least 50% of cycles, and in most women endometrial development is suppressed or adversely affected. Cervical mucus becomes scanty. There are no marked metabolic effects, though studies on lipid metabolism have given inconclusive results. The annual pregnancy rate during the first 5 years is 0.2–1.3%, and the gross cumulative pregnancy rate at 5 years is 2.6 per 100 woman years. Although menstrual irregularities occur, the continuation rate in one clinical trial was over 80% at 1 year and 50% at 4 years, and higher rates have been reported from developing countries (Fotherby 1984, WHO 1985).

About 40% of users report an abnormal bleeding pattern during the first year of use, but the menstrual problems diminish with time. Nevertheless, these problems are the major reason for discontinuation in the first year of use; discontinuation rates due to menstrual irregularities are around 14% at 4 years. It is important that clinical staff are trained to counsel women about these problems. The World Health Organization recommends that until further information is available it is inadvisable to use Norplant as a method of contraception in women undergoing anticoagulation therapy, or with undiagnosed abnormal uterine bleeding, known or suspected pregnancy, hae-morrhagic diathesis, or active hepato-cellular disease.

Vaginal rings

Injectable contraceptives are not immediately reversible, and implants require a small operation in order to be reversed. Vaginal rings, by contrast, can be reversed at any time by simply removing the device. It has been known for many years that drugs can be absorbed through the vaginal epithelium, and in the 1960s it was demonstrated that drugs could be released at a constant rate from polysiloxane tubes, which could therefore be used as a reservoir.

Clinical studies were undertaken in the 1970s, first with medroxy-progesterone acetate and then with other progestogens, at doses sufficient to inhibit ovulation (Fotherby 1984, Elstein & Nuttall 1985). Breakthrough bleeding was a troublesome side-effect with the less potent progestogens such as norethisterone, and further trials have been conducted of rings containing the more potent progestogen, levonorgestrel. If the steroid is uniformly distri-buted through the Silastic, the rate of diffusion drops after the steroid has diffused from outermost layers, and to achieve a constant rate of diffusion the steroid is placed either in a central core or in a layer around the core, beneath the surface of the ring. Most rings are now between 50 and 60 mm in outer diameter and 7.5–9.5 mm thick, and they are pliable and similar to the inert pessaries used in the management of prolapse (Coutinho 1984).

One type of ring (Fig. 16.3) contains both an oestrogen and a progestogen,

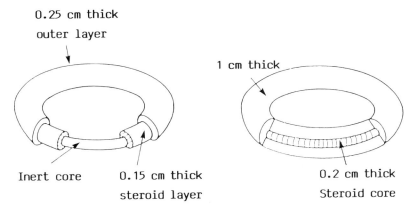

Fig. 16.3   Vaginal rings: shell type (left) and core type (right). The shaded part denotes the steroid-containing layer (from Fotherby 1984, with permission)

usually oestradiol (released at a rate of 160–180 µg/d) and levonorgestrel (released at a rate of 250–300 µg/d). The aim is to inhibit ovulation, and the ring is left in situ for 3 weeks, and then removed for 1 week, in a pattern similar to the COC (Elkik et al 1986).

The other type of ring (Fig. 16.3) releases only a low dose of progestogen, usually levonorgestrel at a rate of 20 μg daily (Landgren et al 1986). These inhibit ovulation in only 50% of users, and exert their contraceptive effect by a local action on cervical mucus and the endometrium. No metabolic changes have been detected (Fotherby 1984). The rings can be left in situ for 3 months, after which time a new ring is fitted. The ring is not removed during intercourse or during menstruation, and does not affect the wearing of tampons.

The World Health Organization has organised a multicentre trial of the levonorgestrel ring. Over 800 women have been admitted to the trial, and 177 have completed 1 year of its use. The continuation rate was 60% and the pregnancy rate 3%. Abnormal bleeding occurred in 15% and expulsions in 20% (Elstein & Nuttall 1985). A study of the social acceptability of the method suggested that the side-effects are well tolerated if a full explanation is given to the patients: in the centres in which counselling was judged to be poor, discontinuation rates for menstrual disturbance were over 30%, but if the counselling was good the discontinuation rate for this reason was only 10%. Among 108 women studied for 1 year in Beijing, China, the pregnancy rate was 3.7% and the continuation rate 71% (Ji et al 1986).

INTRA-UTERINE CONTRACEPTIVE DEVICES

As with COCs, there has recently been concern about possible adverse effects of the intra-uterine contraceptive device (IUD). The Dalkon shield, which was withdrawn from the market several years ago because of a link with pelvic inflammatory disease, is now the subject of well-publicised litigation in the USA (Snowden 1985), and this may fuel concern about the risks of salpingitis with other devices (Mishell 1985). Production of the 'Gravigard' device has been discontinued because of the high cost of successfully defending it against lawsuits in the USA (Illman 1986). Recent studies have shown that the relative risk of pelvic inflammatory disease among IUD users is only 1.6 for devices other than the Dalkon shield; the risk is highest in the first month after insertion and is not significantly different from controls after 4 months (Mishell 1985). A study of copper-containing IUDs showed that there was no significant increase in tubal infertility compared with controls (Daling et al 1985), and in a multicentre study there was a marginal increase in tubal infertility in nulliparous users of copper-containing IUDs, but not among parous users (Cramer et al 1985). It is now generally agreed that the IUD is particularly suitable for the older parous woman (Elias 1985).

The IUD is now well established as a method of post-coital contraception. It appears to be more effective than hormonal methods, and can be used for up to 5 days after intercourse, compared with only 3 days for the most commonly used hormonal method (Bromwich 1985). However, IUD insertion carries risks of pelvic infection in the young woman who may have had multiple sexual partners (Yuzpe 1984).

Research is continuing into the use of medicated IUDs containing substances which might either decrease their adverse effects or increase their effectiveness. Progestasert, which contains progesterone, needs to be replaced every year. IUDs containing the more potent progestogen levonorgestrel have been tested (Fig. 16.4) and seem capable of being left in place for up

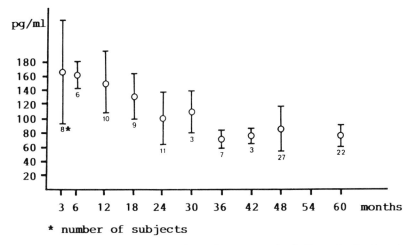

* number of subjects

Fig. 16.4   Mean ± SD, plasma concentrations of levonorgestrel at 3–60 months after insertion of a levonorgestrel-releasing IUD (from Nilsson et al 1986, with permission)

to 6 years (Nilsson et al 1986). It has been suggested on the basis of clinical trials that such devices have a high contraceptive efficacy and cause less alteration of the menstrual pattern than copper-containing devices, but this remains to be confirmed.

ANTIPROGESTINS

Mifepristone (RU486) is a competitive inhibitor of progesterone, acting at the level of the progesterone receptor (Das & Catt 1987), and is capable of interrupting early pregnancy when given either before or after the first missed period. In a study in Paris 100 women were given RU486 within 10 days of their missed period; 85 aborted, of whom 18% had prolonged vaginal bleeding, though curettage was not required. The remaining 15 women required evacuation of the uterus (Couzinet et al 1986). Other studies have included women treated during the luteal phase of the menstrual cycle. In a Dutch study 22 women were treated between days 24 and 27 of the cycle, and all menstruated by day 28 except one who had an anovulatory cycle (Haspels 1985). In America a similar study, carried out on monkeys, indicated that RU486 may be a safe and effective 'once a month' contraceptive (Nieman et al 1987).

'Epostane' is a compound that inhibits an enzyme involved in progesterone synthesis, and it can also interrupt pregnancy, though in order to do so it has to be given for 4 days and may not be successful in all cases (Birgerson et al 1986).

CONDOMS

The condom, one of the oldest methods of contraception, is now being strenuously promoted in the UK in an effort to prevent an epidemic of acquired immune deficiency syndrome (AIDS). (The impact of the advertising campaign quickly became noticeable in the readiness of patients to use the word 'condom'; until recently patients were uncertain about the acceptable terminology for this method of contraception.) The importance of condoms in reducing the spread of sexually transmitted disease was already being emphasised before AIDS became an important issue (Goldsmith 1986), particularly once it was demonstrated that herpes virus could not pass through condoms. It was subsequently confirmed that an AIDS-associated retrovirus cannot pass through condom membranes (Conant et al 1986), and the commonly used spermicide nonoxynol-9 inactivates human immuno-deficiency virus (HIV) in vitro at low concentrations (Wellings 1986). Some doubts have been raised as to whether natural condoms (made from sheep intestinal membranes) are as protective as latex rubber condoms, but natural condoms account for only 1% of the market (Minuk et al 1986, Grimes 1986). Doubts have also been expressed about the efficacy of condoms in preventing the transmission of HIV infection because of their tendency to fail occasionally (Goedert 1987, Kelly & St Lawrence 1987), but initial surveys of patterns of transmission suggest that condoms have an important role in reducing the spread of AIDS (Krogsgaard et al 1986, Mann et al 1987, Tovey 1987).

VAGINAL SPERMICIDES

Most chemical vaginal spermicides use a surfactant or detergent, which acts by disrupting the cell membrane and the midpiece of the sperm, causing rapid loss of motility. The most commonly used is nonoxynol-9, but although this compound is effective in the vagina, it does not impair sperm motility in cervical mucus; by contrast, chlorhexidine, which is now being studied as a spermicide, is effective in cervical mucus (Sharman et al 1986). The new vaginal contraceptive compound, ORF 13904, is a polystyrene polymer and appears to be more effective than nonoxynol-9. It seems to act by agglutinating spermatozoa, altering sperm–mucus interaction and inhibiting sperm acrosin (Foldesy et al 1986).

Side-effects

The question of whether spermicidal contraceptives can cause miscarriage or congenital abnormalities has been the subject of much discussion in the

USA. Extensive epidemiological studies have found no association between spermicides and congenital abnormalities (Bracken 1985, Mills & Alexander 1986), but litigation in America has been successful in spite of this clear scientific evidence (Mills & Alexander 1986).

Propranolol

The beta-blocker, propranolol, inhibits sperm motility in vitro and acts as a spermicide when administered vaginally (Zipper et al 1983). Orally administered propranolol is not concentrated in seminal plasma, and probably does not inhibit sperm motility (Mahajan et al 1984), but when given to women it is concentrated in cervical mucus, possibly because of 'pH trapping'. When an 80 mg tablet of D-propranolol was given to women by mouth, the maximal concentration in cervical mucus was similar to the concentration that inhibits sperm motility in vitro (Pearson et al 1984), but the contraceptive implications of this have not yet been investigated.

SPONGES

It had been hoped that the vaginal sponge, impregnated with nonoxynol-9, might become the female equivalent of the condom, but the failure rate of the 'Today' sponge in an American study was 17 per 100 woman years (Edelman et al 1984) and in a British study was up to 25% (Infield 1985, Skrine 1985). Research on a collagen sponge has now been discontinued because it was inconvenient to both partners, relatively ineffective and possibly unsafe (Chvapil 1985). An increased risk of toxic shock syndrome in sponge users has been suggested by an American study (Faich et al 1986), though the risk of death from this cause has been calculated to be as low as 0.1–0.6 per 100 000 woman years (Reingold 1986). A randomised cross-over study among prostitutes in Bangkok concluded that sponge users have less risk of infection with chlamydia or gonorrhoea but a higher risk of vaginal infection with candida (Rosenberg et al 1987).

CONTRACEPTIVE VACCINES

Immunisation against pregnancy is an attractive idea but difficult to achieve in practice. Theoretically a woman could be immunised against spermatozoa, or against the zona pellucida of the oocyte, or against chorionic gonadotrophin. Immunisation against spermatozoa is difficult to achieve (Voisin 1984). Immunisation against the zona pellucida is possible because cross-reactivity between the human zona and the zona of cows and sheep would allow hetero-immunisation (Aitken et al 1984). However, it is not known whether resting oocytes in primordial follicles are entirely devoid of antigens; if not, high antibody titres could damage these oocytes and lead to irreversible infertility.

Immunisation against chorionic gonadotrophin is the most promising of the 'vaccination' techniques, and antibodies have been raised in a variety of species. When a small number of women in India were immunised against beta-hCG, antibodies appeared after a lag of 6–8 weeks and the response lasted for over 1 year in some subjects, though antibody levels declined during this time (Thanavala et al 1984). Animal studies suggest that as antibody titres decline, conceptions can occur, followed by recurrent miscarriages which occur progressively later in pregnancy (Thanavala et al 1984). Current attempts at making a more effective vaccine include immunisation against the beta subunit of hCG together with its receptor (Saxena et al 1984), the linking of sheep luteinising hormone with tetanus toxoid (Talwar et al 1986) or the use of vaccine against only the C-terminal portion of the hCG molecule (Thanavala et al 1984). Using the third of these approaches, an antigen has been developed, coupled to diphtheria toxoid, and successfully tested in animals (Stevens 1986). This vaccine, which was developed with the help of the World Health Organization, is undergoing safety checks in trials involving sterilised human female volunteers in Australia (Jones et al 1988).

MALE CONTRACEPTION

Research is continuing into methods of suppressing spermatogenesis without affecting libido, but a 'male pill' remains a distant prospect because effective regimens are still too toxic or inconvenient for routine use.

GnRH analogues

In men, as in women, superactive analogues of gonadotrophin-releasing hormone (GnRH) produce 'downregulation' of pituitary receptors, and inhibit gonadotrophin secretion after an initial period of hyperstimulation (Leading Article 1987, Fraser & Baird 1987). They were initially administered by nasal spray, but implants or long-acting injectable forms are becoming available. GnRH analogues alone are unsuitable as male contraceptives because testosterone concentrations are reduced with a consequent loss of libido, and because spermatogenesis is not completely suppressed (Linde et al 1981). Attempts to combine agonistic and antagonistic analogues in order to suppress spermatogenesis completely have not so far been successful (Heber et al 1984). However, GnRH agonist administration, combined with testosterone therapy, may be able to blockade spermatogenesis while retaining normal libido (Tremblay et al 1984), and long-term trials of such regimens are in progress (Doelle et al 1983, Nillius 1984).

Steroids

Androgens produce a fall in gonadotrophin concentration through negative feedback, and this causes a fall in the sperm count, but high doses are required and this may lead to toxic effects. The anabolic steroid, 19-nortestosterone, however, may suppress spermatogenesis without side-effects or loss of potency (Knuth et al 1985). Androgens combined with oestrogens effectively suppress gonadotrophin secretion, but side-effects such as gynaecomastia make this combination unacceptable. Progestogens seem more satisfactory (Jackson & Schnieden 1982), and combinations of testosterone enanthate and levonorgestrel can produce oligospermia (Donaldson 1985), though azoospermia is produced in only 50% of cases (Knuth & Nieschlag 1987). However, the androgen has to be given by injection, and the effectiveness of the combination remains uncertain.

Anti-androgens

Anti-androgens produce a dose-dependent inhibition of spermatogenesis, and cyproterone acetate can inhibit spermatogenesis completely if given in sufficiently high dosage (Neumann 1984). Cyproterone acetate is thought to act on the epididymis, though there is evidence for an action on the Sertoli cells (Neumann 1984, Fredricsson & Carlstrom 1981). However, potency and libido are impaired.

Gossypol

In the 1950s, reports appeared that cooking with crude cottonseed oil caused infertility in males, and subsequent studies conducted mainly in China showed that gossypol—a pigment obtained from the cotton plant—is an effective anti-fertility agent. It appears to affect the development of spermatids and epididymal spermatozoa (Baccetti et al 1986). Trials of gossypol as an oral contraceptive began in 1972, and so far over 8000 men have been included. A dose of 20 mg/day for 75 days will produce infertility in 99% of subjects, and thereafter a maintenance dose of 50 mg/week is given. However, its clinical usefulness is limited by side-effects which include fatigue, gastrointestinal effects and hypokalaemia, and by the slowness of recovery after treatment is stopped (Jackson & Schnieden 1982). Recovery from gossypol treatment is time- and dose-related however (Hoffer & Lisser 1984), so an acceptable regimen may eventually be found (Liu et al 1986).

CONCLUSION

Refinements in the COC and the IUD, and better understanding of the relative contraindications to their use, have now made these methods extremely safe. New long-acting systems for delivering progestogens are very effective, but will probably be more popular in developing countries than in Britain. Anti-progestins may well be viewed with caution by the public because they act after implantation has begun. The 'male pill', though technically possible, seems unlikely to become popular. Contraceptive vaccines are still at an early stage of clinical testing. In the short term, the most likely change in contraception is increased use of condoms as protection against sexually transmitted disease. However, the pregnancy rate associated with the condom is 4% among highly motivated couples, and between 6 and 22% among less motivated users (Vessey & Mackintosh 1987), and it remains to be seen whether explicit public education will increase the contraceptive efficacy of the condom or make women less inclined to use more effective methods of contraception.

REFERENCES

Aitken R J, Richardson D W, Hulme M 1984 Immunological interference with the properties of the zona pellucida. In: Crighton D B (ed) Immunological aspects of reproduction in mammals, Butterworths, London, pp 305–325
Anonymous 1986 Professional confidence: doctors advised to assess child's maturity. British Medical Journal 292: 570
Baccetti B, Bigliardi E, Burrini A G, Renieri T, Selmi G 1986 The action of gossypol on rat germinal cells. Gamete Research 13: 1–17
Birgerson L, Odlind V, Johansson E D B 1986 Effects of Epostane on progesterone synthesis in early human pregnancy. Contraception 33: 401–410
Bowen-Simpkins P 1984 Contraception for the older woman. British Journal of Obstetrics and Gynaecology 91: 513–515
Bracken M B 1985 Spermicidal contraceptives and poor reproductive outcomes: the epidemiologic evidence against an association. American Journal of Obstetrics and Gynecology 151: 552–556
Bromwich P D 1985 Post-coital contraception. Practitioner 229: 427–429
Cancer and Steroid Hormone Study of the Centers for Disease Control 1986 Oral-contraceptive use and the risk of breast cancer. New England Journal of Medicine 315: 405–411
Chvapil M, Droegemueller W, Heine M W, MacGregor J C, Dotters D 1985 Collagen sponge as vaginal contraceptive barrier: critical summary of seven years of research. American Journal of Obstetrics and Gynecology 151: 325–329
Conant M, Hardy D, Sernatinger J, Spicer D, Levy J A 1986 Condoms prevent transmission of AIDS-associated retrovirus. Journal of the American Medical Association 255: 1706
Coutinho E M 1984 The vaginal pill and other new methods of contraception. Journal of Obstetrics and Gynecology 4(suppl 1): S11–S15
Couzinet B, Le Strat N, Ulmann A, Baulieu E M B, Schaison G 1986 Termination of early pregnancy by the progesterone antagonist RU486 (Mifepristone). New England Journal of Medicine 315: 1565–1570
Cramer D W, Schiff I, Schoenbaum S C et al 1985 Tubal infertility and the intrauterine device. New England Journal of Medicine 312: 941–947
Dalen J E, Hickler R B 1981 Oral contraceptives and cardiovascular disease. American Heart Journal 101: 626–639
Daling J R, Weiss N S, Metch B J et al 1985 Primary tubal infertility in relation to use of an IUD. New England Journal of Medicine 312: 937–941
Das C, Catt K J 1987 Antifertility actions of the progesterone antagonist RU486 include direct inhibition of placental hormone secretion. Lancet ii: 599–601
Doelle G C, Alexander A N, Evans R M et al 1983 Combined treatment with an LHRH agonist and testosterone in man. Journal of Andrology 4: 298–302
Donaldson D 1985 Male contraception—a review. Journal of the Royal Society of Health 105: 91–98
Drife J O 1986 Breast development in puberty. Annals of the New York Academy of Sciences 464: 58–65
Drife J, Guillebaud J 1986 Hormonal contraception and cancer. British Journal of Hospital Medicine 35: 25–29

Drug and Therapeutics Bulletin 1986 Medical factors in contraceptive choice. Drug and Therapeutics Bulletin 19: 73–76

Dyer C 1985 Contraceptives and the under 16s: House of Lords ruling. British Medical Journal 291: 1208–1209

Edelman D A, McIntyre S L, Harper J 1984 A comparative trial of the Today contraceptive sponge and diaphragm. American Journal of Obstetrics and Gynecology 150: 869–876

Elder MG 1984 Injectable contraception. Clinics in Obstetrics and Gynaecology II: 723–741

Elias J 1985 Intra-uterine contraceptive devices. Practitioner 229: 431–436

Elkik F, Basdevant A, Jackanicz T M et al 1986 Contraception in hypertensive women using a vaginal ring delivering estradiol and levonorgestrel. Journal of Clinical Endocrinology and Metabolism 63: 29–35

Elstein M, Nuttall I D 1985 The progestagen releasing vaginal ring. Journal of Obstetrics and Gynaecology 5(suppl 2): S51–S57

Faich G, Pearson K, Fleming D, Sobel S, Anello C 1986 Toxic shock syndrome and the vaginal contraceptive sponge. Journal of the American Medical Association 255: 216–218

Foldesy R G, Homm R E, Levinson S L, Hahn D W 1986 Multiple actions of a novel vaginal contraceptive compound, ORF 13904. Fertility and Sterility 45: 550–555

Fotherby K 1984 A new look at progestogens. Clinics in Obstetrics and Gynaecology 11: 701–722

Fotherby K 1985 Oral contraceptives, lipids and cardiovascular disease. Contraception 31: 367–394

Fraser H M, Baird D T 1987 Clinical applications of LHRH analogues. Baillière's Clinical Endocrinology and Metabolism 1: 43–70

Fredricsson B, Carlstrom K 1981 Effects of low doses of cyproterone acetate on sperm morphology and some other parameters of reproduction in normal men. Andrologia 13: 369–375

Goedert J J 1987 What is safe sex? New England Journal of Medicine 316: 1339–1342

Goldsmith M F 1986 Sexually transmitted diseases may reverse the 'revolution'. Journal of the American Medical Association 255: 1665–1667, 1672

Grimes D A 1986 Reversible contraception for the 1980s. Journal of the American Medical Association 255: 69–75

Haspels A A 1985 Interruption of early pregnancy by an anti-progestational compound, RU486. European Journal of Obstetrics, Gynecology, and Reproductive Biology 20: 169–175

Havard J D J 1986 Teenagers and contraception. British Medical Journal 292: 508–509

Heber D, Dodson R, Peterson M, Channabasavaiah K C, Stewart J M, Swerdloff R S 1984 Counteractive effects of agonistic and antagonistic gonadotropin releasing hormone analogs on spermatogenesis: sites of action. Fertility and Sterility 41: 309–313

Hoffer A P, Lisser S P 1984 Recovery of normal testicular ultrastructure and sperm mobility after cessation of gossypol treatment in rats. Journal of Andrology 5: 416–423

Illman J 1986 Implications of the Copper 7's demise, GP November 28, p 37

Infield J 1985 Barrier methods of contraception. Journal of Obstetrics and Gynaecology 5(suppl 2): S58–S59

Jackson H, Schnieden H 1982 Aspects of male reproductive pharmacology and toxicology. Reviews in Pure and Applied Pharmacological Sciences 3: 1–81

Ji G, Hong-zhu S, Gui-ying S, Li-yuan M 1986 Clinical investigation of a low-dose levonorgestrel-releasing vaginal ring. Fertility and Sterility 46: 626–630

Jones W R, Bradley J, Judd S J et al 1988 Phase 1 clinical trial of the W.H.O. birth control vaccine. Lancet i: 1295–1298

Kay C R 1980 The happiness pill? Journal of the Royal College of General Practitioners 30: 8–19

Kelly J A, St Lawrence J S 1987 Cautions about condoms in prevention of AIDS. Lancet i: 323

Khoo S K 1986 Cancer risks and the contraceptive pill. Medical Journal of Australia 144: 185–190

Knuth U A, Nieschlag E 1987 Endocrine approaches to male fertility control. Baillière's Clinical Endocrinology and Metabolism 1: 113–131

Knuth U A, Behre H, Belkien L, Bents H, Nieschlag E 1985 Clinical trial of 19-nortestosterone-hexoxyphenylpropionate (Anadur) for male fertility regulation. Fertility and Sterility 44: 814–821

Krogsgaard K, Gluud C, Pedersen C et al 1986 Widespread use of condoms and low prevalence of sexually transmitted diseases in Danish non-drug addict prostitutes. British Medical Journal 293: 1473–1474

Landgren B M, Aedo A R, Cekan S Z, Diczfalusy E 1986 Pharmacokinetic studies with a vaginal delivery system releasing levonorgestrel at a near zero order rate for one year. Contraception 33: 473–485

Leading Article 1986 Oral contraceptives and breast cancer. Lancet ii: 665–666

Leading Article 1987 LHRH analogues for contraception. Lancet i: 1179–1181

Linde R, Doelle G C, Alexander N et al 1981 Reversible inhibition of testicular steroidogenesis and spermatogenesis by a potent gonadotropin-releasing hormone agonist in normal men. New England Journal of Medicine 305: 663–667

Liu G Z, Lyle K C, Cao J 1986 Experiences with gossypol as a male pill. Paper presented at 12th World Congress on Fertility and Sterility, Singapore

Longstreth W T, Swanson P D 1984 Oral contraceptives and stroke. Stroke 15: 747–750

Loudon N B 1985 Progestogen-only pills. In: Loudon N B, Newton J R (eds) Handbook of family planning, Churchill Livingstone, Edinburgh, pp 99–113

Loudon N B, Kirkman R J A, Dewsbury J A, Lee B, Tolowinska I 1988 Multicentre study comparing the efficacy, cycle control and tolerance of a new oral contraceptive, Femodene, and Microgynon 30 for six cycles. British Journal of Family Planning (in press)

Mahajan P, Grech E D, Pearson R M, Ridgway E J, Turner P 1984 Propranolol concentrations in blood serum, seminal plasma and saliva in man after a single oral dose. British Journal of Clinical Pharmacology 18: 849–852

Mann J, Quinn T C, Piot P et al 1987 Condom use and HIV infection among prostitutes in Zaire. New England Journal of Medicine 316: 345

McEwan J 1985 Hormonal contraceptive methods. Practitioner 229: 415–423

McPherson K, Drife J O 1986 The pill and breast cancer: why the uncertainty? British Medical Journal 293: 709–710

Meirik O, Lund E, Adami H O, Bergstrom R, Christoffersen T, Bergsjo P 1986 Oral contraceptive use and breast cancer in young women: a joint national case-control study in Sweden and Norway. Lancet ii: 650–654

Mills J L, Alexander D 1986 Teratogens and 'litogens'. New England Journal of Medicine 315: 1234–1236

Minuk G Y, Bohme C E, Bowen T J, Hoar D I, Cassol S 1986 Condoms and the prevention of AIDS. Journal of the American Medical Association 256: 1442–1443

Mishell D R 1985 Current status of intrauterine devices. New England Journal of Medicine 312: 984–985

Neumann F 1984 Effects of drugs and chemicals on spermatogenesis. Archives of Toxicology 7(suppl): 109–117

Nieman L K, Choate T M, Chrousos G P et al 1987 The progesterone antagonist RU486: a potential new contraceptive agent. New England Journal of Medicine 316: 187–191

Nillius S J 1984 Luteinising hormone releasing hormone analogues for contraception. Clinics in Obstetrics and Gynaecology 11: 551–572

Nilsson C G, Lahteenmaki P L A, Luukkainen T, Robertson D N 1986 Sustained intrauterine release of levonorgestrel over five years. Fertility and Sterility 45: 805–807

Paul C, Skegg D C G, Spears G F S, Kaldor J M 1986 Oral contraceptives and breast cancer: a national study. British Medical Journal 293: 723–726

Pearson R M, Ridgway E J, Johnston A, Vadukul J 1984 Concentration of D-propranolol in cervicovaginal mucus. Lancet ii: 1480

Pike M C, Henderson B E, Krailo M D, Duke A, Roy S 1983 Breast cancer in young women and use of oral contraceptives: possible modifying effect of formulation and age at use. Lancet ii: 926–930

Realini J P, Goldzieher J W 1985 Oral contraceptives and cardiovascular disease: a critique of the epidemiologic studies. American Journal of Obstetrics and Gynecology 152: 729–798

Reingold A L 1986 Toxic shock syndrome and the contraceptive sponge. Journal of the American Medical Association 255: 242–243

Rosenberg M J, Rojanapithayakorn W, Feldblum P J, Higgins J E 1987 Effect of the contraceptive sponge on chlamydial infection, gonorrhea, and candidiasis. Journal of the American Medical Association 257: 2308–2312

Sartwell P E, Stolley P D 1982 Oral contraceptives and vascular disease. Epidemiologic Reviews 4: 95–109

Saxena B B, Landesman R, Gupta G N, Singh M, Rathnam P, Dattatreyamurty B 1984 New approaches in fertility regulation. Journal of Obstetrics and Gynaecology 4(suppl 1): S16–S22

Segal S 1983 The development of Norplant implants. Studies in Family Planning 14: 159–163

Sharman D, Chantler E, Dukes M, Hutchinson F G, Elstein M 1986 Comparison of the action of nonoxynol-9 and chlorhexidine on sperm. Fertility and Sterility 45: 259–264

Shearman R P 1986 Oral contraceptive agents. Medical Journal of Australia 144: 201–205

Skrine R L 1985 Barrier methods of contraception. Practitioner 229: 441–446

Snowden R 1985 Is the Dalkon shield more dangerous than other IUCDs? British Medical Journal 291: 1203–1204

Stevens V C 1986 Use of synthetic peptides as immunogens for developing a vaccine against human chorionic gonadotropin. In: Porter R, Whelan J (eds) Synthetic peptides as antigens (CIBA Foundation Symposium 119), Wiley, Chichester, pp 200–225

Talwar G P, Singh O, Singh V et al 1986 Enhancement of antigonadotropin response to the beta-subunit of ovine luteinizing hormone by carrier conjugation and combination with the beta-subunit of human chorionic gonadotropin. Fertility and Sterility 46: 120–126

Thanavala Y M, Hay F C, Roitt I M 1984 Fertility control by immunization against hCG. In: Crighton D B (ed) Immunological aspects of reproduction in mammals, Butterworths, London, pp 327–343

Tovey S J 1987 Condoms and AIDS prevention. Lancet i: 567

Tremblay Y, Belanger A, Lacoste D, Giasson M, Labrie F 1984 Selective inhibition of spermatogenesis in the presence of normal libido following combined treatment with an LHRH agonist and testosterone in the dog. Contraception 30: 585–598

Vessey M P 1980 Female hormones and vascular disease—an epidemiological overview. British Journal of Family Planning 6(suppl): 1–12

Vessey M P, Mackintosh L V 1987 Condoms and AIDS prevention. Lancet i: 568

Vessey M P, Lawless M, McPherson K, Yeates D 1983 Neoplasia of the cervix uteri and contraception: a possible adverse effect of the pill. Lancet ii: 930–934

Vessey M P, Lawless M, Yeates D 1984 Oral contraceptives and stroke: findings in a large prospective study. British Medical Journal 289: 530–531

Voisin G A 1984 Active immunization against sperm and sperm autoantigens. In: Crighton D B (ed) Immunological aspects of reproduction in mammals, Butterworths, London, pp 291–303

Wellings K 1986 AIDS and the condom. British Medical Journal 293: 1259–1260

Wellings K, Mills A 1984 Contraceptive trends. British Medical Journal 289: 939–940

World Health Organization (WHO) 1985 Facts about an implantable contraceptive: memorandum from a WHO meeting. Bulletin of the World Health Organization 63: 485–494

Yuzpe A A 1984 Postcoital contraception. Clinics in Obstetrics and Gynaecology 11: 787–797

Zipper J, Wheeler R G, Potts D M, Rivera M 1983 Propranolol as a novel, effective spermicide: preliminary findings. British Medical Journal 287: 1245–1246

Diseases of prostitutes

HISTORICAL INTRODUCTION

Prostitution is often called the 'oldest profession'. However, although it has certainly existed since ancient times (Bess & Janus 1976), it would be more accurate to describe it as a service industry. As such, sexually transmitted infections constitute the prostitutes' industrial diseases. The high incidence of sexually transmitted disease (STD) and their sequelae in female prostitutes first attracted organised medical interest in the UK during the early nineteenth century. The compulsory medical inspection of prostitutes was first performed in an attempt to reduce the prevalence of syphilis, the public concern of which had given rise to the maxim: 'One night with Venus, and a lifetime with Mercury' (Burnham 1971). However, the system of compulsory medical examinations did not flourish as more liberal attitudes in both the UK and the USA developed in the latter part of the nineteenth century. Although eminent London physicians such as William Acton (1857) and military doctors argued strongly in favour of compulsory inspection to reduce the spread of venereal disease, the belief in individual morality combined with better access to individual treatment has prevailed until the present day. Moreover, despite the efforts of Acton in London and Sanger (1858) in New York, the medical care of prostitutes in the nineteenth century in both the UK and the USA failed to contribute significantly to the knowledge of venereal diseases.

The medical care of prostitutes is dependent on the resources available and the inclination of the women to first seek and then accept treatment. Thus the legal and social attitudes towards prostitution determine the standard of care which can be given as well as the facilities for research. Although since 1916 in the UK there has been a free and confidential service for the treatment of venereal diseases, no special provisions have been made for female prostitutes. Other European countries, notably Holland and West Germany, have legislated to provide regular medical examinations for female prostitutes, but their medical care in the UK remains fragmented, with many women seeking treatment in the private sector. The only official statistics available are of convictions for soliciting, which are dependent on the vigour of the police to arrest and the magistrates to convict. Although such figures are increasing, they fail to provide an accurate assessment of the current numbers of women engaged in prostitution, and give no information whatsoever of their medical and social problems. The recent World Health Organization (WHO) guidelines for the control of sexually transmitted diseases (WHO 1985) include female prostitutes amongst the priority groups to which targeted control activities should be directed. Although the spread of infection with human immunodeficiency virus (HIV) has polarised the medical, political and public awareness of the role of the prostitute as a possible vector for infection, history shows that the recognition of this role for other diseases has failed to lead to appropriate action in the past.

DEFINITION OF A FEMALE PROSTITUTE

Female prostitution has been defined as 'the practice in which a woman surrenders her body for some gainful consideration to someone who otherwise is not entitled to have sexual intercourse with her' (Batria 1967), or 'any sexual exchange where the reward for the prostitute is neither sexual or affectionate' (James 1977), or those who 'habitually gain their livelihoods ... by the proceeds of sexual relations' (Acton 1857). Although these definitions are both value-laden and incomplete, they serve to reflect societal attitudes towards prostitution. However, it is essential to ensure that any research into the diseases of female prostitutes carefully defines its study group to exclude, and allow comparison with, the role of 'promiscuous amateurs' in the epidemiology of STD (Rosenthal & Vandow 1958).

FEMALE PROSTITUTION AND STD

The results of studies of the prevalence of STD in female prostitutes show marked geographical variation, depending on the reliability of the diagnostic tests used, the efficacy of the therapeutic regimens given, the number of unprotected sexual exposures, the prevalence of STD in their clients, and the transmissibility of the pathogens to which they are exposed (Darrow 1984).

The earliest study to demonstrate the role of the prostitute as a reservoir for STD was performed in 1832 by Parent-Duchatelet (1857) in Paris. This showed that, of the 3558 registered prostitutes, 936 had been compulsorily treated for syphilis. Moreover, the comparative case rates for syphilis were 1.9 per 100 public prostitutes, 3.7 per 100 brothel inmates, 1.1 per 100 freelance prostitutes and 22.3 per 100 unregistered prostitutes. Meanwhile, in London, Acton (1857) was referring to over 1500 women 'spreading abroad a loathsome poison ...', and in New York, Sanger (1858) had described

29% of female prostitutes as having had syphilis and 14% as having had gonorrhoea. However, more reliable figures had to wait for the turn of the century and improvements in diagnostic techniques, such as the Gram stain and the identification of the gonococcus by Neisser, and the observation of the treponeme by Schaudinn and Hoffman.

The primacy of the role of the female prostitute as an important vector for the transmission of STD was unquestioned until 1958, when Rosenthal and Vandow concluded that although prostitutes accounted for 10% of the STD amongst military personnel in New York, over 80% was acquired from casual sexual contact with 'promiscuous amateurs'. The main STD occurring in both groups was gonorrhoea, with the marked decline in the incidence of syphilis in the post-penicillin era. Similar conclusions were drawn by Willcox (1962), after he had reviewed the international incidence of prostitute-derived STD for a WHO study. He noted that less than 20% of the STD in the UK and USA was acquired from prostitutes, whereas 30% in France and over 80% in Asia was derived from this source. Furthermore, he noted that the recipients of the STD from prostitutes in all these countries tended to be travellers, migrant workers and military personnel rather than the indigenous population.

In an attempt to ascertain the effects of the 1959 Street Offences Act on the prostitutes of Sheffield, Turner & Morton (1976) assessed their socio-legal, as well as their medical problems. They found that the legislation had not resulted in a reduction in the numbers of practising female prostitutes. Furthermore, their study group of 60 women accounted for one-sixth of all the cases of locally acquired gonorrhoea in men, this figure being increased at times of intense police endeavours to control prostitution by increased arrests. This study also noted that female prostitutes suffered from an increased incidence of salpingitis associated with gonorrhoea. They concluded that prostitutes constituted a group which needed a special contact tracing and health education approach to reduce their role as a reservoir for *Neisseria gonorrhoeae* infections. This view was shared by an American study (Potterat et al 1979) which showed that 27% of urethral gonorrhoea in men in Colorado Springs was acquired from just 56 female prostitutes. In Central Africa, over 50% of the 86 female prostitutes studied were infected by cervical gonorrhoea, with 90% of these being asymptomatic (Meheus & De Clerq 1974). These findings support the epidemiological model proposed for the transmission of gonorrhoea (Morton 1977) based on a core of highly sexually active individuals acting as both the reservoir and primary vectors for infection. The arguments that the identification and treatment of this group would significantly reduce the incidence of gonorrhoea in the overall population have gone unheeded in the UK.

With the increasing availability of accurate diagnostic techniques for STD, several studies of the prevalence of conditions other than gonorrhoea and syphilis have been performed on female prostitutes. In a study in Iran, where prostitutes were compulsorily registered and medically examined, Darougar et al (1983) found 94% of the women tested had serological evidence of infection with *Chlamydia trachomatis*, although only 7% of cervical swabs taken from the same women resulted in culture of this organism. They concluded that female prostitutes were acting as a reservoir for this infection, and explained the discrepancy in their results by the common practice of self-medication with antibiotics in their study group causing failure of the cell cultures.

In 1972, Duenas et al described twice the prevalence of herpes simplex virus (HSV) infection in female prostitutes compared with women attending an STD clinic; moreover, they noted a higher incidence of recurrent genital infection in the former group. At the time of this study, their findings were used to explain the increased occurrence of cervical carcinoma in female prostitutes which had been previously recognised (Peryra 1961, Moghissi et al 1968). However, although subsequent work (Singer et al 1976, Campion et al 1985) now implicates human papillomavirus infection as the primary aetiological factor for the development of cervical neoplasia, genital HSV infection may still be an important cofactor (Fish et al 1982). Despite evidence that prostitutes were at 4.7 times the risk of developing cervical cancer (Rojel 1953), a survey of 750 prostitutes in Taipei failed to show an increased risk (Sebastian et al 1978). This may have been because the mean coitarche of the women studied was at the comparatively late age of 18 years, or because of the absence of cofactors (e.g. smoking tobacco), or because of the high use of condoms by their clients which may have resulted in the relatively low rate of gonorrhoea (8%) in the women studied.

Following the recognition that hepatitis B may be acquired by sexual transmission (Hersh et al 1971), studies of the prevalence of the hepatitis B serological profiles of female prostitutes gave support to the importance of this mode of transmission. Frosner et al (1975) found a significant three-fold increase in the prevalence of hepatitis B surface antibody in prostitutes compared with age-matched controls in West Germany. Moreover, there was a strong positive association between the duration of prostitution, the frequency of other STD and the acquisition of hepatitis B infection. In a similar study by Papaevengolou et al (1974) of Greek female prostitutes, the results again showed a significant 2.5 times risk of the acquisition of hepatitis B by this group. However, neither study compared the female prostitutes against a group of equally promiscuous non-prostitute women, nor was any comparison made between prostitutes who did and did not have a history of parenteral drug abuse.

In an attempt to investigate whether the increased prevalence of STD in Chinese prostitutes was related to an inherited immunological susceptibility, Chan et al (1979) examined the HLA profile of 148 unrelated female prostitutes and compared this with their STD history. The results suggested that the possession of the A11–B15 gene locus was associated with a reduced acquisition of syphilis and gonorrhoea. Although their sample was too small to attribute statistical significance to these results, further research into the immunological status of female prostitutes including careful comparisons with control groups are needed.

Recent studies

Although many of the aforementioned studies yielded interesting data on various groups of female prostitutes, there was a lack of any data compiled on the follow-up of a group of prostitutes over a period of time. Most studies have involved measuring the number of cases of a particular STD in a group of female prostitutes at the time of screening.

The problems of recruiting a group for the longitudinal study of all the sexually transmitted infections as well as for the social and psychological characteristics of female prostitutes have recently been tackled by several research groups.

Firstly, Donovan (1984) surmounted the problem of waiting for self-recruitment to his project by persuading the manager of a massage parlour in Sydney, Australia, that it was in his best interests to allow regular on-site check-ups of the women in his establishment. To this end, the investigator performed weekly screening of 70 women for syphilis, gonorrhoea and trichomoniasis. New gonococcal infections occurred in 10% of these women each week, but the women affected were not predictable on the basis of clinical symptoms or signs. Donovan argues that as the incidence of gonorrhoea amongst new prostitutes was 44%, the lower figure of 10% amongst women already on his study demonstrates the beneficial effects of the screening and treatment programme that he was conducting. In addition, he collected many interesting data on the lack of contraceptive use, the high incidence of unwanted pregnancy and the social problems faced by female prostitutes in Sydney. The limitation of this study was the lack of easily transportable diagnostic facilities to the massage parlour, and hence the absence of tests for *C. trachomatis* and HSV infection.

Secondly, a study (Nayyar et al 1986) performed in New York City, the USA and Rotterdam, Holland, extended the range of screening for STD to include several pathogens not previously reported to have an increased incidence in female prostitutes. Their results showed that the incidence of *N. gonorrhoeae* infection had not declined since 1958, and that genital *C. trachomatis* infections are numerically a more serious problem than gonorrhoea in prostitutes. Furthermore, the high incidence of cervical isolates of *Mycoplasma hominis* and *Ureaplasma urealyticum* in female prostitutes corroborated the association of these organisms with a high frequency of sexual partners (McCormack et al 1983). It was also noted that the incidence of trichomoniasis amongst these women was low, and this was attributed to the habit of douching with antiseptics between partners. Although this study widened the spectrum of STD that it was testing for, it was confined to women in brothels and did not involve follow-up.

In an attempt to combine the screening of a wider range of STD with the longitudinal documentation of the behaviour of female prostitutes, a study at the Praed Street Clinic, London, was carried out (Barton et al 1986). Fifty women were examined fortnightly for up to 1 year. The inherent bias of recruitment from patients attending this STD clinic was weighed against the value of long-term follow-up. The subgroups of prostitutes attending were representative of the different types of prostitute in London (Paterson-Brown & Finnerty 1986), categorised by their site of work, i.e. street based, escort agency based, brothel based, advertised private flat based and nightclub based. During the period of the study 28% of the women had at least one episode of gonorrhoea, and 46% had at least one episode of urogenital infection by *C. trachomatis*. The prevalence of genital warts was 6%, but 10% of the women had cytological evidence of cervical intra-epithelial neoplasia. Moreover, four cases of asymptomatic cervical shedding of HSV type 2, six cases of pediculosis pubis and one case of secondary syphilis were diagnosed during the study period.

A major feature of this study was the attempt to investigate the prevalence of HIV infection in London prostitutes, as studies from elsewhere (see Table 17.1) had shown widely varying levels of seropositivity. During the study

Table 17.1   Prevalence of HIV antibody in female prostitutes

Location	Total tested	% positive	Reference
Rwanda	33	88	Van de Perre et al (1985)
Seattle	92	5	CDC (1985)
Florida	25	40	CDC (1985)
Athens	200	6	Papaevengolou et al (1985)
Paris	56	0	Brenky-Fadeux & Fribourg-Blanc (1985)
Pordenone	14 (IVDA)	71	Tirelli et al (1985)
	10 (non-IVDA)	0	

IVDA = intravenous drug abuser

period one woman was found to be infected by HIV; she was asymptomatic but had used intravenous heroin with shared needles and had a history of hepatitis B. Other studies (Tirelli et al 1985, Brenky-Fadeux & Fribourg-Blanc 1985) have also demonstrated that, in Europe, female prostitutes who are not intravenous drug users are not yet at an increased risk of having acquired HIV infection.

However, this apparent absence of current infection does not mean that prostitutes without a history of intravenous drug abuse are not at a high risk of acquiring HIV infection in the future. In particular, the epidemic curve used to estimate the future number of AIDS cases (McEvoy & Tillett 1985) may not yet have reached the gradient of increase needed to result in sufficient transmission to new cases to allow detection except by mass screening. For this reason, all female prostitutes have continued to be classified as a high-risk category for the acquisition of HIV infection (Pinching & Jeffries 1985, Minkoff & Schwarz 1986, Johnson 1988).

PSYCHOSEXUAL CHARACTERISTICS AND PROBLEMS IN FEMALE PROSTITUTES AND THEIR CLIENTS

James and Meyerding (1977) found evidence that female prostitutes enter this occupation because of negative sexual experiences during their childhood. The street prostitutes studied showed a pattern of a lack of parental guidance leading to early, casual sexual intercourse. There was also a high incidence of incest and rape during their adolescence, and an early formation of the belief that sex could be used to gain social status. The early coitarche of prostitutes was also noted by Duenas et al (1972) to be 15.3 years compared with 18.8 years in controls. There is strong evidence that childhood prostitution itself is becoming increasingly common in most large cities in Europe and America (Sereny 1985).

Although female prostitutes have multiple sexual partners, this does not exclude them from experiencing problems during intercourse with their non-client partners. Some evidence of this was gained in the Praed Street Clinic (PSC) study (Barton et al 1986), with 80% of the women studied experiencing deep dyspareunia on a regular basis and 50% needing to use vaginal lubricants. However, 50% of the women had experienced orgasm during sexual intercourse with a client, and 12% of these had only experienced orgasm with clients, despite having regular boyfriends. Both sexual and psychological problems were more common in the women who worked from the street, and lowest in escort agency based prostitutes. The finding that most of the psychopathology associated with prostitution is concentrated in street-based workers was first proposed by Exner et al in 1977. Further studies into these problems are in progress, especially whether the deep dyspareunia noted above is due to a psychosexual cause or the more likely result of pelvic adhesions formed as the sequelae of pelvic infection.

The clients

Further study of the clients of prostitutes was performed in 1960 by Gibbens and Silberman. They found that only 15% of their sample ever used the same prostitute more than once, and that in making their choice on the street, clients showed a preference for girls who appeared 'motherly'. Most importantly, they noted the great difficulty in obtaining accurate histories from such men. This problem accounts for the continued paucity of data on the characteristics and rates of STD in the clients of female prostitutes. A recent study by Donovan (1984) had to abandon screening the male clients of his study group for similar practical reasons; however, he did detect five cases of asymptomatic urethral gonorrhoea in this group. Further details about the clients of massage parlours emerged from a study (Simpson & Schill 1977) in Illinois which showed that 58% were married, 75% initiated the sexual contact and 38% were unable to reach orgasm within 5 minutes of intercourse.

IMPROVED MANAGEMENT OF THE DISEASES OF FEMALE PROSTITUTES

Better identification

In order to improve the delivery of health care to female prostitutes, it is essential to be able to identify the women themselves. In the UK this has relied on women attending STD clinics and declaring their occupation or being arrested by the police and submitted to a compulsory medical examination. However, many female prostitutes are seen in STD clinics without stating their true occupation, hence appropriate diagnostic tests or counselling may be omitted. Moreover, although Conrad et al (1981) have demonstrated that screening convicted prostitutes is an effective way of identifying untreated cases of STD, the more assiduous pursuance of prostitutes by the police has been shown to result in an increase in the cases of STD in their clients (Turner & Morton 1976). Over 90% of the prostitutes in the PSC study (Barton et al 1986) supported the introduction of compulsory medical examinations for all prostitutes, and 80% felt that it should be made an offence for a prostitute to work whilst she knew she had an infectious STD. However, to introduce compulsory medical examinations would require the registering or licensing of prostitutes; although 68% of the PSC study supported the formation of licensed brothels, only 38% said that they would work in them. It is essential that if the WHO (1985) recommendation of directing health screening and education specifically towards female prostitutes is to be implemented, a system of licensing or registering will have to be introduced in association with the decriminalisation of prostitution. Until that time, medical contact with prostitutes should be fostered by discussion with the representative groups (e.g. The English Prostitutes Collective) formed by prostitutes themselves. A lead in the official recognition of such groups has been made by the European Parliament, who hosted the Second World Whores Congress in October 1986.

Better diagnostic facilities

The availability of quicker diagnostic tests for STD are of special benefit to prostitutes. The delay in waiting for a confirmatory culture to exclude an STD or confirm the efficacy of treatment is a major problem for prostitutes. Advice from doctors to avoid sexual intercourse until a result is known would mean lost earnings, and often goes unheeded. The recent introduction of direct monoclonal antibody kits for the diagnosis of infections by *N. gonorrhoeae*, *C. trachomatis* and HSV give the facility for the 'results-while-you-wait' approach to be made more accurate and extensive. The value of instant results and appropriate treatment in this special target group will reduce the problems of poor compliance. Furthermore, the increased availability to gynaecologists of quicker diagnostic tests should allow more comprehensive screening of female prostitutes for STD when they attend with other problems such as unwanted pregnancy, abnormal cervical smears and chronic pelvic pain.

Better health education

Although further studies may reveal valuable data on the prevalence of STD in female prostitutes, the existing information overwhelmingly demonstrates that the female prostitute is a major reservoir and vector for genital infections. Moreover, there is evidence that both hepatitis B and HIV infections do infect female prostitutes by sexual transmission, and thus may be transmitted to their clients. Given that prostitution cannot be eradicated, appropriate health education should be directed at these women to attempt to reduce their chances of contracting new STD. This involves recommending the use of condoms by all their clients, as both HSV and HIV have been shown to be unable to penetrate sheaths (Conant et al 1984, Conant et al 1986), and the associated use of spermicides has been found to hasten the inactivation of HIV (Hicks et al 1985). Moreover, the incidence of gonorrhoea has been shown to be lower in men who correctly used condoms (Barlow 1977). In the PSC study, 60% of the prostitutes claimed that, since they had heard of AIDS, they insisted on condoms for all types of intercourse; however, 80% of these admitted that they made exceptions to this rule for regular clients. In view of the occurrence of asymptomatic gonorrhoea in the regular clients noted by Donovan (1984), these men may constitute an important vector for re-infection. Moreover, the high frequency of ruptured condoms noted by prostitutes, especially during oral and anal intercourse (Barton et al 1985) should lead to improvements in condom design. This protection should reduce the acquisition of new STD, and may also result in a reduction in the number of unwanted pregnancies in these women, although additional hormonal contraceptive measures are advised. Indeed, calls have been made (Wellings 1986) in the UK for the government to provide free condoms—a measure which may encourage prostitutes, amongst others, to use them.

Better informed clients

Public health measures should be directed at the clients of prostitutes to increase their appreciation of the protection afforded by condom use and the need for regular medical examinations. In the PSC study, 80% of prostitutes felt that it should be illegal for a client to have sexual intercourse with them if they knew that they had an infectious STD. Although such a view may seem unrealistic, it emphasises the feeling of prostitutes in this study that 'something must be done' to protect them from HIV infection.

Better resources

All the above measures to improve the medical management of female prostitutes with the goal of reducing the prevalence of STD and associated problems in both them and the whole population are dependent on the recognition that female prostitutes constitute a group meriting special attention. This group needs special resource allocation, medical and social research and health education directed at it. Several studies have demonstrated the willingness of female prostitutes to accept regular screening for STD and also their desire for more comprehensive health education. But although there has been widespread media recognition that HIV infection may be acquired from sexual contact with female prostitutes (Wilsher & Hodgkinson 1986), history has shown us that it is unlikely that there will be a major change in the legal status of these women in the UK. In addition to the problem of HIV infection, other STD such as cervical human papillomavirus infection and chlamydial salpingitis results in the major morbidity of cervical intra-epithelial neoplasia (CIN) and tubal damage respectively. The combined financial burden on society of AIDS, CIN, ectopic pregnancy and tubal infertility may make the improvement in the care of female prostitutes an economic necessity.

CONCLUSION

The epidemiology of HIV merely emphasises the need to be able to identify and communicate with female prostitutes as a group. Health education, screening and the prevention of STD in female prostitutes remains an essential priority for the well-being of the prostitutes, their clients and the public health of society. The acquisition of STD and their sequelae, as well as unwanted pregnancy and psychosexual problems, may result in the female prostitute being seen by a gynaecologist. The recognition of the range of their health problems is essential for the correct management of this special risk group.

REFERENCES

Acton W 1972 Prostitution considered in its moral, social and sanitary aspects, Cassell, London
Barlow D 1977 The condom and gonorrhoea. Lancet ii: 811–813
Barton S E, Underhill G S,. Gilchrist C, Jeffries D J, Harris J R W 1985 HTLV-III antibody in prostitutes (letter). Lancet ii: 1424
Barton S E, Link C M, Underhill G S, Munday P E, Taylor-Robinson D, Harris J R W 1986 A longitudinal study of prostitutes in London, presented to Second World Congress on STD, Paris, France
Batria P 1967 The criminal aspects of prostitution. International Criminal Police Review 206: 80
Bess B E, Janus S S 1976 Prostitution. In: Sadock B J et al (eds) The sexual experience, Williams & Wilkins, Baltimore
Brenky-Fadeux D, Fribourg-Blanc A 1985 HTLV-III antibody in prostitutes (letter). Lancet ii: 1424
Burnham J C 1971 Medical inspection of prostitutes in America in the nineteenth century; the St. Louis experiment and its sequel. Bulletin of the History of Medicine 45: 203–218
Campion M J, Singer A, Clarkson P K, McCance D J 1985 Increased risk of cervical neoplasia in the consorts of men with penile condyloma acuminata. Lancet i: 943–945
CDC 1985 Heterosexual transmission of human T-cell lymphotropic virus type III/ lymphadenopathy-associated virus. Morbidity and Mortality Weekly Report 34(37): 561–563

Chan S H, Tan T, Kamarudin A, Wee G B, Rajan V S 1979 HLA and sexually transmitted diseases in prostitutes. British Journal of Venereal Diseases 55: 207–210

Conant M A, Spicer D W, Smith C D 1984 Herpes simplex virus transmission; condom studies. Sexually Transmitted Diseases 11(2): 94–95

Conant M A, Hardy D, Sernatinger J, Spicer D, Levy J A 1986 Condoms prevent transmission of AIDS associated retrovirus. Journal of the American Medical Association 255: 1706

Conrad G L, Kleris G S, Rush B, Darrow W W 1981 Sexually transmitted disease among prostitutes and other sexual offenders. Sexually Transmitted Diseases 8(4): 241–244

Darougar S, Aramesh B, Gibson J A, Treharne J D, Jones B R 1983 Chlamydial genital infection in prostitutes in Iran. British Journal of Venereal Diseases 59: 53–55

Darrow W 1984 Prostitution and sexually transmitted diseases. In: Holmes K K, Mardh P A, Sparling P F, Weisner P J (eds) Sexually transmitted diseases, McGraw-Hill, New York

Donovan B 1984 Gonorrhoea in a Sydney house of prostitution. Medical Journal of Australia 140: 268–271

Duenas A, Adam E, Melnick J L, Rawls W E 1972 Herpes virus type 2 in a prostitute population. American Journal of Epidemiology 95(5): 483–489

Exner J E, Wylie J, Leura A, Parrill T 1977 Some psychological characteristics of prostitutes. Journal of Personality Assessment 41: 474–485

Fish E N, Tobin S M, Cooter N B E, Papsin F R 1982 Update on the relation of Herpesvirus hominis type II to carcinoma of the cervix. Obstetrics and Gynecology 59(2): 220–224

Frosner G G, Bucholz H M, Gerth H J 1975 Prevalence of hepatitis B antibody in prostitutes. American Journal of Epidemiology 102(3): 241–250

Gibbens T C N, Silberman M 1960 The clients and prostitutes. British Journal of Venereal Diseases 36: 113–115

Hersh T, Melnick J L, Ray D, Goyal R K 1971 Non parenteral transmission of viral hepatitis type B. New England Journal of Medicine 285: 1363–1364

Hicks D R, Martin I. S, Getchell J P et al 1985 Inactivation of HTLVIII/LAV infected cultures of normal human lymphocytes by nonoxynol 9 in vitro (letter). Lancet ii: 1422–1423

James J 1977 Prostitutes and prostitution. In: Sagarin E, Montanino F (eds) Deviants; voluntary actors in a hostile world, General Learning Press, New Jersey

James J, Meyerding J 1977 Early sexual experience and prostitution. American Journal of Psychiatry 134(12): 1381–1385

Johnson A M 1988 Heterosexual transmission of human immunodeficiency virus. British Medical Journal 296: 1017–1020

McCormack N M, Moller B R, Mardh P A 1983 Mycoplasma hominis: a human pathogen. Sexually Transmitted Diseases 10: 160–165

McEvoy M, Tillett H E 1985 Some problems in the prediction of future numbers of cases of the acquired immunodeficiency syndrome in the UK. Lancet ii: 541–542

Meheus A, De Clerq A, Prat R 1974 Prevalence of gonorrhoea in prostitutes in a central African town. British Journal of Venereal Diseases 50: 50–53

Minkoff H L, Schwarz R H (editorial) 1986 AIDS; time for obstetricians to get involved. Obstetrics and Gynecology 68(2): 267–268

Moghissi K S, Mack H C, Porzak J P 1968 Epidemiology of cervical cancer. American Journal of Obstetrics and Gynecology 100: 607–614

Morton R S 1977 Gonorrhoea, W B Saunders, London, p 220

Nayyar K C, Cummings M, Weber J et al 1986 Prevalence of genital pathogens among female prostitutes in New York city and in Rotterdam. Sexually Transmitted Diseases 13(2): 105–107

Papaevengolou G, Trichopolous D, Kremastinou T, Papoutsakis G 1974 Prevalence of hepatitis B antigen and antibody in prostitutes. British Medical Journal 2: 256–258

Papaevengolou G, Roumeliotou–Karayannis A, Kallinikos G, Papoutsakis G 1985 LAV/HTLVIII infection in female prostitutes (letter). Lancet ii: 1018

Parent-Duchatelet A J B 1857 De la prostitution de la ville de Paris, Ballière, New York

Paterson-Brown S, Finnerty S P 1986 Problems of London prostitutes. British Journal of Sexual Medicine 13(9): 260–261

Peryra A J 1961 The relationship of sexual activity to cervical cancer. Cancer of the cervix in a prison population. Obstetrics and Gynecology 17: 154–159

Pinching A J, Jeffries D J 1985 AIDS and HTLVIII/LAV infection: consequences for obstetrics and perinatal medicine. British Journal of Obstetrics and Gynaecology 92: 1211–2117

Potterat J J, Rothenburg R, Bross D C 1979 Gonorrhoea in street prostitutes; epidemiologic and legal complications. Sexually Transmitted Diseases 6(2): 58–63

Rojel R 1953 Interrelation between uterine cancer and syphilis. Acta Pathologica et Microbiologica Scandinavica 97 (suppl): 1

Rosenthal T, Vandow J 1958 Prevalence of venereal disease in prostitutes. British Journal of Venereal Diseases 34: 94–99

Sanger W W 1858 History of prostitution, Harper, New York

Sebastian J A, Leeb B O, See R 1978 Carcinoma of the cervix—a sexually transmitted disease? American Journal of Obstetrics and Gynaecology 131: 620–623

Sereny G 1985 The invisible children, Andre Deutsch, London

Simpson M, Schill T 1977 Patrons of massage parlours. Archives of Sexual Behavior 6(6): 521–524

Singer A, Reid B L, Coppleson M 1976 The role of the high risk male in the aetiology of cervical cancer—a correlation of epidemiology and molecular biology. American Journal of Obstetrics and Gynecology 126: 110–116

Tirelli U, Vaccher E, Carbone A, De Paoli P, Santini G, Monfardini S 1985 HTLV-III antibody in prostitutes (letter). Lancet ii: 1424

Turner E B, Morton R S 1976 Prostitution in Sheffield. British Journal of Venereal Diseases 52: 197–205

Van de Perre P, Carael M, Robert-Guroff M et al 1985 Female prostitutes: a risk group for infection with human T-cell lymphotropic virus type III. Lancet ii: 524–526

Wellings K 1986 AIDS and the condom. British Medical Journal 293: 1259–1260

Willcox R R 1962 Prostitution and venereal disease. British Journal of Venereal Diseases 38: 37–42

Wilsher P, Hodgkinson N 1986 At risk, Sunday Times, 2 Nov

World Health Organization (WHO) 1985 Control of sexually transmitted diseases, WHO, Geneva

Pelvic pain due to venous congestion

INTRODUCTION

Chronic pelvic pain is a common complaint among women, particularly in the reproductive age group. Approximately one-third of the patients attending the gynaecology clinic present with pelvic pain as their major or significant symptom (Morris & O'Neil 1958, Henker 1979). In a survey of the gynaecological laparoscopy conducted by the Royal College of Obstetricians and Gynaecologists (RCOG 1978) over 50% of the diagnostic laparoscopies were done to investigate pelvic pain, which reflects the magnitude of this difficult problem (Table 18.).

Table 18.1 Indication for diagnostic laparoscopy from the survey by the RCOG (1978)

Major indication	number	%
Infertility	9048	43.1
Pain	10825	51.7
Infertility and pain	186	0.9
Menorrhagia	84	0.4
Ovarian enlargement	389	1.9
Lost IUD or other foreign body	156	0.7
Other	283	1.3
Total	20971	100.0

A small number of women attending with chronic pelvic pain have an identifiable gynaecological lesion such as endometriosis or pelvic inflammatory disease. In a very few the pelvic pain can be attributed to a non-gynaecological cause such as recurrent cysto-urethritis, irritable bowel syndrome, ureteric calculus, diverticulitis, chronic ulcerative colitis or referred pain from a lumbo-sacral lesion. The experience of most gynaecologists, however, is that the majority have no obvious organic cause for their pain. The cause of the pain in these women has been uncertain and the objective of this chapter is to clarify the aetiology, pathophysiology, symptomatology and treatment of these women whose condition is described as the pelvic pain syndrome (PPS).

275

The incidence of PPS varies in different studies (Pent 1972, Lundberg et al 1973), but a survey by Gillibrand in 1981 showed that as many as two-thirds of women presenting with pelvic pain have no obvious organic pathology.

Recent research (Beard et al 1984, Hughes & Curtis 1962, Kaupilla 1970) has confirmed that dilated pelvic veins with associated vascular stasis and congestion are commonly found in these women, which is responsible for their pain (Reginald et al 1987).

As early as 1831, Gooch recognised the clinical features of women with this condition. His patients complained of pelvic pain which became worse before the onset of menstruation. Examination revealed an exquisitely tender uterus and cervix which he ascribed to an 'irritable uterus'. He suggested that bodily exertions at times when the uterus is in a susceptible state such as menstruation and puerperium led to this disorder, and recognised 'a morbid state of pelvic blood vessels indicated by their fullness' in these women. He advised these women to maintain a horizontal posture during most of the day and treated them with hip baths, narcotics and by blood letting using leeches.

In spite of the considerable literature over the last 150 years, little advance has been achieved in our understanding of this condition. The clinical picture of symptomatology and signs is confused and, not surprisingly, no convincing explanation for the condition has so far emerged. Perhaps the two main reasons for the slow progress in establishing the nature of this condition have been:

1. the need to perform a laparotomy in order to make a positive diagnosis, and
2. the difficulty of studying the normal pelvic physiology, in particular the pelvic circulation.

In the past many authors have postulated a wide variety of causes and Table 18.2 is the list of the various names they have given to the condition,

Table 18.2 Terminology used over the years by various authors to describe the PPS

Chronic parametritis (Schultze 1875, Opitz 1922)	Pelvic congestion syndrome (Taylor 1949a,b,c, Duncan & Taylor 1952, Allen 1971, Beard et al 1988)
Pelvic sympathetic syndrome (Theobald 1951)	Congestion–fibrosis syndrome (Taylor 1949b)
Broad-ligament neuritis (Young 1938)	
Sclero-cystic ovary (Netter 1953)	Pelvic varicosities (Dudley 1888, Chidikel & Edlundh 1968)
Broad-ligament laceration (Allen & Masters 1955)	Chronic pelvic pain without obvious pathology (Renaer et al 1980)

denoting different aetiologies, and we describe briefly the pathogenesis and the treatment proposed by the advocates of these different theories.

CHRONIC PARAMETRITIS

The concept of 'chronic parametritis', first advanced by Schultze (1875) gained wide acceptance as a cause of chronic pelvic pain. The predominant clinical features of 'chronic parametritis' were tenderness and shortening of the posterior parametrium and the utero-sacral ligaments. This author attributed these findings to the effects of ascending infection from the cervix and uterus causing connective tissue proliferation and contraction in the parametrium and uterosacral ligaments. However, Opitz (1922) and Martius (1939) believed that the shortening was due to the spastic contraction of the smooth muscle fibres of the paracervical tissue, while Frankel (1909) proposed that this was the result of sexual excesses, masturbation, coitus interruptus and lack of sexual satisfaction. Based on the above theories, the treatment included stretching of the parametrium under general anaesthesia, division of utero-sacral ligaments, physiotherapy, injection of alcohol and local anaesthetics into the parametrium, and cervical cautery.

The occurrence of PPS in sexually inactive women and the presence of normal pelvic organs at laparoscopy makes it unlikely that infection is a common cause. Missanelli (1982) was not able to isolate any organism from the fluid in the pouch of Douglas of 50 women with PPS. Although the parametrial and utero-sacral tenderness have been found in the majority of cases of PPS, the shortening of the ligament is not a common accompaniment in most cases (Renaer et al 1980), suggesting that the theory of 'chronic parametritis' is not a satisfactory explanation for PPS.

PELVIC SYMPATHETIC SYNDROME

Theobald (1951) studied a group of women with symptoms consisting predominantly of lower abdominal pain, dyspareunia, backache, dysmenorrhoea and menstrual disturbances for which there was no detectable pathology. He called this 'pelvic sympathetic syndrome' and advanced a hypothesis that these women suffered a lowered pain threshold in one or more sympathetic nerves either in the afferent arc or in the receptor cells of the brain. He suggested that the lowering of the threshold was caused either locally by trauma, inflammation, inordinate or excessive sex, or by mental stress. He believed that the threshold of the affected nerves could be restored to normal by hypnosis or psychotherapy, or achieved locally by blocking the afferent arc via local anaesthesia. He claimed a dramatic success rate (90%) after endometrial cauterisation by silver nitrate—the process he believed stimulated the affected nerves and restored the normal threshold.

Although the above hypothesis attempts to include the divergent theories advanced to explain the syndrome, the results obtained by procedures which might be expected to interrupt afferent nerve pathways carrying the pain impulse, such as the injection of local anaesthetics into the utero-sacral ligament or hysterectomy, are disappointing (Renaer et al 1980).

CHRONIC HYPERAEMIA OF THE OVARY AND SCLERO-CYSTIC OVARIES

It was frequently thought in the past that the ovary was the site of abnormality in women with long-standing pelvic pain (Netter 1953). A clear recognition of ovarian hyperaemia causing pelvic symptoms was first made by Tait in 1883. Chronic hyperaemia and congestion of the ovary was thought to produce proliferation of the connective tissue and fibrosis in the cortex of the ovary, causing interference with ovulation and leading to cyst formation (Sturmdorf 1916). Taylor (1949a,b) demonstrated that the ovaries removed from women with chronic pelvic pain commonly had many peripheral cysts. Although the association of these findings with chronic pelvic pain could not be confirmed, the belief that the ovary was the site of pain led to much unnecessary surgery, with oophorectomy being the commonest gynaecological operation in women with chronic pelvic pain (Taylor 1954). With the advent of laparoscopy, ultrasound and a better understanding of ovarian physiology, gynaecologists have come to recognise the transient nature of such cysts and have increasingly spared the ovaries from surgical assault.

LACERATION OF THE BROAD LIGAMENT

Allen & Masters (1955) studied a group of 28 women whose symptoms and signs were suggestive of PPS. They complained of 'pelvic distress, deep dyspareunia, post sexual ache, dysmenorrhoea and physical fatigue'. More than half of these patients had a history of significant emotional instability. The uterus was tender on examination and ovarian pain was elicited by pressure in the adnexa. At laparotomy, there was no organic lesion but the uterus was slightly enlarged and retroverted, and there was evidence of venous congestion in both the uterus and the infundibulo-pelvic ligaments, and up to 80 ml of serous fluid in the pouch of Douglas. The striking observation was the unilateral or bilateral laceration of the peritoneum and fascia of the broad ligament, with or without a similar tear in the utero-sacral ligaments. They believed that in a proportion of these women the symptoms and signs were due to pelvic hyperaemia and congestion, and advanced an attractive theory explaining the genesis of congestion which was thought to be responsible for the pain. They proposed that fascial and peritoneal laceration resulted in loss of tissue support to the underlying vessels, with resultant venostasis and congestion. This was further exacerbated by retroversion of the uterus. They considered that with the resultant vascular stasis there was extravasation of serum into the pelvic tissues, and hence into the pouch of Douglas, through the laceration. The authors believed that the source of laceration was related to a past obstetrical event such as a traumatic forceps delivery, and recommended surgical repair of the laceration which they claimed produced pain relief in the majority of their patients. Although the explanation is logical, the infrequent observation of broad ligament tears in such women (Renaer et al 1980), the finding of tears in asymptomatic women and the fact that many women with PPS are nulliparous (see Table 18.3) is evidence that it is not a major cause of PPS.

PELVIC VASCULAR CONGESTION

It is apparent from Table 18.2 that disorders of the pelvic vascular system, particularly involving the pelvic veins, form the predominant concept of the pathogenesis of PPS. Gooch (1831) was probably the first to introduce the concept of vascular congestion, but Taylor (1949a,b,c) and Duncan & Taylor (1952) gave a detailed account of the association of pelvic pain with vascular congestion and hyperaemia. Further evidence for vascular disorder is derived from the observation at laparotomy of dilated and congested veins in the broad and infundibulo-pelvic ligaments (Dudley 1888, Emge 1925). With the advent of pelvic venography, Hughes & Curtis (1962), Topolanski-Sierra (1958), Petrucco & Harris (1981), Kaupilla (1970) and Beard et al (1984) have demonstrated abnormal findings in pelvic venograms showing venous dilatation and congestion in women with PPS. Laparoscopy has increased the possibility of detecting these dilated veins, although it must be remembered that dilated veins often disappear rapidly because of the combined effects of raising the intra-abdominal pressure with gas and the head-down tilt used by most gynaecologists.

Stearns & Sneeden (1966) described recognisable pathological changes associated with pelvic congestion. 'The typical uterus weighed 135–150 gm or more with cavity length of 8.5 cm to 10 cm. Sections of the cervix revealed sub-epithelial pale staining band of oedematous fibrous connective tissue containing dilated lymphatics and blood vascular spaces. There was also oedema, lymphangiectasia and telangiectasia in the subserosal area.' Kaupilla (1970) described the pathological changes found in the dilated ovarian plexus of veins as follows: fibrosis of the tunica intima, hypertrophy of the muscular layer of the tunica media, fibrosis of the tunica media, and cellular proliferation of the capillary endothelium with or without fibrosis of the adventitia. These changes were also observed in undilated veins but they were significantly less frequent. Although these histological changes are similar to those found in varicosities in the leg (Ochsner & Mahoner 1939) we refer to pelvic veins as being 'dilated' rather than 'varicose' because we have preliminary evidence that with medical treatment such veins can return to a normal diameter.

Venographic studies

Our studies (Beard et al 1984) have clearly shown the common occurrence of dilated pelvic veins in women with PPS. Forty-five women presenting with the typical symptoms complex of PPS (see below) and a 'normal' pelvis on laparoscopy were investigated further by pelvic venography. A 19-gauge needle with the point protected by a bulbous-ended cannula was passed under direct vision through the cervix to the vault of the uterine cavity. The needle was advanced and after an initial injection of 3 ml of hyaluronidase, 20 ml of Urografin 310 M (Schering) was injected into the myometrium over a period of 30–40 seconds. Spread of dye and disappearance into the pelvic veins was observed by fluoroscopic screening. The results from this group of women were compared with those of two control groups—10 women with other pelvic pathology thought to be the cause of their pain, and 8 women admitted to the hospital for laparoscopic sterilisation who had no pain. Figure 18.1 shows a venogram in a woman with normal pelvic vasculature, in contrast

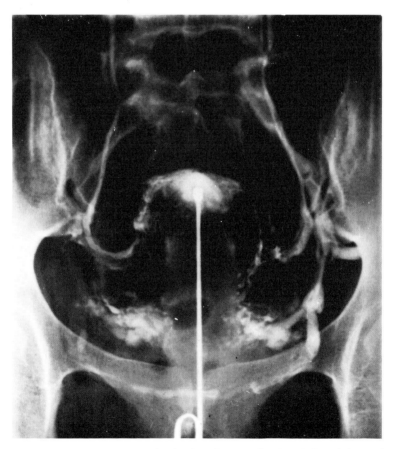

Fig. 18.1 Normal pelvic venogram with tip of needle protruding from bulb-ended cannula into myometrium at fundus of uterus. Film, taken immediately after the end of injection, shows rapid disappearance of dye with small amounts of dye in the broad ligament veins and the ovarian veins clearly outlined

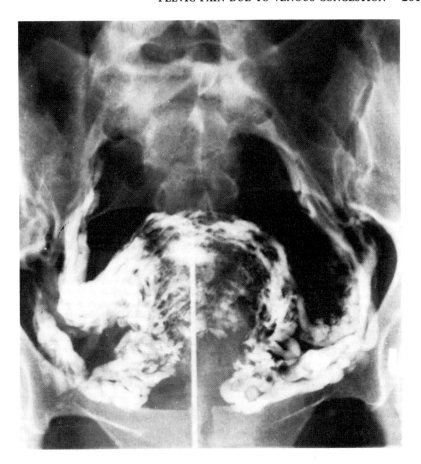

Fig. 18.2 Abnormal pelvic venogram taken immediately after the end of injection. Note the multiple venous channels in the uterus, the congested ovarian plexus and dilated veins in the broad ligament. A markedly dilated right ovarian vein can just be seen

to Figure 18.2 which shows the typical congestion, stasis and venous dilatation. Table 18.3 shows the characteristics and venographic findings in the three groups. The venogram is scored by assessing the extent of stasis and congestion in, and the diameter of, the pelvic veins.

Although, inevitably, the groups are not exactly matched for age and parity, they are all within the reproductive age group, and the combined control groups contain slightly more parous than nulliparous women than in the PPS group. There is clear evidence in the PPS group of abnormally dilated pelvic veins with increased venous stasis and congestion giving a high venogram score, as compared with the two control groups. Pelvic venography, on the basis of a venogram score of 5 or more, gives a sensitivity of 91% and a specificity of 89% in the diagnosis of the pelvic pain syndrome. Parous women were found to have dilated veins more often, but this did not interfere

Table 18.3 Clinical characteristics of patient groups and results of a pelvic venogram study of women with the PPS compared with those with detectable pelvic pathology at laparoscopy and those having a laparoscopic sterilisation

	PPS (n = 45)	Pelvic pathology (n = 10)	Laparoscopic sterilisation (n = 8)
Mean age in years (range)	28 (21–40)	25 (17–33)	33 (29–38)
Parity—nulliparous	21	6	0
—parous	24	4	8
Duration of pain (range in years)	0.5–10	0.5–12	—
Maximum diameter of ovarian vein (mm)	6.73	3.60	3.25
Delayed disappearance of dye (>40 seconds after end of injection)	26	0	0
Congestion of ovarian plexus	38	2	1
Mean venogram score	±6.53	±3.5	±4.0

with the diagnostic potential of venography in the investigation of PPS, nor did the stage of the menstrual cycle when the venogram was done alter the diagnosis. More recent studies have shown that the diameter of the pelvic veins on the side of the developing follicle/corpus luteum is greater than on the contralateral side, showing the ability of pelvic veins to dilate and contract under the influence of hormones throughout the menstrual cycle (see Fig. 18.3).

THE CAUSE OF DILATED PELVIC VEINS

Anatomical factors

The complex venous system of the pelvis comprises many thin-walled, unsupported veins with relatively weak attachments between the adventitia and the supporting connective tissue (von Peham & Amreich 1934). In addition, pelvic veins, unlike those in the leg, are said to be devoid of valves and largely depend on the fascia for their support (Kownatzki 1907). Teleologically, it could be argued that these anatomical characteristics make pelvic veins capable of adapting to the massive increase in blood volume circulating through the pelvis in pregnancy. Hodgkinson (1953) reported that during pregnancy there is a three-fold increase in the dilatation of ovarian veins, with a sixty-fold increase in their capacity. However, in the non-pregnant state these characteristics are liable to make the pelvic veins particularly vulnerable to dilatation, stasis and congestion. Other factors such as weakening of the fascial supports by parturition and, possibly, constitutionally defective veins (Auvray 1924) may also contribute to the venous dilatation. The tendency to dilatation of pelvic veins and its sequelae is further exacerbated by the erect posture causing a rise in the intravenous pressure, resulting in

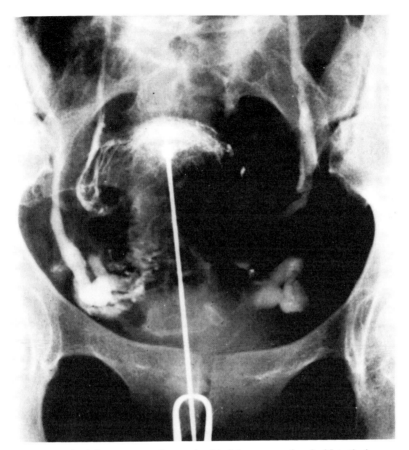

Fig. 18.3   Normal pelvic venogram taken on day 14 of the menstrual cycle. Note the increase in the diameter of the left as compared with the right ovarian vein corresponding with the side of the developing follicle

oedema of the interstitial tissue (Derichsweiler 1934). This fact perhaps explains the worsening of pelvic discomfort on standing and the relief obtained in the recumbent position (Beard et al 1988).

Hormonal factors

Stearns & Sneeden (1966) considered that a hormonal factor was the most likely cause of pelvic congestion. McCausland et al (1963) also reported a 30% increase in venous distensibility a week prior to menstruation and implicated progesterone as the cause, although the role of oestrogen was not ruled out. Barwin & McCalden (1972) demonstrated during in-vitro experiments that the contractions produced by field stimulation on the smooth muscle in the veins of humans could be blocked by 17B-oestradiol and progesterone. McCausland et al (1961) showed the effect of pregnancy on venous distensibility and thought that this was mediated through oestrogen and progesterone on the smooth muscle of the vessel wall. They concluded that increased distensibility contributes to the production of varicosities in pregnancy.

Circumstantial and indirect evidence from our studies and those of others suggests, as follows, that an ovarian hormone(s), probably oestrogen, is the cause of dilated pelvic veins in women with PPS: (1) oestradiol is a potent vasodilator acting on the smooth muscle in veins, (2) PPS is only seen in women of reproductive age, (3) varicose veins of the leg are 3–4 times more common in women than in men, (4) polycystic ovaries, a condition associated with excess oestrogen, is commonly (56%) found in women with PPS (Adams et al 1986), (5) PPS is associated with an increase in ovarian volume, uterine area and endometrial thickness, (6) veins draining the ovary are commonly the most dilated of all the pelvic veins, (7) dilatation of the ovarian veins in normal women occurs on the same side as the developing follicle, and is apparent in the follicular phase of the cycle before progesterone is secreted, (8) suppression of ovarian function results in narrowing of the dilated pelvic veins and shrinkage of the uterus and ovaries (Reginald et al unpublished data), (9) the concentration of oestradiol in ovarian blood is significantly higher than in the periphery (Baird & Fraser 1975). This could explain the progressive dilatation of the ovarian vein on the side of the developing follicle during the menstrual cycle referred to previously.

PSYCHOLOGICAL FACTORS

The early failure to identify an organic component in chronic pelvic pain led to the view that it may be occurring as a response to psychological disturbance. Indeed, many authors (Duncan & Taylor 1952, Benson et al 1959, Beard et al 1977) have reported high levels of distress in this group. The relationship between cause and effect is, however, difficult to establish. The long-term experience of pain may lead to, rather than result from, psychological disorder.

However, in a prospective study by our group, 101 patients with chronic pelvic pain of more than 6 months' duration were assessed on a range of psychological measures (Pearce 1986). No difference was found between the women with obvious pathology at laparoscopy and those with PPS on general measures of personality (Eysenck personality questionnaire, Eysenck & Eysenck 1975) or mood (Profile of mood states, McNair et al 1971). However, specific differences emerge in attitudes to illness as assessed by the illness behaviour questionnaire (Pilowsky 1978), sexual problems and previous exposure to death and illness. Since the groups are of equivalent pain duration it is unlikely that the differences in attitudes that emerge are a simple consequence of chronic pain.

Duncan & Taylor (1952) found that women with PPS reported a greater number of deaths and illness among family members and close friends. They noted that 29 out of 36 women with PPS had an unfavourable family environment, including death of a parent before the age of 12 years. It is possible that exposure to illness leads to greater attention to one's own physical state, hence lowering the threshold for the perception of sensations and labelling them as pain.

However, it is also possible that psychological factors may contribute to the aetiology of pelvic vein dilatation and congestion. Duncan & Taylor (1952), using a thermal conductance technique for measuring blood flow, reported that vaginal blood flow increased in response to the discussion of anxiety-provoking topics during an interview. They proposed that women with PPS reacted to emotional stress with sustained pelvic hyperaemia, leading to congestion, oedema and pain. A further possibility, on the basis of the finding that 60% of women with PPS have polycystic ovaries on ultrasound examination, is that psychological factors may act through the hypothalamus to give rise to an inappropriate release of gonadotrophins from the pituitary, resulting in the formation of polycystic ovaries. If this were the case it would add further support to our concept that dilatation and congestion of the pelvic veins in women with PPS are due to the smooth muscle relaxing effect of prolonged exposure to oestrogen or some other vasoactive substance secreted by the ovaries.

CLINICAL SYMPTOMS AND SIGNS OF WOMEN WITH PPS

Pelvic pain is such a common symptom that there is a real need to try and characterise the symptoms and signs attributable to PPS. To do this, a prospective assessment by questionnaire was undertaken in which 35 women presenting with pelvic pain of more than 6 months' duration and pelvic vein dilatation proven by venography were compared with 22 women with normal pelvic veins but with some other form of pathology found at laparoscopy. These results have been compared with the responses to the same questionnaire obtained from a control group of 36 women admitted for laparoscopic sterilisation.

Typically, the pain complained of by the women with dilated pelvic veins had been present for several years, although occasionally it was of more recent onset. It was described as being a dull ache ('like a bruise') with occasional acute attacks sometimes sufficient to warrant a visit to the doctor or even an emergency admission to hospital. The pain was more often present in the right than the left iliac fossa, but typically it was often described as 'moving' to the other side from time to time. As might be expected of a condition with venous congestion, changes in position and intrabdominal pressure tended to exacerbate or ease the pain. Standing, walking, jumping and bending all make the pain worse, whereas lying down—'relaxation'— usually improved it. Women with PPS are said to be polysymptomatic (Renaer et al 1980), and certainly backache, headache and non-offensive vaginal discharge were common accompanying symptoms. There was no significant increase in varicose veins in the legs. Dysfunctional menstrual bleeding occurred in 54% and congestive dysmenorrhoea in 68% of patients with pelvic pain and venous dilatation (Beard et al 1988). Surprisingly, despite the finding in our ultrasound study of these women that 56% had polycystic ovaries which could account for the menstrual irregularity (Adams et al 1986), there was no evidence of infertility or symptoms commonly ascribed to the polycystic ovary syndrome (Franks et al 1985).

There was frequently a history of suspected pelvic inflammatory disease with repeated courses of antibiotics being prescribed, and because of this many of the single women were convinced that they were infertile. However, in our series of 35 women with dilated pelvic veins, none of the 16 who had been diagnosed elsewhere as having pelvic inflammatory disease had confirmatory evidence on laparoscopy. Other forms of surgical intervention such as appendicectomy and excision of simple cysts of the ovary, particularly in the 16–19 year age group, are commonplace.

Sexual dysfunction is a well-recognised problem amongst women with chronic pelvic pain for which no cause was found, and that was certainly our experience of the 35 women studied by us. Forty-six per cent (17%)* had intercourse less than once a week, 71% (11%) complained of deep dyspareunia and 65% (8%) suffered postcoital ache which was often severe enough to put them off completely from having sexual intercourse.

Women with PPS often appear mildly depressed, particularly those with a long-standing history of emotional disturbance. The interview in itself can be exhausting because patients may be defensive and poor historians, which may lead to misunderstandings with the interviewer when sensitive issues are discussed. On abdominal examination the patient was asked to point to the site of the pain, which was usually one of the iliac fossae. Pressure there usually failed to elicit tenderness, whereas deep pressure over the ovarian point nearly always provoked the pain complained of (the ovarian point is situated at the junction of the upper and middle thirds of a line drawn between the umbilicus and the anterior superior iliac spine). Pelvic venography reveals that the ovarian point is where the ovarian vein crosses the transverse processes of the vertebrae (Beard et al 1984). Compression at this point produced pain, presumably due to back pressure on the distended veins in the hilum of the ovary, particularly on the right side. When the uterus was pushed upwards it was often painful and, even more commonly, compression of one or both ovaries reproduced the pain complained of. This response was so localised that it could clearly be distinguished from the more diffuse tenderness of pelvic inflammatory disease. In the acute case of PPS such a distinction may be more difficult to make because the whole pelvis is usually unbearably tender. These findings, together with the patient's history, are usually diagnostic of the condition.

INVESTIGATION OF PPS

Laparoscopy

This is an essential part of the investigation of all forms of chronic pelvic pain. Although a diagnosis of PPS can virtually be made from the history

* Figures in brackets are the percentages from a control group of 36 women undergoing sterilisation

and physical findings, it is impossible to exclude pelvic endometriosis completely. Dilated pelvic veins and polycystic ovaries can often be visualised through the laparoscope (Adams et al, in preparation). All forms of endometriosis, except for adenomyosis, can be excluded after a thorough examination including lifting up both ovaries to visualise the ovarian fossa.

Pelvic venography

Transuterine pelvic venography is performed as an outpatient procedure and does not require a general anaesthetic. The procedure has been described earlier in this chapter. It has proved to be a highly specific and reliable means of demonstrating dilatation of pelvic veins and congestion.

Pelvic ultrasound

Initial studies (Adams et al 1986) suggest that ultrasound may prove to be the most valuable diagnostic aid. The dilated veins in the uterus, broad ligament and around the ovary can be easily visualised, and the measurement of the uterus and ovaries can be made. This method is non-invasive and could be used at regular intervals to monitor the changes in the veins, uterus and ovaries during and after medical treatment.

TREATMENT OF PPS

Women with PPS are usually told after the diagnostic laparoscopy that their pelvic organs are normal and that no cause could be found to explain their pain. This information is reassuring and occasionally results in a permanent cure (Beard et al 1977), but more often does not. The difficulty of providing effective treatment in the past for women with PPS has been increased by the lack of understanding of the pathology of the condition. The demonstration that these women commonly have pelvic congestion and often polycystic ovaries has resulted in a marked improvement in confidence because they feel that at last a somatic disturbance has been found to explain their pain. It has also led to the development of more specific therapy.

Medical treatment

The fact that the majority of these women with PPS are young and in the reproductive age group (mean age 32 years) means that medical rather than surgical treatment is preferred. The better understanding of the aetiology of PPS, and the relationship of dilated pelvic veins to possible oestrogen excess, has led to attempts to temporarily suppress ovarian activity as the first line of treatment. We have obtained encouraging results from the use of medroxyprogesterone acetate (Provera—Upjohn) 30 mg/day. The effect of this drug is to decrease LHRH release and reduce serum gonadotrophins, testosterone and oestradiol (Worstman et al 1981). Luciano et al (1986) reported that medroxyprogesterone, in doses of 50 mg/day, reduces oestradiol to a level remaining consistent with the early follicular phase of the cycle. The mechanism of action whereby Provera works is probably by narrowing the pelvic veins, thereby improving pelvic blood flow and reducing congestion. With the suppression of ovarian secretion, the dilated pelvic veins return to a normal diameter. If this is so it is likely that the pain will return once ovarian activity returns to normal.

We have so far treated 22 women with PPS using medroxyprogesterone acetate 30 mg/day taken orally for 6 months. Before commencing the treatment the intensity of pain was assessed using a visual analogue scale (Huskisson 1974), and the blood pressure and body weight were recorded. The nature of the treatment was explained to the patients, who were also instructed to maintain a record of vaginal bleeding. They were seen 3 and 6 months after starting the treatment, at which times the blood pressure and body weight were recorded and the intensity of the pain assessed using the visual analogue scale. Of the 22 women treated, 18 women stopped menstruating and all but two showed marked improvement in their pain intensity. The remaining 4 patients continued to have breakthrough bleeding and three of them showed little improvement in pelvic pain, perhaps suggesting adequate ovarian suppression was not achieved. The drug was well tolerated, the major side-effect being intermittent or continuous bleeding in four cases (18%). There was no change in the mean blood pressure and the average weight gain was 3.0 kg. At present a trial of Provera and psychotherapy is under way to assess the combined and individual efficacy in the treatment of PPS.

Surgical treatment

The statement by Taylor in 1957 that 'premature resort to surgery is the characteristic error in present day treatment of women with pelvic pain' is applicable even today. However, the consistent finding of dilated pelvic veins in women with PPS has frequently led gynaecologists in the past to seek a surgical solution. Although the causal relationship between pelvic pain and dilated pelvic veins is difficult to establish, the literature provides clinical descriptions claiming such a relationship. Dudley (1888) and Railo (1968) have resected the ovarian veins in women with PPS with apparently successful outcome. Rundqvist et al (1984) performed retroperitoneal resection of the left ovarian vein in 15 women with a history of PPS. Eight women were completely cured and three others showed considerable improvement. They had only performed retrograde venography to visualise the left ovarian vein and therefore only resected left-sided ovarian veins. They might have achieved better results if the resection of the right ovarian vein was done wherever indicated, as judged by the transuterine venography.

We have no experience in the ligation of the ovarian veins and feel that such attempts will fail because they do not include other veins in the pelvis which can only be successfully ligated by hysterectomy. Oophorectomy with hysterectomy does have a place in treating the older woman who has no further desire for a pregnancy but this needs proper evaluation. Removal of residual ovaries after hysterectomy is also effective when the ovaries have become deeply embedded in adhesions resulting in pain similar to that of pelvic congestion. At present our view is that medical treatment should be offered as the primary treatment before resorting to surgery.

Psychotherapy

Over the 30 years since Taylor's warnings of the dangers of radical surgery for unexplained pelvic pain, there has been intermittent interest in the use of psychological methods for this group of patients. There have been few attempts to evaluate psychological methods systematically, and those studies which have been conducted are generally methodologically inadequate and difficult to interpret. These are reviewed by Pearce & Beard (1984).

One of the earliest papers to discuss psychological treatment approaches to chronic pelvic pain is that of Beard et al (1977). Although no formal outcome measures were taken, several women with PPS apparently responded well to the relaxation training provided by the psychiatrist.

We have recently completed a controlled trial of two behavioural methods— stress analysis and pain analysis—compared with a minimal intervention control group. Women allocated to the stress analysis group received a form of stress management and relaxation training. Discussion of the pain and its associated difficulties and events was discouraged and the focus was directed towards identifying current worries and concerns apart from the pain. Treatment started with a semi-structured interview assessment of potential areas of stress, in which the main problem areas such as financial, marital and housing worries were identified. In addition, patients were asked to keep daily records of the main concerns they had. The therapists' aim throughout was to identify the patients' reactions to identified stressors and to discuss alternative responses. In addition, the use of Jacobsonian relaxation strategies in stressful situations was encouraged. The pain analysis treatment involved the patient in close monitoring of her pain and the associated antecedent and consequent events. The therapists aimed, in collaboration with the patient, to identify patterns associated with pain episodes and to develop alternative strategies for avoiding or reducing pain episodes. These strategies were determined on an individual basis and included both cognitive, behavioural and environmental manipulations. In addition, graded exercise programmes were instituted on an individual basis for each patient. Spouses were encouraged to prompt and reinforce 'well behaviours' and, where possible, were encouraged to become involved in the exercise programme. A range of measures were used to assess outcome, including mood, pain intensity ratings, behavioural disruption and gynaecologists' 'blind' ratings of the extent to which the patient was affected by the pain. On all measures of outcome both treatment groups performed significantly better than the minimal intervention control group at the 6-month follow-up. It can be concluded with reasonable confidence that those patients receiving psychological treatments do better, at least at the 6-month follow-up. The process of change is as yet largely unknown and the integration of psychological and physical methods of treatment is clearly a question for further investigation.

REFERENCES

Adams J, Beard R W, Franks S, Pearce S, Reginald P W 1986 Pelvic ultrasound findings in women with chronic pelvic pain: correlation with laparoscopy and venography. Abstracts of the 24th British Congress of Obstetrics and Gynaecology, Cardiff, April 1986, Royal College of Obstetricians and Gynaecologists, London, p 80
Auvray M 1924 Gazette des hopitaux civils et militaires 97: 481–483, quoted by Taylor (1949)
Allen W M 1971 Chronic pelvic congestion and pelvic pain. American Journal of Obstetrics and Gynecology 109: 198–202
Allen W M, Masters W H 1955 Traumatic laceration of uterine support. American Journal of Obstetrics and Gynecology 70: 500–513
Barwin B N, McCalden T A 1972 The inhibitory action of oestradiol-17B and progesterone on human venous smooth muscle. Proceedings of the Physiological Society, 41 pp
Baird D T, Fraser I S 1975 Concentration of oestrone and oestradiol in follicular fluid and ovarian venous blood of women. Clinical Endocrinology 4: 259–266
Beard R W, Belsy E N, Liebermann M B, Wilkinson J C M 1977 Pelvic pain in women. American Journal of Obstetrics and Gynecology 128: 566–570
Beard R W, Highman J H, Pearce S, Reginald P W 1984 Diagnosis of pelvic varicosities in women with chronic pelvic pain. Lancet ii: 946–949
Beard R W, Reginald P W, Wadsworth J 1988 Clinical features of women with lower abdominal pain and dilated pelvic veins. British Journal of Obstetrics and Gynaecology 95: 153–161
Benson R, Hanson K, Matarazzo J 1959 Atypical pelvic pain in women: gynecologic psychiatric considerations. American Journal of Obstetrics and Gynecology 77: 806–823
Chidikel N, Edlundh K O 1968 Transuterine pelvic venography with particular reference to pelvic varicosities. Acta Radiologica 7: 1–12
Derichsweiler H 1934 Archiv fur Gynakologie 155: 408–414
Dudley A 1888 Varicocele in the female. What is its influence on the ovary? New York Medical Journal 48: 174–177
Duncan C H, Taylor H C 1952 A psychosomatic study of pelvic congestion. American Journal of Obstetrics and Gynecology 64: 1–12
Emge L A 1925 The surgical treatment of varicose veins in the female pelvis. Journal of the American Medical Association 85: 1690
Eysenck H J, Eysenck S B G 1975 Manual of the Eysenck personality questionnaire, Hodder & Stoughton, London
Frankel L 1909 Deutsche Medizinische Wochenschrift 35: 2204–2209
Franks S, Adams J, Mason H, Polson D 1985 Ovulatory disorders in women with polycystic ovary syndrome. Clinics in Obstetrics and Gynaecology 12(3): 605–631
Gillibrand P N 1981 The investigation of pelvic pain. Communication on the scientific meeting on chronic pelvic pain: a gynaecological headache, RCOG, London
Gooch R 1831 On some of the most important diseases peculiar to women, republished by Sydenham Society, London (1859)
Henker F O 1979 Diagnosis and treatment of non-organic pelvic pain. Southern Medical Journal 72: 1132–1134
Hodgkinson C P 1953 Physiology of the ovarian veins during pregnancy. Obstetrics and Gynecology 1: 26–37
Hughes R R, Curtis D D 1962 Uterine phlebography. American Journal of Obstetrics and Gynecology 83: 156–164

Huskisson E C (1974) Measurement of pain. Lancet ii: 1127–1131
Kaupilla A 1970 Uterine phlebography with venous compression. A clinical and roentological
    study. Acta Obstetricia et Gynecologica Scandinavica 49: 33–34
Kownatzki E (1907) Die venen des weiblichen Beckens, Weisbaden, Bergmann
Luciano A A, Turksey R N, Dlugi A M, Carleo J L (1986) Endocrine consequences of oral
    medroxyprogesterone acetate (MPA) in the treatment of endometriosis. Presentation at the
    68th Annual Meeting of the Endocrine Society, Anaheim, California
Lundberg W I, Wall J E, Mathers J E 1973 Laparoscopy in the evaluation of pelvic pain.
    Obstetrics and Gynecology 42: 872
Martius H 1939 Die Kreuzschmerzen der Frau G Thieme, Liepzig
McCausland A M, Holmes F, Trotter A D Jr 1963 Venous distensibility during menstrual
    cycle. American Journal of Obstetrics and Gynecology 68: 640–643
McCausland A M, Hyman C, Winsor T, Trotter A D Jr 1961 Venous distensibility during
    pregnancy. American Journal of Obstetrics and Gynecology 81: 472–478
McNair D M, Lorr M, Droppleman L F (1971) Manual for the profile of Mood States,
    Educational and Industrial Testing Service, San Diego, California
Missanelli J S 1982 Chronic pelvic pain: intrapelvic fluid as a possible aetiological factor. Journal
    of the American Osteopathic Association 7: 492–495
Morris N, O'Neil D 1958 Outpatient gynaecology. British Medical Journal 2: 1038
Netter A 1953 l'Ovarite sclero-kystique, l'Expansion Scientifique Francaise, Paris, pp 1–185
Ochsner A, Mahoner H R 1939 Varicose veins, Mosby, St Louis
Opitz E 1922 Die uberregbarkeit der glattern muskulatur der weiblichen geschlechtsorgane.
    Zentralblatte fur Gynaekologie 40: 1594–1598
Pearce S A (1986) A psychological investigation of chronic pelvic pain in women, PhD thesis,
    University of London
Pearce S, Beard R W 1984 chronic pelvic pain. In: Broome A, Wallace L (eds) Psychology
    and gynaecological problems, Tavistock Publications, London, pp 95–116
Pent D 1972 Laparoscopy: its role in private practice. American Journal of Obstetrics and
    Gynecology 113: 459
Petrucco D M, Harris R D (1981) Pelvic pain: the disease with twenty different names. In:
    Dennerstien L, Burrows G D (eds) Obstetrics, gynaecology and psychiatry. Proceedings of
    the 8th Annual Congress of the Australian Society for Psychosomatic Obstetrics and
    Gynaecology, York Press, Victoria, Australia, pp 111–118
Pilowsky I 1978 Psychodynamic aspects of the pain experience. In: Sternbach R A (ed) The
    psychology of pain, Raven Press, New York, pp 203–217
Railo J E 1968 The pain syndrome in ovarian varicocele. Acta Chirurgica Scandinavica 134:
    157–159
Reginald P W, Beard R W, Kooner J S et al 1987 Intravenous dihydroergotamine to relieve
    pelvic congestion with pain in young women. Lancet ii: 351–353
Renaer M, Nijs P, Van Assche A, Vertommen H 1980 Chronic pelvic pain without obvious
    pathology in women. Personal observations and a review of the problem. European Journal
    of Obstetrics, Gynecology, and Reproductive Biology 10: 415–463
RCOG 1978 Gynaecological laparoscopy. In: Chamberlain G, Brown J C (eds) Report of the
    working party of the confidential enquiry into gynaecological laparoscopy, London
Rundqvist E, Sandholm L E, Larsson G 1984 Treatment of pelvic varicosities causing lower
    abdominal pain with extra peritoneal resection of the left ovarian vein. Annales Chirurgiae
    et Gynaecologiae 73: 339–341
Schultze B S 1875 Archiv fur Gynakologie 8: 134–180, quoted by Taylor (1949a)
Stearns H C, Sneeden U D 1966 Observations on the clinical and pathological aspects of the
    pelvic congestion syndrome. American Journal of Obstetrics and Gynecology 94: 718–732
Sturmdorf A 1916 Tracheloplastic methods and results. Surgery, Gynecology and Obstetrics
    22: 93–104
Tait L 1883 The pathology and treatment of the diseases of the ovaries, William Wood, New
    York
Taylor H C 1949a Vascular congestion and hyperemia. I. Psychologic basis and history of the
    concept. American Journal of Obstetrics and Gynecology 57: 211–230
Taylor H C 1949b Vascular congestion and hyperemia. II. The clinical aspects of the
    congestion–fibrosis syndrome. American Journal of Obstetrics and Gynecology 57: 637–653
Taylor H C 1949c. Vascular congestion and hyperemia. III. Etiology and therapy. American
    Journal of Obstetrics and Gynecology 57: 654–668

Taylor H C 1954 Pelvic pain based on a vascular and autonomic nervous system disorder. American Journal of Obstetrics and Gynecology 67: 1177–1196

Taylor H C 1957 The problem of pelvic pain. In Meigs J V, Samers H S (eds) Progress in gynecology, vol III, Grune & Stratton, New York, pp 191–208

Theobald G W 1951 Pelvic sympathetic syndrome. Journal of Obstetrics and Gynaecology of the British Empire 58: 733–761

Topolanski-Sierra R 1958 Pelvic phlebography. American Journal of Obstetrics and Gynecology 76: 44–52

Von Peham H, Amreich J 1934 Operative gynaecology, vol 1, Lippincott, Philadelphia

Worstman J, Singh K, Murray J 1981 Evidence for the hypothalamic origin of the polycystic ovary syndrome. Obstetrics and Gynecology 58: 137–141

Young J 1938 Lower abdominal pains of cervical origin, their genesis and treatment. British Medical Journal 1: 104–111

Videolaseroscopy for the treatment of endometriosis

INTRODUCTION

Lasers have been used in many fields of medicine for approximately two decades. Laser techniques have evolved rapidly over the past few years in a number of specialties. Of the many lasers that have been used in various surgical fields, three have been used thus far in gynaecology—carbon dioxide, argon and neodymium:yttrium–aluminium–garnet (Nd:YAG) lasers. In this chapter we will discuss the properties of these lasers and in addition we will take a look at some of the new lasers that are being tested and are becoming clinically available.

Recent advances in endoscopic surgery have enabled the gynaecological surgeon to treat an increased number of diseases of the reproductive organs with the use of the laser. In this chapter we will introduce a new modality of treatment in gynaecological surgery called videolaseroscopy. This presentation will include our results from a study of 631 patients who have undergone videolaseroscopy for the treatment of endometriosis (stages I–IV of the American Fertility Society) and other diseases of the reproductive organs.

SURGICAL LASERS

Laser is an acronym for 'light amplification by stimulated emission of radiation'. A laser produces and amplifies visible and near visible light, creating intense, coherent electromagnetic energy which is passed through air and reflected off mirrors to bring it to a precise point (Daikuzono & Joffe 1985).

The three main types of lasers used in surgery are carbon dioxide, argon and neodymium:yttrium–aluminium–garnet. Their properties are listed in Table 19.1. Developmental work involves krypton, punable dye, excimer and potassium-titanyl phosphate (KTP) crystal lasers.

The carbon dioxide laser

The CO_2 laser is most commonly used for vaporization as a part of either ablation or excision. The depth of vaporization is directly related to the time

Table 19.1 Comparative properties of surgical lasers

Property	Laser		
	CO_2	Nd (YAG)	Argon
Wavelength	10.6 μm	1.06 μm	0.5 μm
Type	Gas	Gas	Crystal
Colour dependency	No	Yes	Yes
Coagulation	Low	High	Fair
Cutting ability	++++	++	+
Pass through flexible fibres	No	Yes	Yes
Absorption	Water	Tissue protein	Pigmented tissue
Depth of penetration	+	++++	++

used to make the incision. Ablation of the tissue is complete vaporization into a smoke plume (Nezhat et al 1987). Excision of the tissue is vaporization of an underlying area to lift off the lesion so that it can be sent for pathology evaluation.

The CO_2 laser is a gas molecular laser that emits light in the infra-red range of 10 600 nm (Nezhat et al 1986). It is absorbed by non-reflective solids and liquids, particularly water-containing tissue. The absorption is not dependent upon the colour of the tissue and has minimal scattering.

The CO_2 laser also has the property of coagulation of the surface peritoneum. This is most useful in performing cuff salpingostomies. With this technique the laser can be used in a very low-power density of about 10–50 W/cm² to coagulate and contract the serosal surfaces of the hydrosalpinx. This turns the hydrosalpinx back in a cuff fashion.

The radiation of the CO_2 laser is similar to the radiant energy that can be absorbed when sitting in front of the fireplace. Bruhat first reported the use of the CO_2 laser at laparoscopy with the beam through the channel of an operative laparoscope (Bruhat et al 1979).

The argon laser

The argon laser produces up to 10 lasing wavelengths in the blue/green portion of the spectrum. The argon laser has the greatest absorption occurring in pigmented tissue, including the retina of the eye.

The argon laser can pass through the covering peritoneum over endometriosis and coagulate the deep endometriotic tissue without causing surface disruption. It offers the advantage of selective damage of the endometrial implants with little or no damage to surrounding or underlying tissues (Keye 1986). Since the argon laser is passed through flexible quartz fibres, it can be used through endoscopes.

The neodymium:yttrium–aluminium–garnet (YAG) laser

YAG lasers are solid-state lasers that utilize an artificially grown crystal. The YAG lasers have the greatest penetration and coagulation, but also create a great amount of scatter with the potential to damage anything in the vincinity of the scattered beam.

The YAG laser can penetrate up to 4 mm in depth. As with the argon laser, the YAG laser may be passed through flexible fibres. It is now being used through a hysteroscope, for lasering of endometrium, and through the laparoscope to laser endometriosis (Lomano 1983).

The major limitations are that these fibres are used for non-contact surgery. This type of surgery is imprecise and the tips may burn off and melt if they touch blood or tissue. Because of these problems a system has been developed to perform contact photocoagulation and tissue vaporization with the Nd:YAG laser. This allows direct contact with the fibre tip and the tissue. These new tips allow for vaporization and incision as well as for coagulation. The contact probe decreases the amount of scatter, therefore allowing for increased precision. Less smoke is produced with the laser when using these tips because the same tissue effect can be achieved with less wattage output.

A new laser with potential in gynaecology

A new laser which is now being used in clinical trials in gynaecology as well as in other specialties is the KTP crystal laser.

The advantage of this laser through the laparoscope is that it can be passed through a flexible fibre which can be easily directed under laparoscopic control and placed close to the tissue to be vaporized or incised. Clinical investigations of this laser are currently being conducted in cases of endometriosis and adhesions. This laser is generated by a frequency-doubled YAG laser. It can be used under fluids, is colour-dependent (similar to the argon laser), and has a wavelength of 532 nm. It is in the green spectrum with properties similar to the argon laser.

As laser equipment is continually updated, this will help to ensure that the surgeon has the laser available in the operating room that is best suited for treating the patient, whatever the disease may be.

VIDEOLASEROSCOPY: A NEW MODALITY

Recent advances in laparoscopic surgery have enabled the gynaecological surgeon to treat an increased number of diseases of the reproductive organs with the use of the laser through the laparoscope.

Operating directly through the laparoscope has some disadvantages, including severe back strain during long procedures. In addition, because the surgeon is the only one who can view the operating field, other members of the surgical team may become inattentive. Because of these disadvantages we have introduced a new modality called videolaseroscopy.

Methods and materials

This method involves the development and refinement of a new laser video-monitoring technique incorporating the use of a video-camera, a video-recorder and a high-resolution video-monitor in conjunction with the laser laparoscope.

Videolaseroscopy allows the surgeon to operate in an upright position directly from the video-monitor, reducing back strain and fatigue, as encountered in operating directly through the laparoscope. The surgeon can use both eyes while operating. The camera also allows the surgeon to 'zoom' in on endometriosis or other pathology, regardless of how deep in the pelvis it might be, helping to ensure that the whole disease is eradicated. By magnifying the tubes and ovaries one can perform microsurgery with videolaseroscopy. In addition, the camera enables the surgeon to operate from almost any angle and position by rotating the camera. For example, we have treated numerous cases of anterior abdominal-wall endometriosis which traditionally had been missed and not treated at laparotomy or laparoscopy. Every case is video-taped so that a permanent record may be kept on each patient. This is especially helpful in patient teaching follow-up with endometriosis, and if there is a referring doctor, it provides them with a tape of the procedure. Also, this is an excellent method for teaching residents.

The laser we predominantly have used thus far in our videolaseroscopy treatment has been the CO_2 laser. We have also used the argon and KTP-532 lasers in certain cases of endometriosis.

One advantage of the CO_2 laser is the focal point of the beam, which is 0.2–0.8 mm in diameter and allows precise controlled tissue distribution. In addition, because of the CO_2 laser's collimated beam, there is no lateral damage on impact.

The CO_2 laser beam is totally absorbed by water in soft tissue up to a depth of 0.1 mm from the point of impact, leaving underlying tissue unharmed and allowing a rapid dispersion of heat. Therefore, there is low risk of thermal damage to underlying or surrounding tissue. In addition to precision, the laser can make a bloodless incision. Defocusing the beam enables the surgeon to coagulate (0.5 mm) blood vessels (Nezhat et al 1986). The beam can be defocused by increasing the distance of the scope to the tissue being lasered.

The CO_2 laser, as previously stated, is a very precise laser, having been used for the treatment of several diseases of the reproductive organs by laparotomy and laparoscopy. Videolaseroscopic treatment of endometriosis and other diseases of the reproductive organs can be relatively simple and inexpensive, especially if it is effected at the same time as diagnostic laparoscopy.

For the procedures discussed herein, the CO_2, argon and KTP (Cooper 500, Cooper-Lasersonics Inc., Santa Clara, CA) lasers were used. The CO_2

laser is used through the operating channel of the laparoscope. A direct coupler is used and attached to the laparoscope (Nezhat Coupler, Cabot Medical, Langhorne, PA).

In our present study we have reviewed the cases of 631 patients who have undergone videolaseroscopy for the treatment of endometriosis. The only contributing factor to infertility in this patient group was endometriosis. Other causes of infertility (hormonal, male factor, etc.) had been eliminated as the probable cause of the patients' infertility.

Preoperatively, the possibility of laparotomy, and more extensive additional procedures like colostomy or hysterectomy, were discussed with the patient. Before treating a large endometrioma, careful laparoscopic assessment was done to reduce the chance of draining a pelvic malignancy. The cysts that had the appearance of endometriomas were first aspirated for cytology. Peritoneal washing would have been performed if suspicion of malignancy existed.

The procedures were performed under general endotracheal anaesthesia with patients placed in the lithotomy position. The bladder was drained and a cervical cannula was placed for manipulation of the uterus and for intraoperative injection of diluted indigo carmine. Each patient received 1 g of Mefoxin intravenously preoperatively, and again in the recovery room as a prophylactic dosage.

After pneumoperitoneum induction, the operating laparoscope is inserted intra-umbilically. A 5.5 mm second-puncture trocar is then inserted in the midline approximately 2–4 cm above the symphysis pubis. A Nezhat suction–irrigator probe is then introduced through the second puncture site. This probe has two trumpet valves that can be regulated by the surgeon's finger. By pushing one trumpet valve, the surgeon can easily irrigate as this is connected by tubing to an intravenous bag on a pole with a pressurized cuff around the bag at 300 mmHg. The irrigation fluid consists of 5000 units of heparin in 1 litre of lactated Ringer's solution. By pushing the other trumpet the surgeon can easily suction off any drainage or smoke generated by the laser. This is connected to the suction tubing. This enables the suction and irrigation to be easily available through one probe. When necessary, a third incision is made along the suprapubic line 5–10 cm from the second trocar. This allows other ancillary instruments to be inserted, such as a titanium rod or an atraumatic alligator grasping forceps, that may be required during surgery. All instruments used must be titanium- or sand-blasted when used with the laser to prevent reflection of the laser from shiny surfaces.

A focused beam of $6000-24\,000\,W/cm^2$ (0.5 mm spot-size at a 15–60 W setting) was employed to vaporize endometriosis implants from the ovary, pelvic side-wall, cul-de-sac, tubes, uterosacral ligaments, bladder flap, and peritoneum or capsule of endometriomas. The superpulse mode of the CO_2 laser is used. Endometriomas up to 15 cm in diameter and any peritubal or peri-ovarian adhesions were also treated by laser lysis.

When the cavity is opened, the internal wall is examined for excrescent tumour. If one is found, a frozen section is performed. Larger endometriomas are aspirated and irrigated several times with a Wolf needle and then with the Nezhat suction irrigator probe after fluid is gathered for cytology. The endometriomas are bivalved, the capsule is dissected and as much as possible is removed. The base of the capsule is then vaporized to make the ablation of the capsule complete, helping to ensure that the endometrioma does not persist and to seal off small blood vessels.

After an area of endometriosis is vaporized it is important to irrigate several times. This enables the surgeon to check that all endometriosis has been removed. It is also crucial to remove the charcoal material from sites that have been vaporized as remaining charcoal may cause adhesions. This can be accomplished by washing the area numerous times. At the conclusion of the procedure, thorough irrigation helps to ensure that there is no bleeding as the fluid in the pelvic cavity should be clear, leaving a clean pelvis before closing.

Videolaseroscopy gives the surgeon the ability to closely evaluate the ovaries to help ensure that all adhesions are lasered during the procedure. Lasering any adhesions on the ovary will aid in the egg release. After all adhesions appear to have been vaporized, a final check is made by filling the pelvic cavity with the irrigation solution until the ovary is floating in clear fluid. If any adhesions remain they will flower out from the ovary in the fluid. This enables the surgeon to see and laser any persisting adhesions that otherwise might be missed.

The patients are routinely discharged approximately 4 hours after surgery. Of the 631 patients who underwent videolaseroscopy of endometriosis, we have had no major side-effects and the minor complications have been gas pain and bruises of the abdominal wall associated with laparoscopy.

At the end of the procedure much care is taken to remove as much smoke plume and CO_2 as possible. After removing the laser and coupler from the laser laparoscope, the Nezhat suction irrigator is used in the abdomen for the final time, pushing the remaining smoke and gas out through the suction as well as through the top of the laser laparoscope. This appears to help with postoperative discomfort caused by remaining gas.

Results

In the present study, a total of 631 patients underwent videolaseroscopy for the treatment of their endometriosis. Of these, 441 patients presented with a complaint of infertility and 190 patients had pelvic pain or a pelvic mass. Out of 441 infertility patients with endometriosis, 181 patients had at least one additional factor contributing to their infertility; in 260 patients, endometriosis was the only factor (Nezhat et al 1986).

Of the 260 above-mentioned patients with endometriosis as the sole factor contributing to infertility, 156 have been followed for at least 18 months. The classification and pregnancy rate of these 156 patients are as follows (Table 19.2): of 31 patients who had stage I American Fertility Society (AFS)

Table 19.2 Classifications and pregnancy rate in 156 patients with endometriosis and infertility after 18 months follow-up

Stage (AFS)	No. of patients	No. of pregnancies	%
I	31	24	77
II	63	39	62
III	41	25	61
IV	21	14	66
Total	156	102	65

endometriosis (1985), 24 achieved pregnancy, resulting in a pregnancy rate of 77%; of 63 patients who had moderate or stage II AFS endometriosis, 39 (or 62%) became pregnant; of 41 patients who had severe stage III AFS endometriosis, 25 (or 61%) conceived; and, finally, of 21 patients who had extensive or stage IV AFS endometriosis, in 14 (or 66%), pregnancy resulted.

In summary, 102 out of 156 patients (or 65%) achieved pregnancy; 52 (or 51%) of 102 pregnancies occurred in the first 6 months after surgery; 40 (or 39%) of the patients conceived between 6 and 12 months after surgery; and 10 (or 10%) of 102 pregnancies followed 12–18 months after videolaseroscopy (Table 19.3).

Table 19.3 Length of time required to achieve pregnancy after surgery

No. of months	No. of patients	% success in achieving pregnancy
6	52	51
6–12	40	39
12–18	10	10
6–18	102 (out of 156 total)	65

Among the 190 endometriosis patients with pelvic pain, figures for AFS endometriosis were as follows: 67 had stage I, 73 had stage II, 27 had stage III and 23 had stage IV endometriosis.

In these women, the percentages for pain relief were as follows (Table 19.4):

Table 19.4 Percentage of pain relief in the 1–12 months following videolaseroscopy in 190 patients with endometriosis

No. of months	Patients with total relief	Patients with partial relief	Patients with no relief
1	185 (97%)	5 (3%)	0 (0%)
6	167 (89%)	18 (9%)	5 (3%)
9	160 (84%)	23 (12%)	7 (4%)
12	155 (82%)	25 (13%)	10 (4%)

Total relief: 185 (or 97%) in 1 month; 167 (or 89%) in 6 months; 160 (or 84%) in 9 months; and 155 (or 82%) in 12 months;

Partial relief: 5 (or 3%) in 1 month; 18 (or 9%) in 6 months; 23 (or 12%) in 9 months; and 25 (or 13%) in 12 months;
No relief: 5 (or 3%) in 6 months; 7 (or 4%) in 9 months; and 10 (or 11%) in 12 months.

Discussion

Management and treatment of infertility because of endometriosis may be effected surgically or medically (Guzick & Rock 1983, Buttram et al 1985, Puleo & Hammond 1983, Greenblatt & Tzingounis 1979, Kelly & Roberts 1983, Martin 1985, Buttram 1979, Chong & Baggish 1984).

Danazol has been considered one of the best methods for medical treatment of endometriosis when no significant peritubal or peri-ovarian adhesions are present. Danazol therapy is advantageous in that it avoids major surgery while providing excellent pregnancy rates in mild (stage I AFS) to moderate (stage II AFS) endometriosis (Buttram et al 1985, Puleo & Hammond 1983, Greenblatt & Tzingounis 1979). Treatment with danazol (Buttram et al 1985, Puleo & Hammond 1983, Greenblatt & Tzingounis 1979), however, is expensive and prolonged, lasting for up to 9 months. In addition, undesirable side-effects, including menstrual irregularities, weight gain, nervousness, depression, acne, etc., have been reported. A case of bilateral sensorineural hearing loss has been associated with this therapy (Enyear & Price 1984).

In comparison with hormonal therapy, videolaseroscopic treatment of endometriosis can be relatively simple and inexpensive, especially if it is effected at the same time as diagnostic laparoscopy.

In terms of efficacy of treatment, this study shows favourable results compared with published pregnancy rates for different stages of endometriosis (Buttram 1979) treated with drugs or conservative surgery. Of particular interest is the conception rate for patients with endometriosis classified as severe (stage III AFS) and extensive (stage IV AFS).

Mild, moderate and severe endometriosis have been treated before with laparoscopy using non-laser techniques (Eward 1978, Sulewski et al 1980, Hasson 1979, Daniell & Christianson 1981, Frangeheim 1978). Frangeheim (1978) treated large endometriomas laparoscopically by aspirating the contents. Of the punctured cysts, 60% did not refill, but 40% did refill and required subsequent surgical removal.

When the CO_2 laser is used through the videolaseroscope, the surgeon's line of vision and the beam are almost coincident. They are almost coincident because the line of vision and the line of the CO_2 laser beam emerge from two different channels. This is an important point for one to consider to prevent any inadvertent tissue damage.

We have avoided the significant back strain associated with operating directly through the laparoscope by refining video-monitoring techniques. With videolaseroscopy we are able to excise endometriomas of up to 15 cm in size and stage IV AFS endometriosis.

The use of the video-camera, video-recorder and video-monitor in conjunction with laser procedures provides two benefits. Firstly, fatigue brought on by long, complicated procedures can be minimized as the surgeon works in a more comfortable, upright posture, with increased magnification by the monitor rather than direct eye contact with the scope. Secondly, a video-recording of the procedure is available for future reference. Storz's video-camera (Karl Storz Endoscopy America, Inc., Culver City, CA) and the Wolf Video Camera (Richard Wolf Medical Instruments Corp.) were used interchangeably. Both of these cameras provide good resolution and good quality video-tapes.

The advantages of videolaseroscopy over lapartotomy are a faster recovery period and a shorter hospital stay. Following videolaseroscopy the average hospital stay is 4–6 hours after the patient is brought to the recovery room, with the maximum stay being 24 hours after surgery (a one-night stay). This compares with a routine hospital stay of 3–5 days for laparotomy patients and in some cases as long as 7 days.

Due to very minimal handling of the tissue through laparoscopy, there is less trauma to the abdominal tissues. The incisions made are only big enough to accommodate a 10 mm primary trocar at the umbilicus and as many as 1–3 smaller incisions to accommodate ancillary instruments 5.5 mm in diameter along the pubic hairline. Having smaller incisions and decreased handling, trauma and manipulation of the tissue creates other advantages of videolaseroscopy. Less exposure of the abdominal cavity to the air, thereby reducing secondary dryness of tissue, the elimination of glove powder, less blood loss and suturing of tissue, and overall less chance of contamination to the air along with the formation of postoperative adhesions, are probably all factors that are diminished compared with laparotomy.

Furthermore, susceptibility to bacterial contamination and oozing from the abdominal wall incision may be increased by laparotomy in comparison with laparoscopy and may enhance adhesion formation. The use of the laser in preference to cautery or surgical excision of endometrioma may forestall the formation of postoperative adhesions, to which the ovaries are vulnerable.

Finally, use of the laser can preclude the formidable complications associated with the use of cautery. The energy of the CO_2 laser is focused very precisely, so the tissue beyond 100 μm in depth is unaffected. This precision allows destruction of endometriosis close to the vital structures such as the ureter, bowel or blood vessels when the surgery is performed by an experienced laser surgeon. This precision is not possible with cautery. The addition of the video-camera improves the surgeon's visibility with additional magnification, thereby complementing an already efficacious system.

It must be emphasized that videolaseroscopy be performed only by experienced operative laparoscopists. This requires the surgeon to have extensive training and experience with the laser. It should not be attempted by inexperienced laparoscopists who are not comfortable with multiple puncture techniques. More advanced disease should be treated only when the surgeon thinks the procedure can be done as well or better than if it were done via laparotomy.

We believe videolaseroscopy is an excellent choice for treatment of most diseases of the reproductive organs, particularly endometriosis.

SUMMARY

In our opinion, mild to extensive endometriosis should be treated when infertility or pain is a concern. Furthermore, it is our opinion that conservative surgical management of endometriosis should involve the videolaserscope.

We believe that when conservative surgical management of endometriosis is indicated, videolaseroscopy offers definite advantages to the surgeon, and comparable, if not improved, results to the patient when compared with other modalities of therapy.

In our opinion videolaseroscopy is efficacious and, with its other previously discussed advantages, may be superior to the other surgical therapies for endometriosis. In 102 (or 65%) out of 156 patients with endometriosis, pregnancy was achieved, and 155 out of 190 patients had no pain after 1 year when treated by videolaseroscopy.

Most surgery departments in large hospitals now have at least one or two CO_2 lasers and many are getting YAG or argon lasers too. Laser manufacturers are currently working on developing a laser that will allow the surgeon to switch from CO_2 to argon or YAG by pushing a button on one machine, or on a way to have each type of laser available by plugging into the wall for the laser that is desired, just as wall suction is available in the operating room, so that the surgeon would have the ability to switch from CO_2 to argon to YAG during the same case if so desired. As the laser laparoscopists are becoming more experienced, they are using the CO_2 laser close to the ureters, bladder, bowel or blood vessels and can now open large endometriomas. As these other types of lasers become more readily available, they will give the surgeon another option for ablation or coagulation of the capsule with the advantage of not producing as much smoke as the CO_2 laser.

Because advances in laser equipment are appearing at such a rapid pace, it is important to keep up-to-date on these matters so that the surgeon can have the best equipment and modality possible to treat the patient at hand.

The surgical laser is not a panacea. This adjunctive surgical device in the hands of an experienced laparoscopist can broaden his/her abilities and subsequently improve fertility rates.

In our opinion, conservative surgical management of mild to extensive endometriosis should involve videolaseroscopy.

REFERENCES

The American Fertility Society 1985 Classification of endometriosis. Fertility and Sterility 32: 633

Bruhat M, Mage C, Manhes M 1979 Use of the CO_2 laser via laparoscopy. In: Kaplan I (ed)

Laser surgery III. Proceedings of the Third International Society for Laser Surgery, International Society for Laser Surgery, Tel Aviv, p 275

Buttram V C Jr 1979 Surgical treatment of endometriosis in the infertile female: a modified approach. Fertility and Sterility 32: 635

Buttram V C Jr, Reiter R C, Ward S 1985 Treatment of endometriosis with danazol: report of a 6-year prospective study. Fertility and Sterility 43: 353

Chong A, Baggish M 1984 Management of pelvic endometriosis by means of intraabdominal carbon dioxide laser. Fertility and Sterility 41: 14

Daikuzono N, Joffe S N 1985 Artificial sapphire probe for contact photocoagulation and tissue vaporization with the Nd:YAG laser. Medical Instruments 19(4): 173–178

Daniell J F, Christianson C 1981 Combined laparoscopic surgery and danazol therapy for pelvic endometriosis. Fertility and Sterility 35: 521

Enyear T J Jr, Price W A 1984 Bilateral sensorineural hearing loss from danazol therapy. Journal of Reproductive Medicine 29: 5

Edward R D 1978 Cauterization of stage I and II endometriosis and resulting pregnancy rate. In: Phillips J M (ed) Endoscopy and gynecology, American Association of Gynecologic Laparoscopists, Downey, California, p 276

Frangeheim H 1978 Endoscopy and gynecology. In: Phillips J M (ed) The range and limits of operating laparoscopy in the diagnosis of sterility, American Association of Gynecologic Laparoscopists, Downey, California, p 282

Greenblatt R B, Tzingounis V 1979 Danazol treatment of endometriosis: long-term follow-up. Fertility and Sterility 32: 518

Guzick D S, Rock J A 1983 A comparison of danazol and conservative surgery for the treatment of infertility due to mild or moderate endometriosis. Fertility and Sterility 40: 580

Hasson 1979 Electrocoagulation of pelvic endometriosis lesions with laparoscopic control. American Journal of Obstetrics and Gynecology 128: 128

Kelly R W, Roberts D K 1983 CO_2 laser laparoscopy: potential alternative to danazol in the treatment of stage I and II endometriosis. Journal of Reproductive Medicine 28: 638

Keye W 1986 The present and future application of lasers to the treatment of endometriosis and infertility. International Journal of Fertility 31(2): 160–164

Lomano J M 1983 Laparoscopic ablation of endometriosis with the YAG laser. Lasers in Surgery and Medicine 3: 179

Martin D C 1985 CO_2 laser laparoscopy for the treatment of endometriosis associated with infertility. Journal of Reproductive Medicine 30: 409

Nezhat C 1986 Videolaseroscopy: a new modality for the treatment of endometriosis. Endometriose Symposium, Clermont-Ferrand, France, November

Nezhat C, Crowgey S R, Garrison C P 1986 Surgical treatment of endometriosis via laser laparoscopy. Fertility and Sterility 45(6): 778–782

Nezhat C, Winer W K, Nezhat F, Forrest D, Reeves W 1987 Smoke from laser surgery: is there a health hazard? Lasers in Surgery and Medicine 7: 376–382

Puleo J G, Hammond C B 1983 Conservative treatment of endometriosis externa: the effects of danazol therapy. Fertility and Sterility 40: 164

Sulewski J M, Crucia F D, Brenitskey C 1980 The treatment of endometriosis at laparoscopy for infertility. American Journal of Obstetrics and Gynecology 128: 128

20

B. V. Lewis

Hysteroscopy

INTRODUCTION

Visual examination of the uterine cavity is an old technique. Pantaleoni, in 1865, was the first to examine the uterus using a small tube inserted through the external os of the cervix with a kerosene lamp or a candle for a light source (Lindemann 1973).

This first examination was performed on a 60-year-old woman with intractable post-menopausal bleeding, and it was reported that polyp-like growths were found.

Many technical advances in the optical systems were developed in Europe at the turn of the century (Frangenheim 1987), but only in the last 25 years have fibre-optic light sources and the Hopkins lens system made hysteroscopy a practical diagnostic out-patient procedure.

INSTRUMENTS

A simple hysteroscope consists of a telescope within a sheath.

The telescope is usually 4 mm in diameter with a 5–6 mm sheath so that the instrument can be inserted through the cervix with minimal dilatation.

The telescope has a 25–30° fore-oblique view with a Hopkins lens system consisting of special glass rods placed at intervals along the axis of the telescope. This unique system provides high resolution and contrast, with natural colour tones and a wide viewing angle. The fibre optic light transmission produces a bright image from a proximal high intensity light source so that still photography or closed circuit television is possible. A beam splitter allows simultaneous observation by an assistant with a minimal loss of illumination— a facility which is very valuable for teaching purposes.

The sheath has a proximal valve through which gas or fluid can be insufflated to distend the uterine cavity—an essential requirement before adequate visualisation of the cavity of the uterus is possible.

This simple system is adequate for panoramic examination of the uterine cavity.

If intra-uterine surgery is needed, the 4 mm telescope should be enclosed in an operating sheath which contains a separate channel for instruments. This channel is wider than the non-operating sheath (21 French, Wolf, 7 mm Storz). These flexible instruments are narrow in diameter, but there is a wide range of biopsy forceps, grasping forceps and scissors.

ATTACHMENT TO THE CERVIX

When gas or fluid is used to distend the uterine cavity, some escapes through the cervix. A small leak does not matter, and often, the telescope and sheath block the endocervical canal. However, if leaking is troublesome, the cervix can be occluded by a specially designed portio adaptor, which is attached to the ectocervix by suction. The telescope is then inserted through the adaptor.

CONTACT HYSTEROSCOPY

If the lens of the telescope is in contact with the endometrium or the epithelium of the endocervical canal, a magnified view is obtained, but the field of vision is restricted. A magnified view allows study of the glandular epithelium, and at higher magnification the cellular and microvascular structure can be examined. These additional contact instruments are the Hamou micro-colpo-hysteroscope (Storz) or the cervico-hysteroscope (Wolf).

Contact hysteroscopy is of value in women with positive cervical smears in whom the upper edge of the dysplastic epithelium lies within the endocervix. Direct visualisation of the transformation zone within the canal becomes possible, especially with differential staining of the squamous and columnar epithelium using Lugol's iodine and Waterman's blue dye.

THE HAMOU MICRO-HYSTEROSCOPE

The contact micro-hysteroscope consists of a 4 mm Storz telescope with a direct occular and an offset occular each offering two magnifications (Hamou 1981). Direct vision allows conventional panoramic hysteroscopy at unit magnification. When a small lever is depressed, the offset occular comes into use and the uterine cavity can be examined at × 20 magnification. When the tip of the telescope is placed in direct contact with the epithelium, the magnification increases to × 60 with the direct occular, and to × 150 with the offset occular. At these very high magnifications individual capillaries can be examined in detail, but it must be admitted that interpretation of the pictures requires considerable experience and expertise. Panoramic hysteroscopy is a much easier technique to learn and should be the first priority for the beginner.

The Hamou II (Storz) and the microview telescope (Wolf) do not have a second eye-piece laterally offset from the instrument axis. Both these telescopes have a focusing wheel which can be altered to adjust the focus, and thus the magnification, for each different object/lens distance. The possible magnification is inversely proportional to the distance from the lens to the object to be examined. Thus, maximum magnification is obtained when the tip of the telescope is in contact with the endometrium or cervical canal.

PORTABLE OUT-PATIENT HYSTEROSCOPES

The Van de Pas hysteroscope

Ambulatory hysteroscopy means that the procedure is performed on an out-patient basis. Usually, no premedication, analgesia or anaesthesia is needed, so the operation can be performed in the consulting room, and on completion of the procedure the patient can immediately return home. The Van de Pas system (Van de Pas 1983) was designed for single-handed out-patient use and consists of a portio adaptor and a 4 mm telescope with a 30° angle of vision and a 70° field of vision. The unique feature of the instrument is the sliding mechanism operated by the surgeon single-handed which enables the telescope to be advanced slowly and safely into the uterine cavity for a maximum of 7 cm, therefore reducing the risk of perforation of the fundus.

The Parent self-contained out-patient system (Wolf)

This hysteroscope consists of a 4 mm lumina telescope in a sheath held by a completely self-contained unit which provides both illumination and gas for distending the uterine cavity (Parent et al 1985).

Gaseous distension is provided by a replaceable cartridge of CO_2 gas at a maximum flow rate of 100 ml/min, the gas entering the uterus from a hole in the sheath near the tip of the telescope. Each cartridge contains about 4 litres of gas under pressure, which allows about 10 hysteroscopies or a flow of about 1 hour and 20 minutes at a flow rate of 50 ml/min. Illumination is provided by three rechargeable batteries placed in the handle of the unit. While this light source is adequate for panoramic views, it is not bright enough for photography. It is, however, a simple process to connect the telescope to a high intensity light source via a fibre optic cable. The great advantage of the Parent system is that it is completely self-contained and portable, so it can be transported from office to hospital without the need for a heavy light source or a special gas insufflation.

SPECIALISED HYSTEROSCOPES

The flexible hysteroscope

All the hysteroscopes so far considered are rigid. However, flexible hysteroscopes are being developed and may provide some advantages. The flexible instrument is a modified choledochoscope that is 6 mm in diameter (KeyMed—Olympus). The telescope, with its channel for gas or fluid insufflation, is introduced through the cervix after minimal dilatation, and the tip can be angled through 180° by a wheel on the proximal end. Although the view is more 'grainy' than a rigid telescope because of the large number of fibres, the view, especially into the cornua, may be better than that provided by conventional hysteroscopy, and this could be of advantage for the insertion of intra-tubal devices for sterilisation. Much development work still needs to be done.

The hysteroser

This instrument was developed in France (MTO, Paris). It has a unique telescope consisting of a rod of optical glass which ends in a concave mirror. An ingenious and unique device of mirrors and diaphragms traps and concentrates ambient light so that no external light source is required, illumination being provided by daylight or the reflected light from a theatre lamp. This makes the unit completely portable. However, it can only be used as a contact hysteroscope. This does mean that bleeding into the uterine cavity is not a contraindication for the procedure, and further, no distension of the uterine cavity with gas or fluid is required.

However, no panoramic view is possible and this restriction does limit its use. Although ingenious, it cannot replace the simple standard technique of panoramic hysteroscopy (Baggish 1979).

DISTENDING THE UTERINE CAVITY

The anterior and posterior walls of the uterine cavity are normally adherent and must, therefore, be separated before panoramic hysteroscopy. This is achieved by allowing gas, usually carbon dioxide or fluid (normally 32% dextran or 5% dextrose), to flow into the uterus via a side channel in the telescope sheath. The distending medium may be prevented from leaking around the cervix because of the tight fit between the telescope and the endocervix or by the application of a portio applicator onto the endocervix. Some of the fluid or gas will inevitably leak into the peritoneal cavity through the tubal ostium, but if the flow rate is low and the examining time is short, the volume which enters the peritoneum is insignificant.

Gaseous distension

Carbon dioxide is the gas of choice to distend the uterus because it is easily absorbed and inert.

Carbon dioxide is delivered from a Hysteroflator (Storz) or a Metromat (Wolf). Both these machines deliver gas at a flow rate of not more than 100 ml/min under low pressure. At all times the pressure and flow rate are visible on clear dials and the flow rate can be reduced in increments. It cannot be emphasised too strongly that the pneumoperitoneum apparatus used for laparoscopy must not be used for hysteroscopy because the high pressure and flow rate are dangerous.

Fluid distension

The media used most often today are high molecular-weight dextran (Hyskon), or 5% dextrose in water (Taylor and Hamou 1983).

If dextran is preferred, about 20–30 ml are slowly injected into the uterus via a syringe attached to the perfusion channel in the sheath. Hyskon has the advantage of being non-miscible with blood, which forms globules in the medium. Hyskon is viscous and if it is allowed to dry on the instrument, all the moving parts will block. At the completion of each examination, the telescope and sheath must be disconnected and carefully washed in warm water.

Five per cent dextrose in water can be used as an alternative to distend the uterine cavity. The dextrose should be used in a continuous flow and is especially useful if the examination is carried out in the premenstrual phase of the cycle or when there is intra-uterine bleeding. Blood passes into solution and is washed out through the cervix. If dextrose is used, the expensive gas insufflating machines are not required. Instillation of dextrose is achieved by wrapping a 500 ml plastic bag in a blood pressure cuff inflated to about 100 mmHg.

ILLUMINATION

For panoramic hysteroscopy, adequate illumination is obtained using an 150 W light source and a fibre optic cable. More recently, fluid cables allow even brighter images.

If photography or closed circuit television is being used, a xenon light source is preferable, but this is much more expensive.

THE TECHNIQUE OF PANORAMIC HYSTEROSCOPY

Hysteroscopy is best performed in the immediate postmenstrual phase because blood obscures the view. However, with modern equipment this is less essential than previously, but even so, hysteroscopy is best avoided during menstruation. If bleeding is present, distension of the uterine cavity with a fluid rather than a gaseous medium will wash the blood away and allow more detail to be seen.

The patient should be asked to empty her bladder and is then placed in a modified lithotomy position using the Lloyd-Davies stirrups. A Sims' speculum is inserted into the vagina and the cervix is washed with an antiseptic. A single-toothed vulsellum is used to steady the cervix and a uterine sound is introduced to measure the depth of the cavity. In premenopausal women the telescope can be introduced through the external os with no dilatation of the cervix, but some times minimal dilatation to 5 or 6 Hegar is necessary. In postmenopausal patients moderate dilatation is usually required, but the dilators should not be introduced to the fundus of the uterus because this may stimulate bleeding and therefore obscure the view. If a cervical cap is being used, it should now be placed on the cervix and held in place with a vacuum. If no cap is used, the telescope is gently introduced through the os and advanced under direct vision through the endocervical canal into the cavity of the uterus. The distending fluid or gas slowly opens up the uterine cavity. The uterus is inspected systematically and the cornual orifice on each side is examined. When the lens approaches close to the cornua, the view is magnified.

The main point at issue is whether hysteroscopy should be carried out without analgesia, with a paracervical block, or under a light general anaesthetic. All the European authorities insist that no anaesthetic is necessary in the majority of patients, and only a small number of women need analgesia or a paracervical block.

While this is undoubtedly true, it is more difficult to operate through the hysteroscope without anaesthesia, except for simple retrieval of IUDs. A formal curettage requires anaesthesia. However, hysteroscopy should be regarded generally as an out-patient procedure.

INDICATIONS FOR HYSTEROSCOPY

Hysteroscopy can be performed in all patients in whom a curettage is indicated. Indeed, it is probable that the traditional 'D and C' should now be replaced by 'H and C'. Thus, hysteroscopy is indicated in menstrual irregularity due to dysfunctional bleeding, post-coital bleeding, intermenstrual bleeding and postmenopausal bleeding. In dysfunctional bleeding, the uterine cavity looks normal. Specific indications for hysteroscopy include recurrent abortions to exclude congenital abnormality or a submucous fibroid, and suspected Asherman's syndrome. Adenomyosis and endometrial hyperplasia present a non-specific appearance, and the disgnosis may not be certain on hysteroscopy without histological confirmation.

More recently, the indications for hysteroscopy have been extended to include examination under magnification of the transformation zone in cases of incomplete colposcopy and in operative hysteroscopy for sterilisation or laser ablation of the endometrium. The recovery of a lost coil is often easier when the device can be seen.

Pregnancy is normally considered a contraindication to the operation, but the new technique of chorionoscopy suggests that, even in pregnancy, direct examination of the uterine cavity may be of value. In puerperal bleeding, hysteroscopy may reveal a placental fragment.

The two main contraindications, however, are pregnancy and acute pelvic sepsis.

THE NORMAL APPEARANCE

In premenopausal women, the appearance of the endometrium depends on the phase of the menstrual cycle.

As the telescope passes through the external os, the folds of the endocervical epithelium come into view and rapidly change to the smooth, narrow cervical canal. The tip of the telescope next passes the internal os to enter the uterine cavity, which distends as the gas or fluid medium flows into it.

In postmenopausal women, an uninterrupted view is almost invariable. The endometrium appears as a light pink or red colour, which becomes more prominent as the lens approaches the endometrium and the intensity of illumination increases. In premenstrual women, blood may obscure the view. If gas is the distending medium, blood and gas bubbles can be troublesome, but by manipulating the telescope a clear view of the cavity is obtained. The endometrium is much redder and more vascular. If hysteroscopy is performed during menstruation, the degenerating endometrium can be seen peeling off the basal layer. A fluid medium is of advantage at this time because the blood passes into solution and is washed out through the cervix, or forms globules in the Hyskon.

The cornual orifice on each side is usually visible and indeed becomes a prominent feature in the field of view as the telescope is advanced and magnification increases. It then becomes relatively easy to catheterise the proximal 1 cm of the tube or to insert an intra-tubal device.

With increasing experience it becomes possible to date the endometrium by its appearance, and this opinion correlates well with histology (Stevens & Van Herendael 1986).

In postmenopausal women, the endometrium is atrophic, white and featureless. The cornua, however, are smaller.

As the telescope is rotated, the uterine cavity can be examined completely. When the panoramic view is complete, the telescope is withdrawn and the endometrium and endocervix may be examined at × 20 magnification. This is the time at which biopsy can be carried out if an operating sheath is used.

The operation occupies 5–7 minutes or less, and the amount of gas or fluid which enters the peritoneum through the cornua is small.

ABNORMALITIES SEEN ON HYSTEROSCOPY

Benign polyps

Benign mucous polyps are frequently seen in women with abnormal uterine bleeding. They float in the cavity as the pressure of the distending medium varies, but must be distinguished from strips of dislodged endometrium, especially if the women is premenstrual (Taylor & Hamou 1983).

Fibroid polyps

A fibroid polyp is easily seen and recognised by its pedicle, smooth surface and white appearance. The finding of a fibroid polyp by hysteroscopy in a young woman with menorrhagia is a very satisfying diagnosis which cannot be made with such precision by any other technique.

Lost intra-uterine devices

Ultrasound can confirm that a missing device is in the uterus rather than the peritoneum, but even curettage can be difficult, especially when the device is buried in the endometrium or is penetrating the myometrium. At hysteroscopy the device can be seen, examined in full, and grasped prior to removal with forceps. If a piece of the coil is missing, hysteroscopy allows confirmation that a fragment remains in the uterus (Neuwirth 1975).

Endometrial carcinoma

The majority of patients with endometrial adenocarcinoma of the uterus are postmenopausal and present with bleeding. Hysteroscopy is useful in these patients. A clear view of the uterine cavity has the following advantages:

1. The tumour can be seen and the diagnosis confirmed by biopsy;
2. The size and extent of the growth can be recorded, or invasion of the endocervix can be excluded. This is an important observation because it enables the cancer to be accurately staged (Walton & MacPhail 1986);
3. Dual pathology, such as an associated fibroid, can be excluded.

Hysteroscopy cannot diagnose the depth of invasion into the myometrium, and the procedure has been criticised because of the theoretical risk of dissemination of the cancer into the peritoneum by the action of the flushing medium (Joelsson et al 1971). However, a wide experience throughout the world's literature has failed to reveal a single case where hysteroscopic spread of tumour cells has been confirmed, probably because the superficial cells of the tumour are non-viable. Parent et al (1985) report on a series of 30 hysteroscopies in endometrial carcinoma just prior to surgery. They did not recover any neoplastic cells from fluid in the pouch of Douglas.

Adhesions or synechae

Intra-uterine adhesions (Asherman's syndrome) usually result from previous uterine surgery, especially curettage, septic abortions or pelvic sepsis following delivery, and present with oligomenorrhoea or secondary amenorrhoea. Minor degrees of intra-uterine adhesions may have no symptoms or may present with secondary infertility or dysmenorrhoea (Sugimoto 1978).

Traditionally, the diagnosis is made by hysterosalpingography, but hysteroscopy allows a more precise diagnosis and can distinguish between flimsy adhesions and more solid, thick bands of tissue (Taylor & Hamou 1983).

Even minor adhesions can be responsible for recurrent first-trimester abortions.

When the diagnosis is established, treatment is usually by dilatation and curettage followed by the insertion of an intra-uterine device to maintain the endometrial cavity. An alternative way of managing this condition is by the endoscopic division of adhesions, which is usually followed by spontaneous menstruation. Surgery can be performed by division of the adhesion using a fine pair of scissors under vision via the operating sheath of the telescope. Alternatively, an easier method is to use the bevel of the telescope to separate the adhesions, and this simple technique is of especial value when the adhesive bands are fine. Some authorities recommend that adhesiolysis be followed by therapy with Premarin and Provera to stimulate withdrawal bleeding. Alternatively, clomiphene therapy may induce spontaneous ovulation or menstruation.

Congenital abnormalities of the uterus

Bicornuate uterus or a uterine septum is best diagnosed with the hysteroscope. It is important to note that the normal uterine cavity, when distended with carbon dioxide, shows a 'saddle-shaped' appearance which could be mistaken for a minor fusion defect. However, the main differential diagnosis is from synechae. It is probable that all patients with recurrent mid-trimester pregnancy loss should now be investigated by hysteroscopy to exclude congenital malformations. The method is more accurate and less uncomfortable to the patient than hysterosalpingography.

Adenomyosis and endometrial hyperplasia

Patients with menstrual irregularity may well be suffering from adenomyosis, cystic glandular hyperplasia of the endometrium or atypical hyperplasia. These conditions are much more difficult to recognise at hysteroscopy, but detailed descriptions are given by Parent et al (1985). Extensive polypoidal or generalised hyperplasia is unmistakable, but diffuse endometrial hyperplasia is more difficult to distinguish from the premenstrual endometrium. It is important, therefore, to examine the endometrium in the immediate postmenstrual phase of the cycle when bleeding is less and hyperplasia more obvious. The diagnosis must be confirmed by biopsy or histology.

Postmenopausal endometritis

In some women with postmenopausal bleeding who do not have endometrial cancer, the atrophic endometrium becomes vascularised by fine capillaries which often coalesce to form bleeding vascular patches. This characteristic appearance of menopausal atrophy and bleeding capillaries may explain the cause of bleeding in many postmenopausal women.

COMPLICATIONS OF HYSTEROSCOPY

The complications of this procedure are few and most frequently related to the use of general anaesthesia. When performed without anaesthetic or with paracervical block, the risks are small (Lindemann & Mohr 1976).

Anaesthesia

The main complications of general anaesthesia are anoxia and regurgitation. Local anaesthesia is safe provided it is not injected directly into a blood vessel; otherwise, convulsions can occur.

Perforation of the uterus

No perforations were observed by Lindemann and Mohr (1976) in more than 1245 diagnostic hysteroscopies, although two perforations were recognised in a group of 450 tubal sterilisations. The most likely causes of perforation are failure to recognise a retroverted uterus, inserting the telescope to the fundus of the uterus without direct visualisation, any hysteroscopic procedure combined with intra-uterine surgery, and hysteroscopy in the post-abortal, or puerperal, uterus.

The best method of avoiding perforation is to perform a preliminary bimanual examination and then introduce the telescope through the external os under vision so that the surgeon can see when the lens is close to the fundus.

Infection

Pelvic inflammatory disease is a contraindication for hysteroscopy because of the risk of spread of sepsis into the abdomen. The only exceptions to this rule are when pelvic sepsis is associated with a lost intra-uterine device, or if a placental fragment is retained.

Complications due to the distending medium

There is a very small risk of anaphylactic reactions if dextran is used to distend the uterus.

Complications can occur with the use of CO_2 as a distending medium, but only if the volumes of gas used are very high or the gas is insufflated under high pressure. This is almost impossible if the correct insufflating apparatus is used and the pressure and flow rates are continuously monitored. With the correct machine there is no change in the ECG, blood gases or pH, even if the operation time exceeds 20 minutes (Lindemann & Mohr 1976). Experiments in dogs showed minimal changes in the ECG and respiratory rates, with CO_2 flows of 400 ml/min, and significant changes only occurred when the flow increased to 1000 ml/min. This is more than 10 times the maximum value permitted by the modern insufflating machines (Lindemann & Mohr 1976).

HYSTEROSCOPIC SURGERY

Biopsy

Endometrial biopsy using specially designed fine biopsy forceps, which pass down the operating channel of the hysteroscope, remains the easiest hystero-scopic operation (Wamsteker 1983). Grasping forceps are used for lost IUDs or to remove small polyps.

Adhesiolysis

Fine adhesions can be separated by pressure with the tip of the telescope, but thicker bands may require incision with scissors.

Sterilisation

Hysteroscopic sterilisation may become the method of choice in the future. Several methods are now being developed which combine simplicity with efficiency and which have the major advantage of being reversible.

The first method to be developed was transuterine electrocoagulation of the cornua, but this method has now been abandoned because of the risks of perforation of the uterus or electrical burns of the bowel. In addition, the method has a high pregnancy rate (Lindemann & Mohr 1976).

Chemical caustics, especially the use of mepacrine (quinacrine), have been instilled into the uterus in the hope that they would cause fibrous occlusion of the cornua, but the results were unreliable.

The current methods of sterlisation involve the use of intra-tubal devices. These devices obstruct the tubal lumen so that conception becomes impossible. De Maeyer (1983) uses a liquid silicone mixture which solidifies when inserted into the cornua. It also incorporates a tail so that the device can be removed by traction, thereby restoring fertility.

An alternative method involves the insertion of preformed solid plugs into the cornua (Brundin 1983). The efficiency of all these methods is under current review.

Laser vaporisation of the endometrium

There has been considerable recent interest in the use of the Na:YAG laser to destroy the superficial layers of the endometrium in patients with severe menorrhagia (Goldrath et al 1981). The procedure is performed under general or spinal anaesthesia, and endometrial photo vaporisation is performed under direct vision. Using a power output of 55–60 W, the endometrial surface is destroyed systematically. Early results of this new technique are promising, but large volumes of irrigating fluids are required and this can cause electrolyte disturbances.

PHOTOGRAPHY

Photographic records of hysteroscopy are important for both teaching and recording clinical results.

Still photography requires a high-intensity xenon light source or a halogen lamp. Alternatively, an endocomputer flash unit attached to an Olympus O.M. II camera body by an objective lens allows automatic computer-controlled exposure, and thus perfect still pictures.

It is usual to use 400 ASA film, but the ASA on the camera body must be changed according to the specifications of the telescope. A figure of ASA 1600 is usual.

There are several systems which use a chip camera to permit closed circuit television (Storz, Wolf, KeyMed), all of which allow simultaneous observation of hysteroscopic procedures by other personnel in the operating theatres.

FUTURE DEVELOPMENTS

The main areas where further development in hysteroscopy are taking place are in the use of flexible hysteroscopes, and laser surgery. Sterilisation using intra-tubal devices offers exciting prospects for a safe, simple and efficient method of reversible birth control. However, panoramic hysteroscopy and colpomicrohysteroscopy of the transformation zone have reached such a degree of technical excellence that they should now be regarded as a standard method of investigation in gynaecology. In the very near future we can expect to see hysteroscopic examination of the uterus as daily procedure in hospital practice.

ACKNOWLEDGEMENTS

The author is grateful to Karl Storz—Endoscopie who have generously provided the funding for printing the colour plates.

REFERENCES

Baggish M S 1979 Contact hysteroscopy. Obstetrics and Gynecology 54: 350–354
Baggish M S, Barbot J 1980 Contact hysteroscopy for easier diagnosis. Contemporary Obstetrics and Gynaecology 16: 3–11
Bardot J, Parent B, Dubuisson J B 1980 Contact hysteroscopy. American Journal of Obstetrics and Gynecology 136: 721–726
Brundin J 1983 P-block as a contraceptive method. In: Hysteroscopy, MTP Press, Boston, pp 137–141
De Maeyer J F D E 1983 Trancervical hysteroscopic sterilisation. In: Hysteroscopy. MTP Press, Boston, pp 191–199
Frangenheim H 1988 The history of laparoscopy. In: Gordon A, Lewis B V (eds) Gynaecological endoscopy, Chapman Hall, London
Goldrath M H, Fuller T A, Segal S 1981 Laser photovaporisation of the endometrium for the treatment of menorrhagia. American Journal of Obstetrics and Gynecology 140: 14–19
Hamou J 1981 Microhysteroscopy. Journal of Reproductive Medicine 26: 375–382

Joelsson I, Levine R U, Moberger G 1971 Hysteroscopy as an adjunct in determining the extent of carcinoma of the endometrium. American Journal of Obstetrics and Gynecology 111: 696–702

Lewis B V 1984 Hysteroscopy in gyanecological practice. Journal of the Royal Society of Medicine 77: 235–237

Lindemann H J 1973 Historical aspects of hysteroscopy. Fertility and Sterility 24: 230–242

Lindemann H J, Mohr J 1976 CO_2 hysteroscopy. American Journal of Obstetrics and Gynecology 124: 129–133

Neuwirth R S 1975 Hysteroscopy: major problems in obstetrics and gynaecology, vol 8, W B Saunders, London

Parent B, Guedj H, Barbot J, Nodarian P 1985 Hysteroscopie panoramique, Maloine, Paris

Stevens M J, Van Herendael 1986 Dating of the endometrium by microhysteroscopy. Proceedings of the 2nd European Congress of Hysteroscopy, Antwerp

Sugimoto O 1978 Diagnostic and therapeutic hysteroscopy for traumatic intra-uterine adhesions. American Journal of Obstetrics and Gynecology 131: 539

Taylor P J, Hamou J E 1983 Hysteroscopy: clinical perspectives. Journal of Reproductive Medicine 28: 359–389

Van de Pas H 1983 Hysteroscopy, MTP Press, Boston, pp 39–48

Walton S M, MacPhail S 1986 The value of hysteroscopy in post menopausal bleeding. Proceedings of the 24th British Congress of Obstetrics and Gynaecology, Cardiff

Wamsteker K 1983 Hysteroscopic surgery. In: Hysteroscopy, MTP Press, Boston, pp 165–171

21

Utero-vaginal prolapse

Despite a tendency to smaller family size over the past few decades, utero-vaginal prolapse remains a common gynaecological problem, predominantly of middle and old age. The initial damage generally occurs during childbirth, with a second attack on the pelvic floor integrity occurring around the time of oestrogen deprivation at the climacteric.

AETIOLOGY

The pelvic floor muscles, comprising the levatores ani and coccygei with their fascial attachments, are inserted into the bony pelvis and penetrated by the urethra, vagina and anal canal. Although under normal circumstances the pelvic floor is able to withstand any rise in intra-abdominal pressure such as may be introduced by straining, pushing or coughing, if its integrity has been damaged by vaginal delivery there may be a tendency for prolapse of the genitalia to occur, particularly around the menopause when there is a second insult to the integrity of the pelvic floor consequent upon oestrogen withdrawal. Utero-vaginal prolapse is thus essentially a problem of multipara and particularly the 'grande multip'.

Prolonged labour and high forceps delivery, particularly if prolonged traction is required, have always been reasonably blamed as aetiological factors in the development of utero-vaginal prolapse. The use of the partogram, and when appropriate, augmentation of labour (Duignan 1985), have fortunately greatly diminished the incidence of prolonged labour, and earlier recourse than previously to caesarean section has reduced the incidence of difficult high forceps delivery. Because of the time spans involved (and because studying prolapse does not seem to attract much attention), statistics are not at present available, but it seems likely we will see less prolapse due to these factors in the future.

The author has been unable to find any evidence that the considerable stresses imposed on the pelvic floor during a 'squatting' labour might increase the risk of subsequent prolapse, and prolapse is indeed *less* common in those parts of the world where such labours are the norm; women in these countries do of course commonly return to considerable degrees of physical activity soon after labour, which could be protective, and the same may not apply in this country. There is no evidence that rest after labour lessens the risk of prolapse; the converse is probably more likely.

'Bearing down' before full dilatation

This is obviously going to put a tremendous strain on the uterine supports and must contribute to an increased risk of prolapse in later life.

Fundal pressure

This used to be a recommended method of delivery of the placenta, but it could also lead to gross stretching of the uterine ligaments and has now been abandoned in favour of patience, maternal effort and judicious controlled cord traction.

Inadequate postnatal exercises

Although most women are instructed in 'buttock squeezing' and vaginal tightening, it is doubtful if many keep up these exercises for more than a couple of weeks postpartum. Although solid data are difficult to come by it would seem likely that more firm adherence to physiotherapy advice in this context would be helpful in the avoidance of prolapse in later life.

Smoking

Although smoking is overall a less common habit than 10 years ago, men are giving up more than women, and female smoking-related diseases, including bronchitis, show an increase. This may well increase the risk of prolapse.

Prolapse of the vagina after hysterectomy

Post-hysterectomy vaginal prolapse is a fortunately rare, and always distressing, complication for both patient and surgeon. The reason for this unfortunate complication may be inappropriate choice of operation, abdominal hysterectomy in the presence of pelvic floor weakness, or, conversely, vaginal hysterectomy without repair of associated pelvic floor musculo-ligamentous relaxation. In addition, failure to recognise and eradicate an enterocoele at the time of the original operation is probably a significant factor in the aetiology of vault descent.

Utero-vaginal prolapse and urinary tract obstruction

Recurrent urinary tract infection is a common complication of utero-vaginal prolapse and may be due to stasis in the obstructed ureters and bladder (Jones & Evison 1977).

This relationship was first noted by Brettauer and Rubin in 1923 and was re-emphasised in 1984 by Young et al, who described two cases of procidentia associated with hydronephrosis and hydro-ureter. In one case there was a severe urinary tract infection and septicaemia was present. These authors make the point that patients with unexplained disease of the urinary tract should undergo pelvic examination to exclude a prolapse, and furthermore that women with procidentia should undergo tests of renal function to exclude obstruction of the urinary tract. In elderly, frail women, correction of the prolapse and insertion of a ring or shelf pessary may be all that is necessary to reverse urinary obstruction and renal failure (Young et al 1984) (Fig. 21.1).

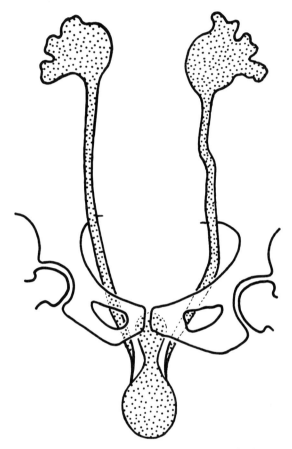

Fig. 21.1 Typical appearance of an intravenous urogram in cases of urinary tract obstructions due to uterine prolapse. Bilateral hydronephrosis is present with dilated ureters, the lower ends of which are displaced out from the pelvis together with the bladder, which has an 'hour-glass' appearance (from Young et al 1984, with permission)

Other risk factors in childbirth possibly relating to the aetiology of utero-vaginal prolapse

Recent electrophysiological tests have shown the underlying functional abnormality in anorectal incompetence to be weakness of the anorectal sphincter and pelvic floor muscles due to partial chronic denervation of these muscles (Swash 1985). It has further been shown by Snooks et al (1984) that obstetric injury can be implicated in both anorectal and urinary incontinence, and they showed that vaginal delivery, but not ceasarean section, can result in damage to the pudendal nerves. This damage is reversible in 60% of patients, more common after forceps delivery, and also related to the length of the second stage and parity. The pudendal nerve terminal motor latency (PNTML) and the external anal sphincter muscle fibre density were studied in a series of 122 pregnant women and a matched series of controls. These studies showed that the fibre density (FD) was increased in the external anal sphincter muscle 2 months after delivery compared with the antenatal measurement. There was no change in the FD in the antenatal and postnatal studies carried out on six women delivered by elective caesarean section, which was similar to the controlled subjects. PNTML and FD were increased in multipara, women delivered by means of forceps and women having a prolonged second stage of labour. Epidural anaesthesia did not seem to be relevant in that there was no significant difference between women delivered by forceps with or without epidural anaesthesia. Perineal trauma does not appear to add to pudendal nerve damage unless the sphincter muscle is involved, but women who sustain third-degree perineal tears were shown to have increased PNTML consistent with injury to the pudendal nerves. There was also noted to be a relationship between birthweight and pudendal nerve damage. Although these studies were mainly carried out to investigate the aetiology of idiopathic anorectal incontinence, there is obviously a correlation with subsequent risk of utero-vaginal prolapse.

In many hospitals a laudable attempt to reduce episiotomy incidence is now being made. Whilst it seems unlikely that superficial perineal tears are relevant to the development of vaginal prolapse in later life, third-degree tears, which *could* be a greater risk if episiotomy is avoided, may on the basis of these studies carry long-term hazards with regard to rectal prolapse, rectocoele and faecal incontinence.

Presentation of uncomplicated utero-vaginal prolapse

80% of patients referred to hospital with genital prolapse complain of 'something coming down' (Fergusson 1984). It is common clinical experience that the degree of prolapse bears little relationship to the presenting symptoms; someone with a major prolapse, or indeed a procidentia, may have few symptoms, whereas others with a small cystocoele may complain vociferously.

Some patients complain of frequency of micturition, incomplete bladder-emptying necessitating digital pressure on a cystocoele, or difficulties in emptying the bowel. It is the author's experience that abdominal and back pain are rare presentations in prolapse. Women complaining of such symptoms are very much more likely to have primary back problems (which may be referable to the abdomen) and they must be counselled to the effect that operating on their prolapse may not in any way help their backache, although of course the enforced rest may be beneficial.

A few patients with decubital ulceration due to ischaemia or the friction of clothing may present with bleeding and discharge (Fig. 21.2), and a small

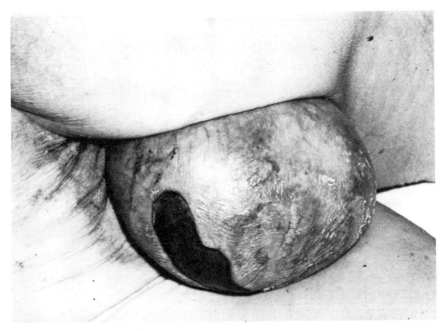

Fig. 21.2 Decubital ulceration

number of patients may complain of coital difficulties consequent upon their altered vaginal anatomy.

EXAMINATION

A full general and abdominal examination are necessary. It is necessary to exclude chronic chest problems, gross obesity and abdominal masses. Patients complaining of prolapse should be examined gynaecologically in the left lateral position using a Sims' speculum. Descent of any part of the lower genital tract can be demonstrated by asking the patient to cough or strain; the cervix can usually be adequately visualised and a cervical smear taken if appropriate. Following inspection and cervical smear taking, bimanual palpation should always be carried out to exclude pelvic masses such as ovarian cysts or large fibroids; large fibroids are of course likely to prevent uterine descent.

Uterine descent is classically divided into three degrees of severity, with the first degree being defined as descent of the uterus within the vagina, the second degree showing descent of the cervix through the introitus on straining, and the third degree showing permanent descent of the uterus.

Cystocoele, urethrocoele, rectocoele and enterocoele are usually merely divided into major or minor degrees of abnormality.

INVESTIGATION

Many patients presenting with prolapse will be elderly and may therefore need medical investigation including chest X-ray, ECG and IVU or renal ultrasonography. If urinary incontinence is a problem in addition to prolapse, a cystometrogram may be indicated prior to planning definitive treatment. A major degree of obesity is frequently present and it may be advisable that a patient loses weight prior to consideration of surgery.

TREATMENT

Prevention

It is to be hoped that we will see fewer prolapses as the years go by, with a tendency to shorter labours and smaller family size, combined with improvements in general health and possibly also increased use of hormone replacement therapy at the menopause. It is possible also that increased attention to physiotherapy might produce a lower incidence of prolapse occurring at the time of the climacteric. The exercises described by Mandelstam (1978), which essentially produce lower vaginal tightening, should be carried out for 6 weeks postnatally.

Hormone replacement therapy (HRT)

In assessing a patient with utero-vaginal prolapse it is frequently noted that considerable atrophic change is present in the vaginal and cervical epithelium. Mild degrees of prolapse may be helped merely by the establishment of the patient on HRT, initially often in the form of an oestrogen-containing cream, and if this proves effective it might well be appropriate to establish the patient on long-term formalised HRT using either oral or implant modes of treatment.

It is unlikely, however, that HRT will help major degrees of prolapse, although this treatment is commonly used preoperatively to improve the condition of the atrophic vaginal and cervical tissues prior to surgery. A 2-week course of any of the proprietary oestrogen-containing creams is adequate for this purpose.

Pessaries

Ring pessaries, shelf pessaries, tampons, pads and all sorts of other supporting devices have a time-hallowed place in the management of prolapse, but a diminishing one for anything other than temporary relief of symptoms. A ring pessary may be useful in the final weeks of pregnancy if there is uterovaginal prolapse with stress incontinence or whilst a patient is awaiting surgery. Rings and shelf pessaries may be used in the very elderly, very frail patient who is unwilling or unfit for anaesthesia, but there are very few such patients these days with modern anaesthetic techniques, including the use of regional blocks.

We have all seen the problems that can arise from ring pessaries, including vaginal ulceration, with bleeding and sepsis and also in some cases complete epithelialisation of the ring if it is neglected for a long period of time. Such rings may need cutting with bone forceps prior to piecemeal removal.

The use of ring pessaries has diminished latterly but still has a place. It is best if they are used only in combination with oestrogen-containing creams to diminish the risk of vaginal ulceration and they should be cleaned and replaced every 6 months.

Formal surgical repair of utero-vaginal prolapse

Surgery remains the definitive form of treatment and the operations used are basically variations of vaginal hysterectomy and repair.

Manchester or Fothergill operation

The aim of the Fothergill or Manchester repair is to produce uterine elevation by approximating shortened cardinal ligaments anterior to the cervix and suturing them to the cervical stump following its amputation. This procedure is combined with anterior colporrhaphy. Some gynaecologists prefer the Manchester repair to vaginal hysterectomy. It may work satisfactorily for all degrees of uterine descent and is obviously chosen if the patient has for any reason decided to keep her uterus. The most commonly carried out operation for utero-vaginal prolapse at the present time is vaginal hysterectomy, combined with vaginal vault support, using the transverse cervical and utero-sacral ligaments, anterior colporrhaphy and also some form of utero-sacral ligament approximating suture to close any space between these ligaments and hence reduce the likelihood of postoperative enterocoele formation. For an elegant and well-illustrated review of the most suitable procedures used in the definitive surgical treatment of utero-vaginal prolapse, the reader is referred to the writings of Feroze (1986) (Fig. 21.3).

Abdominal procedures for utero-vaginal prolapse

A satisfactory degree of eradication for up to moderate degrees of cystocoele can be obtained by means of the modified Burch colposuspension procedure as described by Stanton & Cardozo (1979).

The place of anterior colporraphy alone

It is common clinical experience that a lot of patients present thinking that their uterus has dropped, whereas in fact the bulge they are feeling is due to a cystocoele. In such patients, if there is no uterine descent of any significance and no evidence of urinary stress incontinence, an anterior colporrhaphy alone may suffice. Recent work would seem to indicate that if there is stress

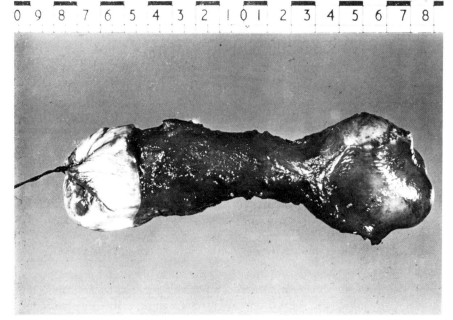

Fig. 21.3   Complete procidentia in a nullipara, showing extensive cervical elongation

incontinence present, some form of colposuspension procedure is more satisfactory (Stanton & Cardozo 1979).

Posterior colporrhaphy

There is a tendency nowadays to perform few posterior colporrhaphies unless
the patient really has marked symptoms attributable to weakness of the posterior vaginal wall; tightening the vaginal wall posteriorly is a potent cause of
dyspareunia and postoperative pain as well as urinary retention (Scott 1976).
It is notable how many patients can tolerate even moderate degrees of rectocoele without any symptoms at all, and particularly if a functional vagina
is required it is best to leave such lesions alone.

Le Fort's operation

This is a rarely performed procedure for major degrees of utero-vaginal prolapse in the elderly, infirm patient or for dealing with vaginal inversion.
It essentially consists of removing rectangular pieces of vagina from the anterior and posterior vaginal walls and then suturing the raw surfaces of the
vaginal walls together to produce partial closure with a narrow lateral canal
on each side; sexual intercourse is impossible afterwards and the operation
also precludes subsequent diagnostic curettage. To a large extent this pro-

cedure has been superseded by vaginal hysterectomy and repair and by abdominal procedures for elevating the vaginal vault in case of post-hysterectomy vault prolapse.

Enterocoele repair

Enterocoele repair, either at the time of colporrhaphy or following either vaginal or abdominal hysterectomy, requires a particular surgical technique as described by Feroze (1986) and Roberts (1977). It is obviously important that an enterocoele sac is sought at the time of every vaginal hysterectomy and repair procedure, and it is re-emphasised that any gap between the utero-sacral ligaments must be occluded by separate suturing at the time of vaginal hysterectomy to reduce the incidence of this particular complication.

Management of patients with post-hysterectomy vaginal prolapse

The management of patients with post-hysterectomy vaginal prolapse has been reviewed recently by Kauppila et al (1985) who reported on the results of operation for post-hysterectomy vaginal prolapse in 22 patients between 1973 and 1982. All the corrective operations were done abdominally, with a combination of sacral colpopexy and enterocoele resection being the most common procedure used. The abdominal approach to the repair of post-hysterectomy vaginal inversion has also been described by Yates (1975) and Grundsell & Larsson (1984). The procedures used all basically involved anchoring the vaginal vault to the promontory of the sacrum with either Mersilene or some alternative artificial mesh, or straps of external oblique aponeurosis (Williams & Richardson 1952). From the most recent reviews of the subject (Kauppila et al 1985, Grundsell & Larsson 1984), fixation of the vaginal vault to the sacrum appears to carry a lower risk of recurrence than anterior fixation of the vaginal vault to the round ligaments—but the numbers reported in these series are small. Some form of sacral colpopexy using mesh or fascia appears to be the procedure of choice, with a lower risk of recurrence than if the vaginal vault is directly sutured to the sacrum (Fig. 21.4).

Operative bleeding may be a problem if the vaginal vault if attached to the hollow of the sacrum (Sutton et al 1981) as opposed to the promontory. Transvaginal fixation of the vaginal vault to the sacrospinus ligament has been described (Birnbaum 1973, Randall & Nichols 1971), but this obviously involves 'blind' suturing and an increased risk of damage to the bowel or ureter.

Combined vaginal and rectal prolapse may occasionally occur in elderly patients with very poor tissues (Fig. 21.5); a combined vaginal approach operation by the gynaecologist and an abdominal operation by the general surgeon will usually be effective.

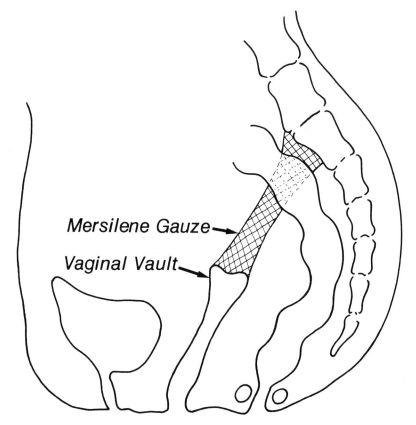

Fig. 21.4   Vaginal vault suspension using Mersilene gauze

Recent developments in postoperative management

The most important development in the last two decades from the point of view of patient comfort, and possibly reduction in urinary tract infection, has been the introduction of suprapubic catheterisation using a Bonnano or similar proprietary device. The use of suprapubic catheters means of course that recurrent urethral catheterisation is avoided, and as far as the author is concerned is now felt to be vastly preferable to urethral catheterisation.

Preoperative antibiotic treatment for vaginal hysterectomy and repair, using metronidazole suppositories which are commenced at the time of premedication and continued for 48 hours postoperatively, and trimethoprim until the catheter is removed, has provided a satisfactory absence of postoperative infective problems.

The use of subcutaneous heparin

Deep venous thrombosis is a fortunately rare complication of vaginal surgery. Avoiding pressure on the calves by putting the patient's legs *inside* the litho-

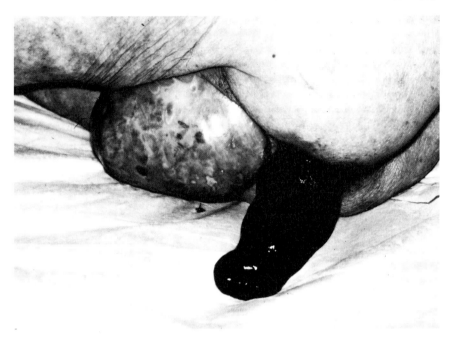

Fig. 21.5   Prolapsed uterus and rectum

tomy poles, using graduated support stockings and mobilising early are sensible, simple precautions, and the use of subcutaneous heparinisation has become commoner, but not fully accepted, as some surgeons have noted an increased risk of preoperative bleeding and postoperative haematoma formation. It is probably best if simple harmless measures such as the physical ones outlined are used in all cases and if the use of heparin is reserved for special cases such as the grossly obese patient or the patient with a past history of thrombo-embolic disease.

Preoperative treatment of procidentia

Admission for bed rest with replacement of an ulcerated procidentia and vaginal packing using a pack soaked in proflavine is frequently beneficial prior to definitive surgery for procidentia; it is surprising how quickly cervical ulceration clears if the anatomy is corrected, and after 2 weeks packing the vaginal tissues may be much more amenable to surgery. The use of topical oestrogen cream may be beneficial in addition.

Recurrent prolapse

Even with expert surgery and faultless postoperative management, recurrence will always occur, especially in the obese, the constipated and the smoker. Recurrence rates of up to 25% are quoted (Fergusson 1984).

SUMMARY

Utero-vaginal prolapse is still providing the gynaecologist with a sizeable workload, although it seems possible that this might diminish with changes in methods of labour management as most prolapses are thought to follow prolonged or difficult labours. As many patients are elderly, careful pre-operative assessment is necessary before the definitive treatment, primarily by means of surgery, and most commonly by means of vaginal hysterectomy and anterior colporrhaphy.

REFERENCES

Birnbaum S J 1973 Rational therapy for prolapsed vagina. American Journal of Obstetrics and Gynecology 86: 693

Brettauer J, Rubin I C 1923 Hydronephrosis and hydroureter: a frequent secondary finding in cases of prolapse of the uterus and bladder. American Journal of Obstetrics and Gynecology 6: 696–708

Duignan N 1985 Active management of labour. In: Studd J (ed) The management of labour, Blackwell, Oxford, p 146

Fergusson I L C 1984 Genital prolapse. In: Contemporary gynaecology, Butterworth, London, pp 211–218

Feroze R M 1986 Colporrhaphy. In: Bonney's Gynaecological surgery, 9th edn, pp 208–216

Grundsell H, Larsson G 1984 Operative management of vaginal vault prolapse following hysterectomy. British Journal of Obstetrics and Gynaecology 91: 808–811

Jones J B, Evison G 1977 Excretion urography before and after treatment of procendia. British Journal of Obstetrics and Gynaecology 84: 304–308

Kauppila O, Punnonen R, Teisala K 1985 Prolapse of the vagina after hysterectomy. Surgery, Gynecology and Obstetrics 161: 9–11

Mandelstam D 1978 Physiotherapy, vol 64, p 236

Randall C L, Nichols D H 1971 Surgical treatment of vaginal inversion. British Journal of Obstetrics and Gynaecology 38: 327–332

Roberts D W T (ed) 1977 Operative surgery (gynaecology and obstetrics), Butterworth, London

Scott J S 1976 Dewhurst C J (ed) Prolapse and stress incontinence of urine in integrated obstetrics and gynaecology for postgraduates, 2nd edn, Blackwell, Oxford, p 651

Snooks S J, Swash M, Henry M M, Setchell M 1984 Injury to innervation of the pelvic floor sphincter musculature in childbirth. Lancet ii: 546–550

Stanton S L, Cardozo L D 1979 British Journal of Obstetrics and Gynaecology 86: 693

Sutton G P, Addison W A, Livengood C H III, Hammond C B 1981 Life threatening haemorrhage complicating sacral colpopexy. American Journal of Obstetrics and Gynecology 140: 836–837

Swash M 1985 Anorectal incontinence: electrophysiological tests. British Journal of Surgery (suppl): S14–S22

Williams G A, Richardson A C 1952 Transplantation of external oblique aponeurosis: and operation for prolapse of the vagina following hysterectomy. American Journal of Obstetrics and Gynecology 64: 552–558

Yates M J 1975 An abdominal approach to the repair of post-hysterectomy vaginal inversion. British Journal of Obstetrics and Gynaecology 82: 817–819

Young J B, Selby P L, Peacock M, Brownjohn A M 1984 Uterine prolapse and urinary tract obstruction. British Medical Journal 289: 41–42

Steroid receptors and gynaecological cancer

INTRODUCTION

It is well recognised that the growth and function of female genital tract organs is dependent on oestrogens and other sex hormones, and that inappropriate oestrogen stimulation can lead to an environment in which neoplasia may develop. A clear understanding of the mechanisms by which steroids exert the effect on target tissues should, therefore, provide some insight into the genesis and continuing development of some tumours of the female reproductive system, and provide an opportunity to assess the effect of manipulation of these mechanisms on tumour initiation and growth. This chapter deals mainly with the incidence of oestrogen (OR) and progesterone (PR) receptors in gynaecological cancers and will explore the correlations of OR and PR with various histological features, stages of disease, response to treatment and eventual prognosis.

MECHANISM OF STEROID ACTION

Transport of steroid hormones in the circulation

Nature has provided a complex but precise system for the transport and delivery of sex steroids to the target cell and their eventual passage to the cell nucleus. Following the biosynthesis of steroid hormones, secretion into the bloodstream is probably modified by the concentration of circulating binding proteins, including sex-hormone binding globulin (SHBG) and serum albumin; perfusion studies in vitro have demonstrated, for instance, that binding proteins facilitate the passage of steroids through capillary walls. The association between steroid and binding-protein is extremely fast and depends on the physico-chemical nature of the steroid and of the specific binding site; for cortisol and progesterone, the half-time of association with cortisol-binding globulin is 57 and 17 milliseconds respectively, which is presumably fast enough to protect these steroids from chemical or enzymatic attack in the unbound state (Westphal 1980).

In the female, only 1–3% of testosterone and oestradiol circulates freely in the plasma: 18% of testosterone is bound to albumin and 80% to SHBG, whilst 38% of oestradiol is bound to albumin and 60% to SHBG (Quinn 1982). Testosterone and oestradiol bind to the same site on SHBG, but testosterone is the more closely bound whereas oestradiol is more strongly bound to albumin. There is general agreement that only unbound steroid hormones are biologically active (Anderson 1974, Nisker et al 1980) and, therefore, anything which alters the concentration of binding proteins will have a profound effect on steroid delivery to the target cell. For instance, if oestradiol production increases, SHBG production is stimulated, causing a differential fall in unbound T; conversely, if testosterone production increases, a fall in SHBG occurs, resulting in an increase in unbound testosterone relative to oestradiol.

In the post-menopausal woman, who is generally at higher risk from genital cancer than her younger counterpart, a variety of physiological factors control SHBG production. Important in this regard is the effect of body weight, with obese women having lower SHBG levels than lean women, a situation which has potentially profound implications for the amount of free hormone reaching the target cell (Nisker et al 1980). Whether protein-bound hormone is selectively released in the region of target cells is unknown, but if so, then circulating binding proteins can be viewed as a reservoir of hormones capable of exerting a homeostatic effect on cell growth according to the needs of a particular target organ. Certainly, the rapid speed of dissociation of hormones from binding proteins makes this a viable possibility. With free oestrogen in the circulation entering cells, SHBG-bound oestrogen becomes displaced, allowing fresh binding sites to be utilised for further oestrogen transport. Binding proteins therefore exert an important influence on the amount of free hormone available for receptor binding and thus, eventually, for cell function and growth.

Metabolic clearance of hormones

A second controlling factor governing the delivery of hormones to target cells is the rate of metabolism and eventual clearance of the hormone from the circulation. A rapid metabolic clearance rate (MCR) reduces the time in which hormones can reach and interact with their receptors and, conversely, a slow MCR will extend the time for homones to interact with their receptors.

In addition, intracellular metabolism will further affect the quantity of hormone available to receptors. For instance, oestradiol and oestrone undergo extensive interconversion in endometrial cytoplasm, and this interconversion is influenced by the presence of progesterone which increases the conversion of oestradiol to oestrone (Tseng & Gurpide 1974).

Steroid uptake by cells

It would appear that the entry of steroids from the extracellular space, across the cell membrane, and into the cytoplasm occurs by simple diffusion and is unselective, i.e. target and non-target cells are exposed to the same initial intracellular concentrations of hormones, with the concentration of free circulating hormone presented to each cell being the most important factor in determining how much diffusion takes place (Peak et al 1973). None the less, facilitated movement across the cell membrane still remains a possibility (Milgrom et al 1973).

Cellular receptors

Target cells, in general, contain two sets of binding sites—type I sites which are of limited number but which have marked specificity and a high affinity for each hormone, and type II sites, which are present in much larger amounts but with considerably less affinity and specificity. The type I sites do not exhibit *absolute* specificity for each class of hormones. For instance, it has been shown that oestrogen receptors have some affinity for all steroids, and in-vitro studies using pharmacological amounts of androgens have demonstrated the ability of large concentrations of androgens to simulate oestrogen action via binding to oestrogen receptors. It should also be noted in this context that the binding of progesterone to its receptor appears to be less specific than that of oestrogen, since physiological amounts of progesterone will bind to androgen and glucocorticoid receptors and, conversely, progesterone receptors will readily bind glucocorticoids.

Binding of steroids to their specific cytoplasmic receptors results in translocation of the steroid–receptor complexes to the cell nucleus, resulting in a depletion of cytoplasmic receptors. Evidence for such translocation includes the observations that, for oestrogen receptors for instance, cytoplasmic and nuclear receptor complexes have similar binding affinities and sedimentation characteristics (Puca & Bresciani 1968, Stancel et al 1973).

Nuclear binding of steroid–receptor complexes occurs at acceptor sites with high affinity (probably non-histone proteins) for the steroid–receptor complex and also at other sites on chromatin, which are more numerous in number but have much less affinity. This latter binding provides for maximisation of steroid–receptor complexes within the nucleus and increases the likelihood that steroid–receptor complexes may reach the specific receptor sites on chromatin.

The binding of receptor–hormone complexes to high-affinity acceptor sites results in the transcription of RNA polymerase, leading to an increase in RNA and protein synthesis. It would seem that steroid–receptor complexes need to be retained within the nucleus for a minimum amount of time to effect an alteration in protein production.

Oestrogens such as oestriol and dimethylstilboestrol, which cause nuclear accumulation of their receptors for less than 6 hours after a single dose, do not cause true uterine growth; this failure is correlated with a rapid loss of nuclear binding sites and may also be due to a lower binding affinity by these oestrogen–receptor complexes with nuclear binding sites. If, however, repeated administration of such oestrogens is effected, their nuclear retention is long enough to promote true uterine growth. Consequently, merely switching on RNA and protein synthesis is not enough for the sustained growth of target tissues, and long-term nuclear retention is required. This is well demonstrated by the effects of non-steroidal anti-oestrogens such as tamoxifen and clomiphene which also exhibit oestrogen agonist activity by causing prolonged nuclear retention of oestrogen–receptor complexes.

Among the proteins synthesised as a result of nuclear oestrogen action are new oestrogen receptors (ER) and progesterone receptors (PR). Thus, continued exposure to oestrogen results in an increased content of cytoplasmic oestrogen receptors via new synthesis and via replenishment of receptors returning to the cytoplasm after stimulating transcriptional events. Thus, endometrial cytoplasmic oestrogen and progesterone receptors will vary in quantity according to the phase of the menstrual cycle and, more importantly, the presence of PR implies an intact biological mechanism for ER. None the less, some breast tumours have been described which grow in the absence of oestradiol, yet their PR falls with oestrogen withdrawal, making them oestrogen-dependent, implying a dissociation between oestrogen-controlled tumour growth and oestrogen-controlled PR synthesis (Horwitz et al 1985). This classical theory that cytoplasmic translocation to the nucleus is necessary for hormones to act on their target organs has been questioned by King & Greene (1984) and Welshons et al (1984), who suggested independently, and using different biochemical techniques, that little, if any, receptors existed in the cell cytoplasm, and that previous findings related to cytoplasmic receptors were due to artefact, possibly disruption of the cell nuclei, during preparation of the tissue for receptor analysis. Whether this is the case or not is probably unimportant in clinical terms, since the presence and quantity of receptors are probably more important in terms of prognosis and response of the tumour to hormonal therapy than their intracellular location.

STEROID RECEPTORS AND GYNAECOLOGICAL TUMOURS

Epithelial ovarian tumours

Table 22.1 depicts the incidence of ER and PR in epithelial ovarian carcinoma, with 59% of tumours being ER-positive and 49% PR-positive. It should be noted that the cut-off value for ER and PR varies markedly between laboratories, with values as low as 1 fmol/mg protein for OR and PR being considered as positive in some series (Galli et al 1981, Toppila et al 1986) and values such as less than 10 fmol/mg protein for ER and less than 50 fmol/mg protein for PR being considered as negative in another series (Sutton et al 1986a). Such a variation obviously profoundly affects the incidence of receptor positivity or negativity. More importantly, perhaps, than absolute positivity or negativity is the absolute value of receptor content,

Table 22.1 Incidence of steroid receptors in ovarian epithelial carcinoma (reported series)

Principal author	Number of tumours	OR+	PR+
Taylor (1973)	8	0	—
Kiang (1977)	5	2	—
Friberg (1978)	4	1	—
Holt (1979)	24	14	5
Dapunt (1979)	57	29	18
Friedman (1979)	34	34	34
Stedman (1980)	11	4	3
Galli (1981)	11	7	6
Creasman (1981)	17	11	4/15
Bergqvist (1981)	11	7	3/8
Schwartz (1982)	30	16	—
Saarikoski (1982)	7	4	2
Kusanishi (1982)	8	8	2
Hahnel (1982)	22	10	3
Quinn (1982)	28	15	9/27
Ford (1983)	39	15	6
Kauppila (1983)	68	60	55
Gronroos (1984)	21	13	12
Lantta (1984)	54	24	22
Richman (1985)	36	26	—
Iversen (1985)	31	16	15
Sutton (1986)	32	22	7/20
Toppila (1986)	100	53	40
Total (%)	658	391 (59%)	246/497 (49%)

since there is strong evidence that the higher the level of hormone receptor, the more likely is the response to hormone manipulation. This is certainly true for breast cancer (McGuire et al 1983) and is probably true for endometrial cancer (Quinn et al 1985a).

Table 22.2 depicts the effect of histological sub-type on the incidence of receptor positivity: 67% of serous and 69% of endometrioid carcinomas are OR-positive compared with only 30% and 22% of mucinous and clear cell carcinomas respectively. A similar situation exists with regard to PR, with 50% of serous and 63% of endometrioid tumours being PR-positive compared with 38% of mucinous and 7% of clear cell carcinomas.

If one performs a X^2 analysis on these incidences (whilst acknowledging the dangers of drawing too many conclusions on a compiled series), it is apparent that serous and endometrioid tumours have similar incidences of ER and PR, with both being significantly more likely to be ER-positive than mucinous and clear cell tumours, and all histological types are significantly more likely to be PR-positive than clear cell tumours.

The effect of tumour differentiation on receptor positivity has been examined by a number of authors with variable findings. Some authors (Quinn et al 1982, Ford et al 1983b, Kauppila et al 1983, Iversen et al 1986) have noted that well-differentiated tumours have an increased chance of being receptor-positive, but others (Holt et al 1979, Creasman et al 1981, Galli

Table 22.2 Effect of histological sub-type on OR and PR in ovarian epithelial carcinoma (reported series)

	Serous		Mucinous	
Principal author	OR+	PR+	OR+	PR+
Holt (1979)	5/7	—	1/1	—
Galli (1981)	2/2	1/2	2/2	1/2
Creasman (1981)	3/5	4/5	—	—
Bergqvist (1981)	4/4	2/2	2/3	1/3
Kusanishi (1982)	5/5	0/5	—	—
Schwartz (1982)	13/19	—	0/2	—
Hahnel (1982)	6/10	2/8	1/4	1/1
Quinn (1982)	13/19	7/19	1/19	2/8
Kauppila (1983)	37/39	35/39	7/11	9/11
Ford (1983)	7/20	2/20	0/11	0/11
Gronroos (1984)	8/9	7/9	3/3	2/3
Lantta (1984)	7/22	12/22	3/6	3/6
Iversen (1986)	10/18	12/18	0/1	0/1
Toppila (1986)	35/54	18/54	4/17	5/17
Total	155/233	102/203	24/80	24/63
	(67%)	(50%)	(30%)	(38%)

	Endometrioid		Clear cell	
	OR+	PR+	OR+	PR+
Holt (1979)	0/1	—	—	—
Creasman (1981)	1/1	0/1	—	—
Bergqvist (1981)	—	—	1/2	0/2
Schwartz (1982)	1/2	—	0/2	—
Hahnel (1982)	3/4	1/4	0/1	—
Quinn (1982)	2/5	2/5	0/1	0/1
Kauppila (1983)	7/9	7/9	—	—
Ford (1983)	8/8	4/8	—	—
Gronroos (1984)	1/1	1/1	0/4	0/4
Lantta (1984)	7/11	5/11	3/6	1/6
Iversen (1986)	4/5	2/5	0/2	0/2
Toppila (1986)	13/21	15/21	—	—
Total	47/68	37/65	4/18	1/15
	(69%)	(57%)	(22%)	(7%)

et al 1981, Schwartz et al 1982, Gronroos et al 1984, Sutton et al 1986a, Toppila et al 1986) have failed to show this association.

The stage of the disease at the time of surgery does not seem to influence receptor status, but Kaupila et al (1983) reported that, although stage was not correlated with the incidence of receptor positivity, recurrent tumour was less likely to contain ER and PR, and even when present, values were lower than in the primary tumour.

Reports on the effect of receptor status on survival are variable. Creasman et al (1981) suggested that the combination of ER-positive/PR-positive conferred a survival advantage compared with ER-negative/PR-negative, and Kauppila et al (1983) reported a mean survival time of 27 months in five patients with ER-positive/PR-positive tumours (>30 fmol/mg protein), compared with a mean survival time of 11.4 months in patients with tumours without these receptor characteristics. Iversen et al (1986) noted that the median survival of patients with PR-positive or ER-positive/PR-positive malignancies was 30 and 31.5 months respectively, compared with 10 and 9 months for those with receptor–negative tumours. In comparison, Schwartz et al (1982) and Richman et al (1985) were unable to show a positive association between the presence of ER and survival. It must be noted that multiple factors influence survival in patients with ovarian malignancy, including age, stage, histology, tumour differentiation, cell ploidy and, perhaps most import- ant of all, amount of residual disease left at the time of surgery. Important in this regard is the finding of Kauppila et al (1983) that patients with advanced tumours with low or absent ER and/or PR were more likely to have residual disease left at the time of the primary operation.

The relationship between receptor status and response to either cytotoxic or hormonal therapy has not been extensively studied. Likewise, the effect of these agents on tumour receptor content has been the subject of few reports. Richman et al (1985) noted little effect on the ER content of chemo-resistant tumours, whereas Sutton et al (1986a) noted three tumours which became ER-negative after cytotoxic therapy had been administered, and reported that in one patient with an endometrioid carcinoma treated with tamoxifen, PR levels more than doubled and ER levels fell from 65 to 4 fmol/mg protein. Gronroos et al (1984) tested the effect of tamoxifen (T) and medroxyprogester- one acetate (MPA) alone, and in combination, on tumour cell growth in vitro, and correlated response with receptor status: ER and PR status pre- dicted the response in 62% of tumours cultured with the combination but in only 38% of tumours exposed to T and 33% of those exposed to MPA, whereas approximately 15% of receptor–negative tumours also responded to these hormones, alone or in combination.

Much of the conflicting data on the incidence of receptors in ovarian carci- noma, the effect of histological type, differentiation and stage, and the relation- ship between survival response to therapy and receptor status may be accounted for by the observation that variation in receptors may be present within primary tumours, between bilateral tumours and between primary and metastatic disease. For instance, Holt et al (1979) noted only two ER- positive metastases in six patients with ER-positive primary tumours, Galli et al (1981) reported a PR-positive secondary tumour in a patient with a PR-negative primary tumour, and Schwartz et al (1982) and Toppila et al (1986) have noted both qualitative and quantitative variations in receptor status between primary and metastatic disease. Our own studies in 44 cases (Quinn et al 1987, unpublished observations) have revealed consistent findings in receptor status in only 56% of cases where multiple sites of the primary tumour have been assayed, and a 50% discrepancy between primary and metastatic tumours, with most (but not all) metastatic disease having lower ER and/or PR than the primary site. When one considers the large volume usually present in patients with ovarian cancer, these findings are not surpris- ing.

Table 22.3 Incidence of steroid receptors in non-epithelial ovarian tumours

Principal author	OR+	PR+
Granulosa-cell tumour		
Galli (1981)	2/2	2/2
Creasman (1981)	0/1	0/1
Holt (1981)	1/4	—
Bergqvist (1981)	0/1	1/1
Hamilton (1981)	1/1	—
Young (1982)	0/1	1/1
Quinn (1982)	2/2	1/2
Meyer (1982)	0/1	1/1
Kauppila (1983)	1/2	1/2
Schwartz (1983)*	1/3	3/3
Lantta (1984)	1/3	0/3
Total	9/21 (43%)	10/16 (63%)
Dysgerminoma		
Hahnel (1982)	0/1	0/1
Quinn (1982)	0/1	0/1
Schwartz (1983)	0/2	2/2
Kauppila (1983)	0/1	0/1
Lantta (1984)	0/2	1/2
Total	0/7	3/7 (43%)
Endodermal sinus tumour		
Schwartz (1983)*	0/4	2/4
Kauppila (1983)	1/1	1/1
Total	1/5 (20%)	3/5 (60%)
Mixed carcinoma/sarcoma		
Galli (1981)	0/1	0/1
Hamilton (1981)	0/1	—
Quinn (1982)	1/1	0/1
Schwartz (1983)	5/7	4/7
Total	6/10 (60%)	4/9 (44%)

* ⩾5 fmol/mg protein (text reads >30 fmol/mg protein receptor rich)

Non-epithelial ovarian tumours

Table 22.3 depicts a literature review of the incidence of steroid receptors in a variety of non-epithelial ovarian malignancies; 43% of granulosa cell tumours are ER-positive and 57% are PR-positive. We have studied a further seven cases since our original report in 1982, two of which were ER-positive and all seven of which were PR-positive. To date, no case of an ER-positive dysgerminoma has been published, and likewise, endodermal sinus tumours have a low incidence of positive ER. Sixty per cent of mixed carcinoma/sarcoma of the ovary are ER-positive and 44% are PR-positive, almost identical incidences to that of ovarian carcinoma alone (see Table 22.1). The study of steroid receptors in these rare ovarian malignancies may yet prove valuable. Schwartz et al (1983) reported a patient with a granulosa cell tumour which was ER- and PR-positive who had stable disease for 10 months on progestogen therapy and stable disease for 4 months on tamoxifen. We have treated a patient with tamoxifen who had a recurrent granulosa cell tumour involving the liver and who had stable disease on scanning for 9 months (Quinn et al 1986, unpublished report).

Endometrial carcinoma

Studies on the steroid receptor content of endometrial cancer have been much more extensive than in any other gynaecological tumour. It is now almost 20 years since Brush et al (1968) first demonstrated the specific binding of radio-labelled 17β-oestradiol to malignant endometrial tissue, and since then over 1000 tumours have been studied (Table 22.4) with, overall, 79% being

Table 22.4 Incidence of positive OR and PR in endometrial cancer (reported series)

Principal author	OR+	PR+
Terenius (1971)	7/9	—
Haukkamaa (1971)	—	4/6
Maas (1972)	6/8	—
Rubin (1972)	6/16	—
Rao (1974)	2/2	0/2
Crocker (1974)	15/16	—
Muechler (1975)	12/17	—
McLaughlin (1976)	—	4/13
Gustafsson (1977)	—	6/10
Grilli (1977)	11/12	5/12
Friberg (1978)	23/50	—
Spona (1979)	16/18	16/18
Hunter (1980)	41/60	12/26
Ehrlich (1981)	54/68	56/95
Saarikoski (1982)	11/13	9/13
Iacobelli (1982)	—	11/18
Billiet (1982)	26/37	—
Genton (1982)	12/15	14/15
Kauppila (1982)	108/123	87/104
Martin (1982)	39/39	32/47
Baulieu (1983)	37/38	32/38
Pollow (1983)	140/145	116/145
Martin (1983)	60/73	43/73
Carlson (1984)	17/25	13/25
Horbelt (1984)	8/18	10/18
Quinn (1985)	120/155	108/148
Creasman (1985)	112/160	86/125
Liao (1986)	68/86	66/86
Total	951/1203 (79%)	730/1037 (70%)

ER-positive and 70% being PR-positive. The vast majority of series report a reduced incidence of ER and PR in poorly differentiated tumours. Table 22.5 is a literature summary of the effect of tumour differentiation on ER and PR incidence. Ninety-two per cent of well-differentiated (G1) tumours are ER-positive compared with 56% of poorly differentiated (G3) tumours, whilst 84% of G1 tumours are PR-positive compared with 44% of G3 tumours.

Table 22.5 Incidence of positive ER and PR according to tumour differentiation (reported series for endometrial carcinoma)

Principal author	ER+			PR+		
	G_1	G_2	G_3	G_1	G_2	G_3
McLaughlin (1976)	—	—	—	2/3	2/8	0/1
Grilli (1977)	7/7	4/5	—	4/17	1/5	—
Friberg (1978)	12/18	9/22	2/10	—	—	—
Spona (1979)	9/10	3/3	4/5	9/10	3/3	4/5
Prodi (1979)	13/13	8/10	0/1	10/11	4/6	0/1
Hunter (1980)	18/16	15/22	8/12	3/7	8/16	1/3
Ehrlich (1981)	18/22	31/37	5/9	27/32	25/45	4/18
Kauppila (1982)★	34/36	21/34	2/8	34/36	21/34	2/8
Baulieu (1983)	22/22	12/13	3/3	19/21	11/13	2/4
Pollow (1983)	56/56	48/48	36/41	56/56	43/48	17/41
Carlson (1984)	4/6	8/11	5/8	3/6	8/11	2/8
Quinn (1985)	64/67	19/24	11/31	54/62	13/23	16/31
Creasman (1985)	55/67	40/56	17/37	47/62	23/28	16/27
Liao (1986)	37/39	22/29	9/18	36/39	22/29	8/18
Total	349/379	240/314	102/183	304/362	184/269	72/165
	(92%)	(76%)	(56%)	(84%)	(68%)	(44%)

★ Values are for 'receptor-rich' tumours (>30 fmol/mg protein)
G_1 = well differentiated
G_2 = moderately well differentiated
G_3 = poorly differentiated

Not only are G1 tumours more likely to be ER- and also PR-positive, but the mean value of ER and PR in these tumours is higher than the mean value of ER and PR in receptor-positive G3 tumours. Quinn et al (1985b) reported on 155 cases of endometrial cancer in which ER was measured, and 148 cases in which PR was measured. The mean value of OR in G_1 and G_2 tumours combined was significantly higher than that of G_3 tumours, and the mean value of PR in G_1 tumours was significantly higher than that of G_2 and G_3 tumours combined. Thus, not only do G_3 tumours have a reduced incidence of positive receptors, but even when receptors are present values tend to be low. The effect of tumour type on ER and PR status has not been reported widely (Table 22.6). Creasman et al (1985) reported a significantly reduced incidence of ER- and PR-positive clear cell and papillary carcinomas compared with other histological types; Quinn et al (1985b) noted no differences in the incidence of ER or PR of adenosquamous or clear cell carcinomas compared with endometrioid adenocarcinomas in toto, but adenosquamous carcinomas were significantly more likely to be ER-positive than G_3 endometrioid adenocarcinomas. In the study of Liao et al (1986), the mean ER and PR level of adenosquamous tumours was 40.6 fmol/mg protein and 74.2 fmol/mg protein respectively, compared with 92.2 fmol/mg protein and 157.1 fmol/mg protein for adenocarcinomas.

The effect of myometrial invasion on receptor content has been studied by Creasman et al (1985) and Liao et al (1986), who found no effect, in contrast to Kauppila et al (1982) who noted a significantly reduced mean PR value in tumours invading more than halfway through the myometrium.

Table 22.6 Incidence of ER and PR according to histological type of
endometrial cancer (reported series)

Principal author	ER+	PR+
Adenosquamous carcinoma		
Quinn (1985)	22/26	20/25
Creasman (1985)	20/28	14/18
Liao (1986)	7/14	5/14
Total	49/68 (72%)	39/57 (68%)
Clear cell carcinoma		
Quinn (1985)	4/7	5/7
Creasman (1985)	3/5	2/7
Total	7/12 (58%)	7/14 (50%)
Papillary carcinoma		
Creasman (1985)	9/17 (53%)	3/11 (27%)

Quinn et al (1985b) have emphasised that since G_1 tumours are more likely to be superficial than G_3 tumours, analysis for the effect of invasion must be performed on each histological variant as well as for endometrial carcinoma as a whole, and found that invasion of greater than two-thirds of the myometrium was associated with a reduced incidence of ER and PR for all tumours analysed together, but that when the analysis was performed on individual histological sub-types, the only effect of invasion on receptor incidence was in G_3 endometrioid tumours. Furthermore, the mean ER and PR content of ER-positive and PR-positive G_1 tumours with less than one-third myometrial invasion was significantly more than that of ER-positive and PR-positive G_1 tumours with more than one-third invasion (Figs 22.1 and 22.2).

The same caution must be applied when analysing stage as an independent variable on receptor status and content, since G_3 and deeply invasive tumours are more likely to have extra-uterine spread at the time of surgery than well-differentiated and/or superficially invasive tumours. Liao et al (1986) used such a multivariate analysis with stage, grade and histology as single variables, but not invasion, and noted significantly lower mean receptor levels of ER and PR with increasing clinical stage, whilst Creasman et al (1985), who included myometrial invasion as a variable, noted a reduced incidence of ER and PR when extra-uterine metastases were documented at surgery, but noted no effect of clinical stage.

The effect of irradiation on endometrial cancer receptor content was noted by Hunter et al (1980) to reduce the incidence of positive ER by 34% and the incidence of positive PR by 44%.

A significantly positive correlation has been noted between ER and PR in endometrial tumours as a whole (Neumannova et al 1983, Creasman et al 1985, Quinn et al 1985b) and also for each histological sub-type (Quinn et al 1985b). Figure 22.3 depicts the relationship of cytoplasmic ER to PR in 148 cases. The presence of this correlation in each histological sub-type suggests that the presence of PR has been as a result of an intact biological

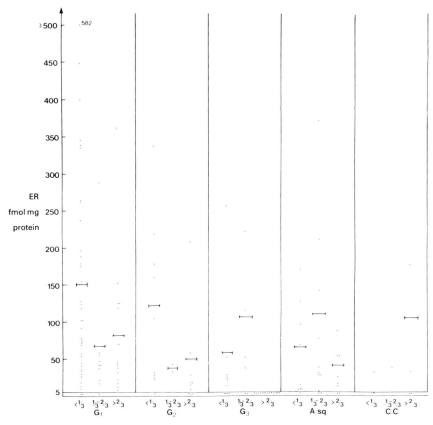

Fig. 22.1   Effect of myometrial invasion on oestrogen receptor content of endometrial carcinoma (from Quinn et al 1985, with permission)

ER mechanism and not via any tumour gene de-regulation, and provides a sound biochemical basis for hormonal manipulation.

The effect of receptor status on survival seems to be independent of stage, grade of tumour, invasion and histology. Kauppila et al (1983) characterised tumours as being 'receptor-poor' (ER and/or PR <30 fmol/mg protein) or 'receptor-rich', and noted for patients with stage I carcinoma a 93% survival at a 3-year follow-up in patients with receptor-rich tumours against an 82% survival in patients with receptor-poor tumours. A similar finding was noted in patients with advanced disease. In a study of 87 women, Martin et al (1983) reported that the survival of patients with an ER-negative tumour was significantly less than that of patients with an ER-positive tumour, independent of stage, histological grade or degree of myometrial invasion. Such a finding has been confirmed by Creasman et al (1985) in 168 cases and by Liao et al (1986) in 86 cases for both ER and PR. We have performed a similar analysis on the effect of ER and PR on survival in 349 patients, and have had similar findings based on whether ER and/or PR were negative

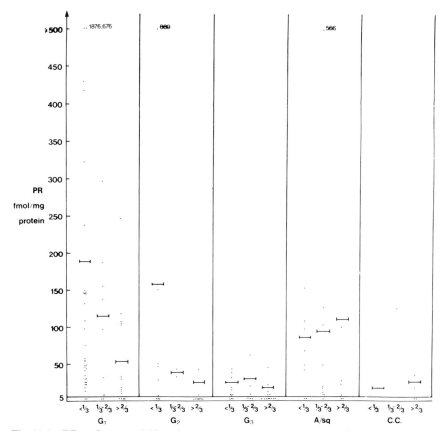

Fig. 22.2 Effect of myometrial invasion on progesterone receptor content of endometrial carcinoma (from Quinn et al 1985, with permission)

or positive; further analysis according to actual receptor levels has revealed an even more significant survival benefit when the tumour had an ER value of greater than 65 fmol/mg protein and a PR value of greater than 30 fmol/mg protein (Quinn et al 1987, unpublished observations).

One of the main hopes in measuring receptors in endometrial tumours is that such information may be valuable in predicting the response of recurrent or residual disease to hormone therapy. Table 22.7 depicts current information as to receptor status and response to progestogens. 139 cases have been evaluated, with 66% of patients with PR-positive tumours responding and only 8% with PR-negative tumours responding, a situation not dissimilar to ER status and breast cancer. In fact, the ER status of tumours in patients with advanced endometrial carcinoma is also an excellent predictor of response, with 63% of patients with ER-positive tumours responding to progestogens and only 6% of ER-negative cases responding. It still remains to be seen if receptor status adds anything to prediction of response to progestogens over and above known predictive factors such as degree of differentia-

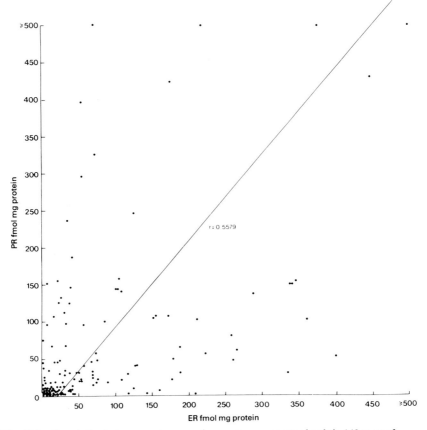

Fig. 22.3   Correlation between oestrogen and progesterone receptor levels in 148 cases of endometrial carcinoma

tion, site of recurrence, number of metastases and the disease-free interval. It certainly seems that the actual value of receptor content rather than being just positive or negative will give a better guide to response, again similar to the situation in breast cancer.

An exciting development in this regard has arisen from the observation of an increase in PR in endometrial tumours in patients treated with tamoxifen (Baulieu et al 1983), which is known to be an effective single agent in patients with recurrent and/or advanced endometrial cancer (Quinn et al 1981). Following ingestion of tamoxifen 40 mg daily for 5–7 days, PR increased in tumour samples from eight patients with PR-positive tumours, and even more interestingly PR appeared in three tumours that were initially PR-negative; no change in PR levels was noted in a further four patients. Ten patients treated with tamoxifen 10 mg at 8 and 4 hours prior to repeat endometrial sampling had no increase in PR noted. It thus seems reasonable to use tamoxifen and a progestogen in combination, which should hopefully improve

Table 22.7   Endometrial carcinoma steroid receptors and response to progestogens

Principal author	Response		No response	Receptor 'cut-off' level (fmol/mg)
Ehrlich (1978)	PR+	4	0	50 (PR)
	PR−	1	9	
Martin (1979)	ER+ PR+	13	1	10 (PR)
	ER+ PR−	1	5	
McCarty (1979)	ER+ PR+	4	1	10 (ER, PR)
	ER− PR−	0	8	
Creasman (1980)	ER+ PR+	3	2	7 (ER, PR)
	ER− PR−	1	7	
Benraad (1980)	ER+ PR+	5	1	10 (ER, PR)
	ER+ PR−	2	0	
	ER− PR−	0	5	
Kauppila (1982)	ER+ PR+	2	2	30 (ER, PR)
	ER− PR−	1	16	
Pollow (1983)	PR+	9	7	
	PR−	0	6	NS
Quinn (1985)	ER+ PR+	2	6	5 (ER, PR)
	ER− PR+	1	1	
	ER+ PR−	0	1	
	ER− PR−	0	12	

NS = not stated

response rates; such an outcome has been reported (Rendina et al 1984). None the less, there are theoretical reasons to suggest that although the two hormones can be used simultaneously, the anti-oestrogen should be administered 7–14 days before the progestogen to maximally induce PR (Horwitz et al 1985), and this approach awaits further clinical trials.

Endometrial sarcoma

Since leiomyomas contain ER and PR which vary according to the stage of the menstrual cycle and which therefore presumably reflect endogenous hormone fluctuations (Soules & McCarty 1982), and since responses to hormonal therapy have been documented in patients with sarcomas, especially endometrial stromal sarcoma (Baggish & Woodruff 1972, Pellillo 1968, Krumholy et al 1973, Lantta et al 1984, Baker et al 1984, Piver et al 1984), it would be expected that sarcomas also contain ER and PR.

The literature concerning receptor levels in these tumours is scanty and the information is further diluted by the wide variety of histological types of tumour (Table 22.8). Two patients with PR-positive endometrial stromal

Table 22.8 Incidence of steroid receptors in uterine sarcomas (reported series)

Principal author	LMS		MMT		ESS	
	OR+	PR+	OR+	PR+	OR+	PR+
Terenius (1971)	0/1	—	—	—	—	—
Ehrlich (1978)	—	—	—	1/4	—	2/6
Hahnel (1979)	—	—	1/4	—	—	—
Prodi (1979)	—	—	0/2	0/2	—	—
Quinn (1984)	4/6	3/6	2/7	2/7	0/1	0/1
Soper (1984)	3/5	1/6	12/22	6/18	1/2	0/1
Tseng (1986)	—	—	3/5	3/5	—	—
Total	7/12	4/12	18/40	12/36	1/3	3/8
	(58%)	(33%)	(45%)	(33%)	(33%)	(38%)

LMS = leiomyosarcoma
MMT = malignant mixed Müllerian tumour
ESS = endometrial stromal sarcoma

sarcoma have failed progestogen therapy (Ehrlich et al 1978), as have two patients with PR-negative mixed müllerian tumours. Endometrial stromal sarcoma, especially, is likely to contain high levels of receptors, and Sutton et al (1986b) have reported on a patient with an ER/PR-positive tumour who had a partial response in the primary and in a lung secondary to tamoxifen. A strong correlation between ER and PR was noted by Soper et al (1984) however, and a response to tamoxifen has been noted in a patient with a mixed müllerian tumour (Gynaecological Group, Clinical Oncological Society of Australia 1986). Of note is the fact that, in general, receptor levels in this group of tumours tend to be low, a situation which reflects their infrequent response to hormone therapy (Quinn 1984, Sutton et al 1986b).

Of interest has been the recent report of Tseng et al (1986) in which aromatose activity was detected in eight mixed müllerian tumours studied in vitro, and in which exposure of cultured sarcoma cells to progesterone caused a large increase in aromatose activity in a receptor-positive tumour. Furthermore, the production of oestrogen within uterine sarcomas was inhibited by aminoglutethimide, which has been shown to be an effective agent in patients with advanced endometrial carcinoma (Quinn et al 1981), suggesting the possibility that such an agent may also be useful in patients with advanced uterine sarcoma.

Carcinoma of the cervix

Endocervical gland secretion is, of course, profoundly affected by changes in circulating steroids during the menstrual cycle, with peak production occurring at the time of the pre-ovulatory burst of oestrogen into the circulation. Both oestrogen and progesterone receptors are present in normal cervical tissue (Sanborn et al 1975, 1976), with 40% of carcinomas being ER-positive and 50% being PR-positive (Table 22.9). The effect of histology on receptor

Table 22.9 Incidence of steroid receptors in carcinoma of the cervix (reported series)

Principal author	ER+	PR+
Terenius (1971)	16/26	—
Martin (1982)	51/185	—
Saarikoski (1982)	—	0/4
Gao (1983)	17/31	23/39
Ford (1983)	11/30	13/30
Soutter (1986)	60/120	19/37
Total	155/392 (40%)	55/110 (50%)

status has not been studied in detail, although Ford et al (1983a) and Martin et al (1986) reported an increased incidence of ER in adenocarcinomas. Likewise, the relationship between receptor presence and stage of disease has provoked little attention; no effect on ER incidence was detected by Martin et al (1982), nor on ER or PR incidence by Gao et al (1983).

An initial suggestion by Martin et al (1982) that patients with ER-positive cancers of the cervix had a better prognosis than patients with ER-negative cancers has not been substantiated when larger numbers of patients were analysed (Martin et al 1986), although Gao et al (1983) suggested that premenopausal patients with PR-positive tumours had a significantly better survival than those with PR-negative tumours; none the less, there were only 20 premenopausal cases in this study and much larger numbers will be required to confirm this initial observation.

The measurement of steroid receptors in cervical cancer is not just an academic exercise: responses of up to 27% of recurrent carcinomas to endocrine therapy have been reported (Briggs et al 1967), and Sugimori et al (1976) reported an improved survival in radiotherapy-treated patients who were also given oestrogens.

CONCLUSION

This chapter has been mainly confined to a review of the current status of receptors in gynaecological cancers and should tempt the reader to explore many unanswered questions about the hormonal control of cell growth. The study of tissue such as endometrium provides a unique model in this regard, with physiological fluctuations of hormonal activity having profound effects on cell proliferation, turnover and regression. Nowhere else in the human anatomy is such an accessible site available for study, and detailed examination of endometrial growth at both a receptor and a chromosomal level will surely lead to many clues about neoplastic growth in general. The observations outlined above provide only a glimmer of what is happening once the neoplastic process is underway and are only static observations of an acutely dynamic process. It should always be remembered that observations of hormone and receptor levels do not reflect the equilibrium which is so necessary for homeostasis, and that therapeutic interventions may in fact be valuable not only for their direct effect at the cell level, but also for their indirect effect of altering biochemical and cellular kinetics. Information has been available for almost a century that an alternation in circulating hormones can reverse tumour cell growth in breast cancer, and this has already been extrapolated to the use of medical adrenalectomy in endometrial cancer (Quinn et al 1981). Therapeutic strategies in this regard must look at the possibility of perhaps not only reducing endogenous oestrogen, but also preventing its access to the target cell.

Since tumour de-differentiation has been shown to be such an important concomitant of reduced hormone receptors, and since tumour de-differentiation is such a poor prognostic factor for a wide variety of tumours, it must be asked whether reduced receptor levels have resulted in tumour de-differentiation or vice versa. Would oestrogen administration in patients with endometrial cancer increase receptor levels, and if so, could differentiation occur? Baulieu's observations on the effect of induction of PR in PR-negative tumours by tamoxifen in this regard are particularly exciting. If oestrogen were able to act in this way, would ER always have to be present or would ER-negative cells still be able to respond by some other mechanism? Horowitz et al (1985) have described a breast cancer cell line which is ER-negative but PR-positive; the growth of this cell line in culture is diminished by the addition of a progestogen and is unaffected by the addition of oestrogens or anti-oestrogens. Such a situation in vivo occurs occasionally, with responses noted to progestogens in anti-oestrogen resistant, ER-negative tumours.

It seems obvious that the accumulation of data on steroid receptors in gynaecological cancer must continue; in particular, the influence of such receptors on survival and response to treatment, no matter what the modality, must be assessed so that a true perspective of the value of their measurement can be defined.

REFERENCES

Anderson D C 1974 Sex-hormone binding globulin. Clinical Endocrinology 3: 69–96
Baggish M S, Woodruff J D 1972 Uterine stromatosis, clinicopathological features and hormone dependancy. Obstetrics and Gynecology 40: 487–498

Baker V V, Walton L A, Fowler W C, Currie J L 1984 Steroid receptors in endolymphatic stromal myosis. Obstetrics and Gynecology 63: 725–745

Baulieu E E, Robel P, Mortel R, Levy C 1983 Estrogen and progesterone receptors in postmenopausal endometrial carcinoma: the potential of a dynamic test using tamoxifen. In: Jasonni V M et al (eds) Steroids and endometrial cancer, Raven Press, New York, pp 61–68

Benraad T J, Friberg L G, Koenders A J M, Kullander S 1980 Do estrogen and progesterone receptors in metastasizing endometrial cancers predict the response to gestagen therapy? Acta Obstetricia et Gynaecologica Scandinavica 59: 155–159

Bergqvist A, Kullander S, Thorell J 1981 A study of estrogen and progesterone cytosol receptor concentration in benign and malignant ovarian tumors and a review of malignant ovarian tumors treated with medroxyprogesterone acetate. Acta Obstetricia et Gynecologica Scandinavica (suppl) 101: 75–81

Billiet G, De Hertogh R, Bonte J, Ide P, Vlaemynck G 1982 Estrogen receptors in human uterine adenocarcinoma: correlation with tissue differentiation, vaginal karyopyknotic index and effect of progesterone or anti-estrogen treatment. Gynecologic Oncology 14: 33–39

Briggs M H, Caldwell A D S, Pitchford A G 1967 Sex hormones in female cancer. Lancet ii: 100

Brush M G, Taylor R W, King R J B, Kalinga H A 1968 The uptake and metabolism of (6,7-^{3}H) oestradiol by human endometrial carcinoma tissues in vivo and in vitro. Journal of Endocrinology 41: xii–xiii

Carlson J A, Allegra J C, Day T G, Wittliff J L 1984 Tamoxifen and endometrial carcinoma: alterations in estrogen and progesterone receptors in untreated patients and combination hormonal therapy in advanced neoplasia. American Journal of Obstetrics and Gynecology 149: 149–153

Creasman W T, Sasso R A, Weed J C, McCarty K S Jr 1981 Ovarian carcinoma: histological and clinical correlation of cytoplasmic estrogen and progesterone binding. Gynecologic Oncology 12: 319–327

Creasman W T, Soper J T, McCarty K S Jr, McCarty K S Sr, Hinshaw W, Clarke-Pearson D L 1985 Influence of cytoplasmic steroid receptor content on prognosis of early stage endometrial carcinoma. American Journal of Obstetrics and Gynecology 151: 922–932

Crocker S G, Milton P J D, King R J B 1974 Uptake of (6, 7-^{3}H) oestradiol-17β by normal and abnormal human endometrium. Journal of Endocrinology 62: 145–152

Dapunt O, Daxenbichler G, Margreiter R 1979 Steroid hormone receptor distribution in breast and genital carcinoma. Cancer Treatment Reports 63: 1186

Ehrlich C E, Cleary R E, Young P C M 1978 The use of progesterone receptors in the management of recurrent endometrial cancer. In: Brush M G, King R J B, Taylor R W (eds) Endometrial cancer, Baillière Tindall, London, pp 258–264

Ehrlich C E, Young P C M, Cleary R E 1981 Cytoplasmic and estradiol receptors in normal, hyperplastic and carcinomatous endometria: therapeutic implications. American Journal of Obstetrics and Gynecology 141: 539–546

Ford L C, Berek J S, Lagasse L D, Hacker N F, Heins Y L, De Lange R J 1983a Estrogen and progesterone receptor sites in malignancies of the uterine cervix, vagina and vulva. Gynecologic Oncology 15: 27–31

Ford L C, Berek J S, Lagasse L D et al 1983b Estrogen and progesterone receptors in ovarian neoplasms. Gynecologic Oncology 15: 299–304

Friberg L G, Kullander S, Persijn J P, Korsten C B 1978 On receptors for estrogens (E2) and androgens (DHT) in human endometrial carcinoma and ovarian tumours. Acta Obstetricia et Gynecologica Scandinavica 57: 261–264

Friedman M, Lagois M, Markowitz A, Jones H, Resser K, Hoffman P 1979 Estradiol (EE) and progesterone (PR) in ovarian cancer. Clinical and pathological correlation. Clinical Research 27: 385A (abstract)

Galli M C, De Giovanni C, Nicoletti G et al 1981 The occurrence of multiple steroid hormone receptors in disease-free and neoplastic human ovary. Cancer 47: 1297–1302

Gao Y L, Twiggs L B, Leung B J et al 1983 Cytoplasmic estrogen and progesterone receptors in primary cervical carcinoma: clinical and histopathological correlates. American Journal of Obstetrics and Gynecology 146: 299–304

Genton C Y, Buchi K A 1982 Are the histological and ultrastructural features of endometrial carcinomas reliable indicators of their steroid receptor content? Gynecologic and Obstetric Investigation 13: 213–225

Grilli S, Ferreri A M, Gola G, Rocchetta R, Orlandi C, Prodi C 1977 Cytoplasmic receptors for 17β-estradiol, 5a-dihydrotestosterone and progesterone in normal and abnormal human uterine tissues. Cancer Letters 2: 247–258

Gronroos M, Kangas L, Maenpaa J, Vanharanta R, Nieminen A L, Johansson R 1984 Steroid receptors and response of ovarian cancer to hormones in vitro. British Journal of Obstetrics and Gynaecology 91: 472–478

Gustafsson J A, Einhorn N, Elfstrom G, Nordenskjold B, Wrange O 1977 Progestin receptor in endometrial carcinoma. In: McGuire W L et al (eds) Progesterone receptors in normal and neoplastic tissues, Raven Press, New York, pp 299–312

Gynaecological Group, Clinical Oncological Society of Australia 1986 Tamoxifen in advanced and recurrent uterine sarcomas: a phase II study. Cancer Treatment Reports 70: 811–812

Hahnel R, Martin J D, Masters A M, Ratajczak T, Twaddle E 1979 Estrogen receptors and blood hormone levels in cervical carcinoma and other gynecological tumors. Gynecologic Oncology 8: 226–233

Hahnel R, Kelsall G R H, Martin J D, Masters A, McCartney A J, Twaddle E 1982 Estrogen and progesterone receptors in tumors of the human ovary. Gynecologic Oncology 13: 145–151

Hamilton T C, Davies P, Griffiths K 1981 Androgen and oestrogen binding in cytosols of ovarian tumours. Journal of Endocrinology 90: 421–431

Haukkamaa M, Karjalainen O, Luukkainen T 1971 In vitro binding of progesterone by the human endometrium during the menstrual cycle and by hyperplastic, atrophic and carcinomatous endometrium. American Journal of Obstetrics and Gynecology 111: 205–210

Holt J A, Caputo J A Kelly M K, Greenwald P, Chorost S 1979 Estrogen and progestin binding in cytosols of ovarian adenocarcinomas. Obstetrics and Gynecology 53: 50–58

Horbelt D V, Freedman R S, Roberts D K, Walker N J, Edwards C L, Jones L A 1984 An ultrastructural comparison of Grade I and II endometrial adenocarcinoma considering estrogen and progesterone receptor status. Gynecologic Oncology 18: 150–156

Horwitz K B, Wei L L, Sedlacek S M, d'Arville C N 1985 Progestin action and progesterone receptor structure in human breast cancer: a review. In: Greep R O (ed) Recent progress in hormone research, vol 41, Academic Press, Orlando, pp 249–308

Hunter R E, Longcope C, Jordan V C 1980 Steroid hormone receptors in adenocarcinoma of the endometrium. Gynecologic Oncology 10: 152–161

Iacobelli S, Longo P, Natoli V, Baroccioni E, Marchetti P, Scambia G 1982 New tools of potential value for predicting hormone responsiveness in human endometrial cancer. In: Fioretti P et al (eds) The menopause: clinical, endocrinological and pathophysiological aspects, Academic Press, London, pp 297–303

Iversen O E, Skaarland E, Utaaker E 1986 Steroid receptor content in human ovarian tumors: survival of patients with ovarian carcinoma related to steroid receptor content. Gynecologic Oncology 23: 65–76

Kauppila A, Janne O, Kujansuu E, Vihko R 1980 Treatment of advanced endometrial adenocarcinoma with a combined cytotoxic therapy: predictive value of cytosol estrogen and progestin receptor levels. Cancer 46: 2162–2167

Kauppila A J I, Isotalo H, Kujansuu E, Vihko R 1982 Clinical significance of female sex steroid hormone receptors in endometrial carcinoma treated with conventional methods and medroxyprogesterone acetate. In: Cavalli F et al (eds) Proceedings of the International Symposium on Medroxyprogesterone Acetate. Excerpta Medica, Amsterdam, pp 350–359

Kauppila A, Vierikko P, Kivinen S, Stenback F, Vihko R 1983 Clinical significance of estrogen and progestin receptors in ovarian cancer. Obstetrics and Gynecology 61: 320–326

Kiang D T, Kennedy B J 1977 Estrogen receptor assay in the differential diagnosis of adenocarcinomas. Journal of the American Medical Association 238: 32–34

King W J, Greene G L 1984 Monoclonal antibodies localize oestrogen receptor in the nuclei of target cells. Nature 307: 745–747

Krumholz B A, Lobovsky F Y, Halitsky V 1973 Endolymphatic stromal myosis with pulmonary metastases. Remission with progestin therapy: report of a case. Reproductive Medicine 10: 85–89

Kusanishi H, Tamaya T, Yamada T et al 1982 Characterization of steroid receptors in human ovarian cancer. Asia-Oceania Journal of Obstetrics and Gynaecology 8: 427–432

Lantta M 1984 Estradiol and progesterone receptors in normal ovary and ovarian tumours. Acta Obstetricia et Gynaecologica Scandinavica 63: 497–503

Lantta M, Kahantaa K, Karkkainen J, Lehtovirta P, Wahlstrom J, Widholm O 1984 Estradiol and progesterone receptors in two cases of endometrial stromal sarcoma. Gynecologic Oncology 18: 233–240

Liao B S, Twiggs L B, Leung B S, Yu W C, Potish R A, Prem K A 1986 Cytoplasmic estrogen and progesterone receptors as prognostic parameters in primary endometrial carcinoma. Obstetrics and Gynecology 67: 463–467

Maas H, Bruemmer P, Egert D et al 1972 On the existence of receptors for estradiol in normal and malignant human tissue and the mode of action of progesterone. Acta Obstetricia et Gynecologica Scandinavica (suppl) 19: 30–34

MacLaughlin D T, Richardson G S 1976 Progesterone binding by normal and abnormal human endometrium. Journal of Clinical Endocrinology and Metabolism 42: 667–678

Martin P M 1982 Endometrial cancer: correlations between oestrogen and progestin receptor status, histopathological findings and clinical responses during progestin therapy. In: Cavalli F et al (eds) Proceedings of the International Symposium on Medroxyprogesterone Acetate. Excerpta Medica, Amsterdam, pp 333–348

Martin P M, Rolland P H, Gammerre M, Serment H, Toga M 1979 Estradiol and progesterone receptors in normal and neoplastic endometrium: correlations between receptors, histopathological examinations and clinical responses under progestin therapy. International Journal of Cancer 23: 321–329

Martin J D, Hahnel R, McCartney A J 1982 Prognostic value of estrogen receptors in cancer of the uterine cervix. New England Journal of Medicine 306: 485

Martin J D, Hahnel R, McCartney A J, Woodings T L 1983 The effect of estrogen receptor status on survival in patients with endometrial cancer. American Journal of Obstetrics and Gynecology 147: 322–324

Martin J D, Hahnel R, McCartney A J, De Klerk N 1986 The influence of estrogen and progesterone receptors on survival in patients with carcinoma of the uterine cervix. Gynaecologic Oncology 23: 329–335

McGuire W L, Osborne C K, Clark G M, Knight W A 1983 Hormone receptors and breast cancer. In: Jasonni V M, Nenci I, Flamigni C (eds) Steroids and endometrial cancer. Raven Press, New York, pp 29–35

Meyer J A, Rad B R, Valdes R, Burstein R, Wasserman H C 1982 Progesterone receptor in granulosa cell tumor. Gynecologic Oncology 13: 252–257

Milgrom E, Atger E, Baulieu E E 1973 Studies on estrogen entry into uterine cells and on estradiol-receptor complex attachment to the nucleus–is the entry of estrogen into uterine cells a protein-mediated process? Biochimica et Biophysica Acta 320: 267–283

Muechler E K, Flickinger G L, Mangan C E, Mikhail G 1975 Estradiol binding by human endometrial tissue. Gynecologic Oncology 3: 244–250

Neumannova M, Kauppilla A, Vihko R 1983 Cytosol and nuclear estrogen and progestin receptors and 17 beta-hydroxysteroid dehydrogenase activity in normal and carcinomatous endometrium. Obstetrics and Gynecology 61: 181–188

Nisker J A, Hammond G L, Davidson B J et al 1980 Sex hormone binding globulin capacity and the percentage of free oestradiol in postmenopausal women with and without endometrial carcinoma. American Journal of Obstetrics and Gynecology 138: 637–642

Peak E J, Burgner J, Clark J H 1973 Estrophilic binding sites of the uterus: relation to uptake and retention of estradiol in vitro. Biochemistry 12: 4596–4603

Pellillo D 1968 Proliferative stromatosis of the uterus with pulmonary metastases. Remission following treatment with a long-acting synthetic progestin. Obstetrics and Gynecology 31: 33–39

Piver M S, Rutledge F N, Copeland L, Webster K, Blumenson L, Suh O 1984 Uterine endolymphatic stromal myosis: a collaborative study. Obstetrics and Gynecology 64: 173–178

Pollow K, Mann B, Grill H-J 1983 Estrogen and progesterone receptors in endometrial cancer, Raven Press, New York, pp 37–60

Prodi C, De Giovannini C, Galli M C et al 1979 17β-Estradiol, 5a-dihydrotestosterone, progesterone and cortisol receptors in normal and neoplastic human endometrium. Tumori 65: 241–253

Puca G A, Bresciani F 1968 Receptor molecules for oestrogens from rat uterus. Nature 218: 967–969

Quinn M A 1982 Endocrine changes in the climacteric and post-menopausal years. In: The biology of aging. NH and MRC Report of a Workshop in Biomedical Research into Aging, Australian Government Publishing Service 131: 41–46

Quinn M A 1984 Is endocrine status relevant to treatment planning in patients with gynaecological cancer? Australian and New Zealand Journal of Obstestrics and Gynaecology 24: 153–157

Quinn M A, Campbell J J, Murray R, Pepperell R J 1981 Tamoxifen and aminoglutethimide in the management of patients with advanced endometrial carcinoma not responsive to medroxyprogesterone. Australian and New Zealand Journal of Obstetrics and Gynaecology 21: 226–229

Quinn M A, Pearce P, Rome R, Funder J W, Fortune D, Pepperell R J 1982 Cytoplasmic steroid receptors in ovarian tumours. British Journal of Obstetrics and Gynaecology 89: 754–759

Quinn M A, Cauchi M, Fortune D 1985a Endometrial carcinoma: steroid receptors and response to medroxyprogesterone acetate. Gynecologic Oncology 21: 314–319

Quinn M A, Pearce P, Fortune D W, Koh S H, Hsieh C, Cauchi M 1985b Correlation between cytoplasmic steroid receptors and tumour differentiation and invasion in endometrial carcinoma. British Journal of Obstetrics and Gynaecology 92: 399–406

Rao B R, Wiest W G, Allen W M 1974 Progesterone 'receptor' in human endometrium. Endocrinology 95: 1275–1281

Rendina G M, Donadio C, Fabri M, Mazzoni P, Nazzicone P 1984 Tamoxifen and medroxyprogesterone therapy for advanced endometrial carcinoma. European Journal of Obstetrics, Gynecology, and Reproductive Biology 17: 285–291

Richman C M, Holt J A, Lorincz M A, Herbst A L 1985 Persistence and distribution of estrogen receptor in advanced epithelial ovarian carcinoma after chemotherapy. Obstetrics and Gynecology 65: 257–263

Rodriquez J, Sen K K, Seski J C, Menon M, Johnson T R, Menon K M J 1979 Progesterone binding by human endometrial tissue during the proliferative and secretory phases of the menstrual cycle and by hyperplastic and carcinomatous endometrium. American Journal of Obstetrics and Gynecology 133: 660–665

Rubin B, Gusberg S B, Butterly H, Han T C, Maralit M 1972 A screening test for estrogen dependence of endometrial cancer. American Journal of Obstetrics and Gynecology 114: 660–669

Saarikoski S, Selander K, Kallio S, Pystynen P 1982 Steroid receptors in normal and neoplastic female reproductive tissue. Gynecologic and Obstetric Investigation 13: 206–212

Sanborn B M, Held B, Kuo H S 1975 Specific estrogen binding proteins in the human cervix. Journal of Steroid Biochemistry 6: 1107–1112

Sanborn B M, Held, B, Kuo H S 1976 Hormonal action in the human cervix. II. Progestogen binding protein in the human cervix. Journal of Steroid Biochemistry 7: 655–672

Schwartz P E, Li Volsi V A, Hildreth N, MacLusky N J, Naftolin F N, Eisenfeld A J 1982 Estrogen receptors in ovarian epithelial carcinoma. Obstetrics and Gynecology 59: 229–238

Schwartz P E, MacLusky N, Sakamoto H, Eisenfeld A 1983 Steroid receptor proteins in nonepithelial malignancies of the ovary. Gynecologic Oncology 15: 305–315

Soper J T, McCarty K S Jr, Hinshaw W, Creasman W T, McCarty K S Snr, Clarke-Pearson D L 1984 Cytoplasmic estrogen and progesterone receptor content of uterine sarcomas. American Journal of Obstetrics and Gynecology 150: 342–348

Soules M R, McCarthy K S Jr 1982 Leiomyomas: steroid receptor content. American Journal of Obstetrics and Gynecology 143: 6–11

Soutter W P, Ginsberg R, Lether V, Sharp F 1986 Cytoplasmic and nuclear steroid receptors in cervical carcinoma. Anti-Cancer Research 6: 339

Spona J, Ulm R, Bieglmayer C, Husslein P 1979 Hormone levels and hormone receptor contents of endometria in women with normal menstrual cycles and patients bearing endometrial carcinoma. Gynecologic and Obstetric Investigation 10: 71–80

Stancel G M, Leung K M T, Gorski J 1973 Estrogen receptors in the rat uterus. Relationship between cytoplasmic and nuclear forms of the estrogen binding protein. Biochemistry 12: 2137–2141

Stedman K E, Moore G E, Morgan R T 1980 Estrogen receptor proteins in diverse human tumours. Archives of Surgery 115: 244–248

Sugimori M, Taki I, Koga K 1976 Adjuvant hormone therapy to radiation treatment for cervical cancer. Acta Obstetrica et Gynaecologia Japonica 23: 77–82

Sutton G P, Senior M B, Strauss J F, Mikuta J J 1986a Estrogen and progesterone receptors in epithelial ovarian malignancies. Gynecologic Oncology 23: 176–182

Sutton G P, Stehman F B, Michael H, Young P C M, Ehrlich C E 1986b Estrogen and progesterone receptors in uterine sarcomas. Obstetrics and Gynecology 68: 709–714

Taylor T W, Brush M G, King R J B 1973 The use of oestradiol uptake and binding-site studies in endometrial and ovarian carcinoma. Postgraduate Medical Journal 29: 77–82

Terenius L, Lindell A, Persson B H 1971 Binding of estradiol-17B to human cancer tissue
   of the female genital tract. Cancer Research 31: 1895–1898
Toppila M, Tyler J P P, Fay R et al 1986 Steroid receptors in human ovarian malignancy.
   A review of four years tissue collection. British Journal of Obstetrics and Gynaecology 93:
   986–992
Tseng L, Gurpide E 1974 Induction of human endometrial estradiol dehydrogenase by
   progestins. Endocrinology 97: 824–833
Tseng L, Tseng J K, Mann W J et al 1986 Endocrine aspects of human uterine sarcoma:
   a preliminary study. American Journal of Obstetrics and Gynecology 155: 95–101
Welshons W V, Lieberman M E, Gorski J 1984 Nuclear localization of unoccupied oestrogen
   receptors. Nature 307: 747–749
Westphal U 1980 How are steroids transported in the blood before they enter target cells?
   In: Wittliff J L, Dapunt O (eds) Steroid receptors and hormone-dependent neoplasia, Masson
   Publ, USA, pp 1–17
Young P C M, Ehrlich C E, Cleary R E 1976 Progesterone binding in human endometrial
   carcinomas. American Journal of Obstetrics and Gynecology 125: 353–358
Young P C M, Grosfeld J L, Ehrlich C E, Roth L M 1982 Progestin- and androgen-binding
   components in a human granulosa-theca cell tumor. Gynecologic Oncology 13: 309–317

A practical approach to colposcopy

Medicine is as subject to fashions as is high couture. Colposcopy was rarely used in Britain until some 10 years ago, and sceptics rightly ask if this alluring technique is destined ultimately to follow the mini-skirt into oblivion. An answer to this provocative question may be found in a consideration of the pathophysiology of cervical squamous neoplasia and its relevance to clinical practice.

THE BASIS OF COLPOSCOPY

Eversion of the cervix

At puberty, during pregnancy or when the combined oral contraceptive pill is taken, the cervix enlarges, probably as a result of oestrogen stimulation. As it does so, there is a tendency to eversion and to the 'exposure' of columnar epithelium on the ectocervix—an event akin to the opening of the petals of a flower in response to the rays of the sun. The thin, columnar epithelium appears red and the result is what is so often erroneously referred to as a 'cervical erosion'. To some degree the 'exposure' is more apparent than real, and the extent of columnar epithelium on the ectocervix can be exaggerated by using a Cusco's speculum and opening the blades widely.

Squamous metaplasia

The columnar epithelium on the ectocervix is replaced gradually by sqamous metaplasia which spreads towards the cervical canal from the squamocolumnar junction. The normal end-result of this process is the replacement of the 'ectopic' columnar epithelium with mature squamous epithelium. If the entrance to a cervical crypt has been covered by squamous epithelium and cells continue to secrete mucus in the depths of the crypt, a nabothian follicle results. This is the only clinical evidence of the prior existence of columnar epithelium in that area. When the cervix becomes smaller in the months and years following pregnancy and after the menopause, it gradually inverts, drawing the new squamocolumnar junction up the endocervical canal.

The transformation zone

The region of the cervix in which this process of metaplasia occurs is called the transformation zone. In some women the transformation zone may extend onto the vaginal walls. A common source of confusion in colposcopy is the loose use of the term 'transformation zone' when referring to that part of the true transformation zone where metaplastic or dysplastic epithelium can be seen colposcopically.

The genesis of squamous cervical neoplasia

Squamous neoplasia result from the disruption of the normal metaplastic process. The earliest recognisable form of this disease—a cervical intra-epithelial neoplasm (CIN) (Table 23.1)—develops as a confluent lesion confined to an area of the cervix contiguous with the squamocolumnar junction. *It is this characteristic localisation which enables the colposcope to be used in the assessment of CIN.*

Table 23.1 Histology of cervical premalignant disease

CIN I	Mild dysplasia
CIN II	Moderate dysplasia
CIN III	Severe dysplasia
	Carcinoma in situ

(CIN = cervical intra-epithelial neoplasia)

INDICATIONS FOR COLPOSCOPY

Prior to the advent of colposcopy, cytologists recommended referral to a gynaecologist only after two, successive, severely dyskaryotic smears were obtained. The reason for this delaying policy was because a knife cone biopsy would be required to determine whether or not there was a premalignant lesion on the cervix and this operation had potentially serious consequences for the future obstetric prospects of the young women in whom these abnormalities were most often found.

That conservative policy is no longer justifiable. With colposcopy, the women who require treatment can be identified and the most appropriate and least traumatic treatment can be chosen. Most women with CIN can be treated in the outpatient clinic with methods that do not prejudice their future fecundity. For those who do require a cone biopsy, the laser can be used, often under local anaesthesia (Bekassy et al 1983, Partington et al 1987). The complications of laser cone biopsy are less than those of knife cone biopsy, the technique is far more precise (Larsson et al 1983) and the distortion of the cervix that results is much less, suggesting fewer problems in any subsequent pregnancies.

Along with the development of less traumatic treatment methods, it has become apparent that a high proportion of women with mildly abnormal smears have far more significant lesions than the cytology would suggest. About 50% of women with mild dyskaryosis and 37% with only mild atypia short of dyskaryosis are found to have CIN II–III (Soutter et al 1986a). For these reasons it is apparent that the indications for referral need to be revised (Table 23.2). It is hoped that nowadays no woman with abnormal cytology is treated without prior colposcopy.

Table 23.2 Management of abnormal cervical cytology

Papanicolaou class	Histology	Action
I Normal	0.1% CIN II–III	Repeat in 3 years (unless clinical suspicion)
II Inflammatory	6% CIN II–III	Repeat in 6 months (colposcopy after 3 abnormal)
Mild atypia	20–37% CIN II–III	Repeat in 4 months (colposcopy after 2 abnormal)
III Mild dyskaryosis	50% CIN–III	Colposcopy
Moderate dyskaryosis	50–75% CIN II–III	Colposcopy
IV Severe dyskaryosis Positive Malignant cells	80–90% CIN II–III 5% invasion	Colposcopy
V Invasion suspected	50% invasion	Urgent colposcopy
Abnormal glandular cells	?Adenocarcinoma cervix or endometrium	Urgent colposcopy

Although the majority of women sent for colposcopy have abnormal smears, a suspicious-looking cervix is sufficient reason for referral, even if the smear is negative. Such women sometimes have invasive cancer.

A PRACTICAL TECHNIQUE

Every colposcopist will develop his/her own routine. The following is suggested as a basis upon which newcomers to the technique may build.

Bimanual examination

I begin with a bimanual examination, touching the end of the cervix as little as possible. The objective is to exclude frank invasive disease of the cervix, or a uterine or ovarian mass, any of which may present with abnormal cervical cytology. Indeed, an endocervical cancer may only be detected in this way.

The smear

I then introduce a bi-valve speculum and take a smear. Deferring the smear until after the colposcopic inspection has some merit. This reduces the risk of removing the epithelium one wishes to study (see below) but may provide a less satisfactory sample for the cytologist. After scraping the cervix around the os with an Ayre's spatula, I wipe the four quadrants of the cervix in turn in case the lesion is placed on the periphery of the cervix. If the os is narrowed or the squamocolumnar junction is out of sight up the canal, I use an endocervical brush (Cytobrush).

The preliminary examination

If the view of the cervix is obscured by a discharge, this should be removed gently with saline. The preliminary inspection should include both the cervix and upper vagina. At this stage of the examination there are three objectives: to identify leukoplakia, to exclude obvious evidence of invasive disease, and to identify viral condylomata.

Leukoplakia must be identified prior to the application of acetic acid, after which it may be impossible to differentiate from acetowhite epithelium. Because the hyperkeratinisation of leukoplakia may conceal invasive disease, biopsy is mandatory.

Invasion is often obvious from the bizarre appearances of the surface of the cervix, which may appear grossly irregular, either raised or ulcerated. This disorganisation of the surface is usually recognisable even when atypical vessels cannot be identified or, as sometimes happens, when the area subsequently fails to turn white after the application of acetic acid.

The atypical vessels seen on invasive lesions may run a bizarre course and are often corkscrew- or comma-shaped. They may be large in diameter, abruptly appearing on and disappearing from the surface. They do not branch dichotomously like normal vessels. It is often said that these vessels can best be seen at this stage of the examination and that they may be obscured by acetic acid. That is not my impression but a careful, if brief, inspection prior to the application of acetic acid is essential.

Condylomata are usually obvious from their regular, frond-like surface, but biopsies should be taken, especially when they are located within the active part of the transformation zone where it is more difficult to be sure of their benign nature.

The application of acetic acid

Having completed the first inspection of the cervix, 5% acetic acid should be applied liberally and gently. This turns abnormal epithelium white, producing the so-called acetowhite changes of CIN. Lower concentrations of acetic acid are often used, but the colour takes longer to develop and is more transient. It is important to put enough acetic acid both on to the whole cervix and into the canal, and to allow sufficient time to elapse for even faintly stained areas to show up. I attempt to achieve these ends by using a small cotton bud to baste the cervix and vaginal fornices with acetic acid taken from the puddle in the posterior blade of the speculum, rather in the way a good cook will baste a chicken—slowly and thoroughly. All the while, I inspect the cervix and vaginal fornices under low power in order to have the widest field of view possible. In this way it is easier to observe areas of faint acetowhite against the contrasting background of normal epithelium.

Identifying the limits of the lesion

After about 30 seconds it is usually possible to proceed. If a lesion has become visible its outer limits should first be determined. When the cervix must be moved to allow a clear view of the lesion or the canal, a 'jumbo Q-tip' or an Ayre's spatula may be pushed gently into the fornix towards which the cervix must be moved to expose the opposite side.

Next the position of the squamocolumnar junction (SCJ) must be ascertained to determine the upper limits of the abnormality. It is this crucial step which gives rise to the most common errors in colposcopy. These are described fully on p. 361. For the moment it is sufficient to say that the *SCJ is marked by the lower limit of normal columnar epithelium, not the upper limit of squamous, as these do not always lie at the same level.* The higher the SCJ appears to lie in the canal, the more difficult it becomes to assess the lesion accurately and, except when the cervix is very patulous, 5 mm represents the limit above which colposcopic evaluation becomes unsafe. In postmenopausal women, ethinyloestradiol 20 mg daily for 7–14 days may bring the SCJ into view.

Determining the nature of the lesion

Having identified the limits of the lesion, the colposcopist must now turn to the most difficult part of his task—determining the nature of the lesion. There are those who set great store by their skill in doing this, but I seek only to decide whether or not a lesion with malignant potential is indeed present and whether invasion may have already occurred. For reasons which will shortly become apparent, I adopt a very conservative approach to the latter objective and tend to regard cases of 'severe' CIN III as being potentially invasive.

Non-malignant epithelium that becomes acetowhite

When determining the significance of a lesion, the colposcopist looks at the colour, the margins and the vascular markings. It should be remembered that not all areas of acetowhite change are malign. Columnar epithelium will blanch markedly but briefly after exposure to acetic acid. It may be identified by its villous or furrowed surface. Squamous metaplasia has a glassy white appearance but can be hard to distinguish from CIN I. After any form of treatment the cervix may develop areas of acetowhite, sub-epithelial fibrosis. This can be recognised by the radial arrangement of lines of fine punctation.

Wart virus lesions

Pure viral lesions are difficult to identify with certainty, especially if they are flat. This is hardly surprising considering the difficulties the histo-pathologist has in differentiating CIN from wart virus lesions. In general, flat viral lesions have faint, very irregular margins and isolated, satellite lesions. In slightly raised areas, looped capillaries in small villi may be seen or the surface may take on a shiny, white, encephaloid appearance. The delicate fronds of fully formed condylomata are usually easy to identify, but all raised lesions on the active transformation zone must be biopsied lest they be invasive cancer. In practice, it is seldom important to make this difficult distinction between CIN and viral lesions on the cervix as both can be treated with relative ease. Indeed, because it is so difficult to differentiate the two by any diagnostic method, both should probably be treated.

Features of CIN

Cervical intra-epithelial neoplasia are usually distinct acetowhite lesions with clear margins. They often show a mosaic vascular pattern with patches of acetowhite separated by red vessels, like red weeds between white flagstones. Where the vessels run perpendicular to the surface, punctation is seen as the vessels are viewed end on. This appears as red spots on a white back-ground. In general, the more quickly and strongly the acetowhite changes develop, the clearer and more regular the margins of the lesion, and the more pronounced the mosaic or punctation the more severe is the lesion likely to be. However, not all features will be equally marked and many CIN III lesions show only a strong matt white colour.

Features of invasion

Frank, early invasion is often suspected before the application of acetic acid (see above), but features suggestive of micro-invasion may not become appar-ent until this stage. A very marked mosaic pattern or coarse punctation (large diameter, widely separated, red spots) may reveal early stromal invasion. Atypical vessels (see above) may be observed. It must be said, however, that even expert colposcopists will fail to identify correctly every case of early invasion (Anderson 1986). This may not matter if the invasive focus is small and superficial, but even more extensive lesions can escape detection

(Grundsell et al 1983, Bekassy et al 1983). Care must be taken to avoid the pitfalls of colposcopy, but even that may not be sufficient to prevent the occasional diagnostic error. A wider use of excisional treatment, providing the whole lesion for histological assessment, would help to reduce this risk. Fortunately, the laser, which has been widely used to vaporise and destroy lesions, can also be used to excise cone biopsies. The advantages are reduced complications in comparison with knife biopsies (Larsson et al 1983, Fenton et al 1986) and an ability to be used in the outpatient department under local anaesthesia in most cases (Partington et al 1987).

PITFALLS OF COLPOSCOPY

The first pitfall—the false SCJ caused by an abrasion

The SCJ should be identified by observing *the lower limit of normal columnar epithelium*, not the upper limit of squamous. The reason for this is the ease with which CIN and metaplastic epithelium can be detached from the underlying stroma by an examining finger, by the insertion of a speculum or, most commonly, by the taking of a smear. This is particularly true at the SCJ where the unwary may mistakenly regard the upper limit of acetowhite change as synonymous with the SCJ. When this happens, careful inspection of the red epithelium at this junction will reveal a flat surface covered by spidery and often whorled blood vessels characteristic of exposed stroma. This abrasion must be distinguished from columnar epithelium. The latter will be recognised by the following features: the surface looks velvety and soft and blanches strikingly (but briefly) when exposed to acetic acid; on the ectocervix it tends to have a villous surface but in the canal the villi coalesce to form longitudinal ridges rather like the furrows in a ploughed field.

The second pitfall—the SCJ in the canal

When the SCJ lies within the endocervical canal, great care must be taken to obtain a clear view of the upper part of the lesion, which must not be inspected from too acute an angle. To do so makes unreliable the assessment of both the length of the endocervical canal involved with CIN and the severity of the lesion. It is impossible to lay down rules as to how far up the canal can safely be evaluated but, in general, it would be unwise to regard an examination as being conclusive when the SCJ is more than 5 mm up the canal. Often, even that figure would be excessive.

The third pitfall—the previously treated cervix

All of the foregoing observations apply only to the unadulterated cervix. When a cervix has been treated previously for an 'erosion' or for CIN by diathermy, cryocautery, 'cold' coagulation or laser or knife cone biopsy, the topography of the transformation zone will have been drastically altered. Areas of metaplasia, CIN or invasive disease in the canal or in the cervical glands may have escaped destruction and may persist as isolated 'iatrogenic skip lesions' surrounded by the columnar epithelium which replaced the area destroyed, or covered by new squamous epithelium.

Using ablative methods to treat CIN in such patients is usually unwise. Both the method and extent of therapy should be guided by a careful consideration of the likely depth of the damage caused by the previous treatment. For example, if a patient has recurrent CIN on the ectocervix following cryotherapy, and the SCJ is easily seen close to the cervical os, it is probably safe to assume that the lower margin of an 'iatrogenic skip lesion' will not lie more than 4–5 mm up the canal (the maximum likely depth of cryotherapeutic destruction). Thus, treatment of the cervix to 10 mm should remove the entire volume at risk with a reasonable margin. *In my opinion, the second treatment should excise this part of the cervix in order to evaluate it histologically.* This can often be done in the outpatient clinic using the laser and intracervical local anaesthesia.

The fourth pitfall—glandular lesions

Although it is often difficult to distinguish adenocarcinoma of the cervix from squamous cancer, and it seems possible that both may arise from the same location on the cervix, it cannot be assumed that the rules of colposcopy apply to women with adenocarcinoma or adenocarcinoma-in-situ (AIS). I am unable to identify AIS colposcopically and believe that a cone biopsy is an essential investigation in the management of a patient with abnormal glandular cells in her smear. A further difficulty in this policy is the very high false-positive rate with such reports. Fortunately, most of these patients also have CIN which requires treatment in its own right. Although isolated areas of AIS may occur some distance above the SCJ, this is probably uncommon, and most lie adjacent to the junction, often close to an area of CIN. I therefore treat most of these patients with a small cone biopsy which removes approximately 15 mm of the endocervical canal above the SCJ.

COLPOSCOPY OF THE VAGINA

Colposcopy of the vagina is complicated by four problems: pre-invasive disease of the vagina is often multifocal; the area to be examined is large and most of it is difficult to view at right angles; many of these patients have already had a hysterectomy so not all of the area involved may be visible; and because the treatment of vaginal intra-epithelial neoplasia (VAIN) is so difficult, it is more important to differentiate viral disease from premalignant lesions.

In general, the colposcopic features of VAIN are similar to those seen in

CIN. The irregular surface of the vagina makes it difficult to identify all of the suspect areas. It is also hard to view the lateral walls of the vagina at anything other than a very acute angle. The colposcope must be moved from side to side to examine the opposite wall, and it sometimes helps to withdraw and rotate the speculum slightly while looking through the blades from the side. The anterior and posterior walls of the lower half of the vagina can be inspected while slowly withdrawing the speculum. I regularly use Lugol's iodine after the inspection with acetic acid to reduce the risk of overlooking an area of abnormality.

If the patient has already had a hysterectomy, not only is it very difficult to inspect thoroughly the vaginal angles, but it is also probable that residual VAIN or invasive cancer may persist concealed above the suture line. The latter problem has obvious, important implications for treatment.

Although small, short-term studies have reported promising results in the treatment of VAIN with 5-fluorouracil (Petrilli et al 1980, Kirwan & Naftalin 1985) or the carbon dioxide laser (Capen et al 1982, Townsend et al 1982), these have not been confirmed by other workers (Sillman et al 1985). In Birmingham, Woodman and his colleagues (1984) used the laser to treat 14 patients with VAIN persisting after hysterectomy. Only six were still free of disease and two had developed invasive cancer. In contrast, 28 patients remained disease-free after surgical excision or radiotherapy (Hernandes-Linares et al 1980). Most had been followed for at least 5 years.

The combination of multifocal disease, difficulty of diagnosis and the poor results of simple, conservative therapy makes the management of VAIN quite different from that of CIN. General anaesthesia is necessary to allow adequate colposcopic assessment in many cases. Full-thickness knife biopsies are often required, especially with VAIN following hysterectomy.

COLPOSCOPY OF THE VULVA

Because of the multifocal nature of vulval intra-epithelial disease (VIN) and the keratinisation of vulval skin, colposcopy of the vulva is difficult and the recognition of early invasive disease more problematical.

A preliminary inspection may reveal areas of pigmentation, ulceration or atrophy. Condylomata may be recognised. Acetic acid must be applied thoroughly for 2 or 3 minutes. A good way of doing this is to soak a gauze swab or sanitary towel and to lay this on the vulva. Many hitherto unnoticed condylomata will appear shining white, displaying their characteristic villous surface. Some areas of VIN will also appear white and may show a faint mosaic or punctation. The vascular patterns are less marked and less reliable than in CIN. I do not use toluidine blue because of the difference in opinions as to its diagnostic value.

On the vulva, the colposcope will indicate the suspicious areas from which biopsies should be taken. It can often give reassurance that invasion is unlikely, but it cannot differentiate between VIN III and early invasion.

COLPOSCOPY IN TREATMENT

The discussion thus far has centred upon the diagnostic value of the colposcope and upon its ability to locate areas of abnormal epithelium on the cervix, vagina and vulva. With these powers it seems self-evident that treatment should be guided by colposcopy too.

Laser vaporisation

Laser vaporisation has always been performed under colposcopic guidance with the laser beam directed by a micromanipulator attached to the colposcope. This has permitted very precise treatment of cervical lesions, not only outlining the abnormal areas accurately but also treating to a carefully measured depth in the stroma. This resulted initially in the treatment being too superficial, but experience showed that increasing the depth of vaporisation to 10 mm improved the success rate without any obvious increase in complications (Soutter et al 1986b).

Careful control of the depth of treatment is obviously important in those cases of vaginal disease selected for laser vaporisation. In the vagina, because there are usually no gland crypts, the epithelium need only be destroyed to just beyond the basement membrane. This can be recognised colposcopically (see below).

It is in treatment of the vulval disease that the colposcopic control of the depth of laser vaporisation is most important. The colposcopic recognition of three surgical planes delineated by the laser has been described by Reid (1985, 1986).

The first surgical plane is recognised by moving the laser beam rapidly in parallel lines until bubbles of silver opalescence can be seen beneath the surface char. This is accompanied by a crackling sound. If this sound disappears the treatment has extended into the dermis. If the correct depth of vaporisation has been achieved the basement membrane may then be exposed by wiping off the char with a moist swab. Further light application of the laser will expose yellowish tissue that looks like a chamois cloth. This is the papillary dermis and marks the second plane. Vaporisation to the first or second surgical planes is sufficient for viral disease or for vulval dystrophy without atypia, causing otherwise intractable pruritus vulvae. Healing is usually complete within 14 days and the cosmetic result is excellent.

The third plane is the superficial reticular dermis and is identified by the presence of whitish fibres like soggy thread. This is the deepest level from which normal healing can take place by epithelialisation from skin appendages in the base of the crater. The fourth plane—the deep reticular dermis—contains most of the hair follicles and apocrine glands. These look like grains of sand when exposed by the laser but are usually largely destroyed by the time they become visible. Skin grafting is necessary if the dermis is destroyed to this level.

The depth of treatment required for VIN is still unclear (Dorsey 1986). In some cases hair follicles may be involved for several millimetres below the surface (Mene & Buckley 1985), but it seems that it is not always necessary to destroy the whole depth of involved appendage (Dorsey 1986). In any case, treatment of the whole vulva to such a depth would result in a third-degree burn which would need skin grafting. A practical policy may be to treat the abnormal areas to the second surgical plane. This will usually heal well after 2–3 weeks. If VIN in a follicle grows onto the surface after this treatment, the localised area of recurrence can be treated more deeply.

Cone biopsy—laser or knife

When CIN is not suitable for destructive therapy, the colposcope can often be used with endocervical forceps to determine the extent of disease in the canal and thus to tailor the length of the cone biopsy required. Where the SCJ cannot be seen with the colposcope, it can be located with the micro-colpohysteroscope (Soutter et al 1984, Fenton et al 1985). If the cone biopsy is performed with the laser under colposcopic control, a very accurately tailored biopsy can be obtained. Even knife cone biopsy can be improved by a preliminary colposcopy in theatre. In this respect the findings in the colposcopy clinic several days or even weeks earlier cannot be relied upon. The cervix undergoes extensive eversion and inversion throughout the menstrual cycle and even the use of a different speculum may alter the apparent length of the canal involved with CIN.

Other ablative methods of treating CIN

One of the disadvantages of cryotherapy (and, I imagine, of cold coagulation) is that the probe cannot be applied to the cervix under colposcopic vision; indeed it obscures the lesion. Radical electrodiathermy applied with a needle can be performed under colposcopic vision provided that a sucker is used to extract the smoke. This may not seem necessary with a modality that causes such extensive destruction, but the zone of thermal damage around the needle entry point may be less extensive than is generally believed and the SCJ may lie further up the canal than it did at the initial evaluation in the clinic (see above).

CONCLUSIONS

With the increasing realisation that many women with mild cytological abnormalities have CIN, a change is necessary in the indications for referral to colposcopy. This will result in an increase in the already heavy workload of colposcopy clinics throughout the country, but the appropriate provisions must be made if the full benefit of screening cytology is to be realised.

Just as laparoscopy has found an enduring place in British gynaecological practice when high-quality instruments became available, so colposcopy has become an essential part of the management of women suspected of harbouring a pre-clinical neoplasm, both in identifying the lesion and in guiding treatment.

REFERENCES

Anderson M C 1986 Are we vapourising microinvasive lesions? In: Sharp F, Jordan J A (eds) Gynaecological laser surgery, Perinatology Press, New York, pp 127–132

Bekassy Z, Alm P, Grundsell H, Larsson G, Asted B 1983 Laser miniconisation in mild and moderate dysplasia of the uterine cervix. Gynecologic Oncology 15: 357–362

Capen C V, Masterton B J, Magrina J F, Calkins J W 1982 Laser therapy of vaginal intraepithelial neoplasia. American Journal of Obstetrics and Gynecology 142: 973–976

Dorsey J H 1986 Skin appendage involvement and vulval intraepithelial neoplasia. In: Sharp F, Jordan J A (eds) Gynaecological laser surgery, Perinatology Press, New York, pp 193–195

Fenton D W, Soutter W P, Sharp F, Mann M 1985 Preliminary experience with microcolpohysteroscopically controlled cone biopsies. Colposcopy & Gynecologic Laser Surgery 1: 167–172

Fenton D W, Soutter W P, Sharp F, James C 1986 A comparison of knife and carbon dioxide laser excision biopsies. In: Sharp F, Jordan J A (eds) Gynaecological laser surgery, Perinatology Press, New York, pp 77–84

Grundsell H, Alm P, Larsson G 1983 Cure rates after laser conisation for early cervical neoplasia. Annales Chirurgiae et Gynaecologiae 72: 218–222

Hernandez-Linarez W, Puthawala A, Nolan J F, Jernstrom P H, Morrow C P 1980 Carcinoma-in-situ of the vagina: past and present management. Obstetrics and Gynecology 56: 356–360

Kirwan P, Naftalin N J 1985 Topical 5-fluorouracil in the treatment of vaginal intraepithelial neoplasia. British Journal of Obstetrics and Gynaecology 92: 287–291

Larsson G, Gullberg B, Grundsell H 1983 A comparison of complications of laser and cold knife conisation. Obstetrics and Gynecology 62: 213–217

Mene A, Buckley C H 1985 Involvement of the vulval skin appendages by intraepithelial neoplasia. British Journal of Obstetrics and Gynaecology 92: 634–638

Partington C K, Soutter W P, Turner M J, Hill A S, Krausz T 1987 Laser excisional biopsy under local anaesthesia—an outpatient technique? Journal of Obstetrics and Gynaecology 8: 48–52

Petrilli E S, Townsend D E, Morrow C P, Nakao C Y 1980 Vaginal intraepithelial neoplasia: biological aspects and treatment with topical 5-fluorouracil and the carbon dioxide laser. American Journal of Obstetrics and Gynecology 138: 321–328

Reid R 1985 Superficial laser vulvectomy. II. The anatomic and biophysical principles permitting accurate control over the depth of dermal destruction with the carbon dioxide laser. American Journal of Obstetrics and Gynecology 152: 261–271

Reid R 1986 Laser vulvectomy—how to assess and control depth. In: Sharp F, Jordan J A (eds) Gynaecological laser surgery, Perinatology Press, New York, pp 197–205

Sillman F H, Sedlis A, Boyce J G 1985 A review of lower genital intraepithelial neoplasia and the use of topical 5-fluorouracil. Obstetrical and Gynecological Survey 40: 190–220

Soutter W P, Fenton D W, Gudgeon P, Sharp F 1984 Quantitative microcolpohysteroscopic assessment of the extent of endocervical involvement by cervical intraepithelial neoplasia. British Journal of Obstetrics and Gynaecology 91: 712–715

Soutter W P, Wisdom S, Brough A K, Monaghan J M 1986a Should patients with mild atypia in a cervical smear be referred for colposcopy? British Journal of Obstetrics and Gynaecology 93: 70–74

Soutter W P, Abernethy F M, Brown V A, Hill A S 1986b Success, complications and subsequent pregnancy outcome relative to the depth of laser treatment of cervical intraepithelial neoplasia. Colposcopy and Gynecologic Laser Surgery 2: 35–42

Townsend D E, Levine R U, Crum C P, Richart R M 1982 Treatment of vaginal carcinoma in situ with the carbon dioxide laser. American Journal of Obstetrics and Gynecology 143: 565–568

Woodman C B J, Jordan J A, Wade-Evans T 1984 The management of vaginal intraepithelial neoplasia after hysterectomy. British Journal of Obstetrics and Gynaecology 91: 707–711

Cervical adenocarcinoma

INTRODUCTION

'The literature on adenocarcinoma of the cervix presents certain problems for the unwary reader' (Shingleton et al 1981). This statement is as pertinent now as when it was first written, for of the many studies published to date on this subject none has been prospective, few have been controlled, and most are small in terms of patient numbers yet large in terms of number of years spanned. As a consequence of these factors, uniformity in nomenclature is poor and treatment schedules have varied.

This chapter attempts to present the available data in a clear and balanced fashion in order that conclusions may be left to the reader. The inconclusive nature of much of the published work frequently renders this task difficult, if not impossible.

EPIDEMIOLOGY

Incidence

The reported frequency of cervical adenocarcinoma is variable (3–34%) (Table 24.1), histological criteria and the time interval studied both contributing

Table 24.1   The frequency of cervical adenocarcinoma

Principal author	Date	Tumour type	Reported incidence (%)
Rombeaut	1966	Pure adeno	3.0
Weiner	1975	Pure adeno	5.0
Hurt	1977	Pure adeno	3.0
Rutledge	1975	Adeno plus mixed	5.9
Mikuta	1969	Adeno plus mixed	6.1
Korhonen	1978	Adeno plus mixed	7.1
Ireland	1985	Adeno plus mixed	8.1
Glucksmann	1956	Adeno plus mixed	13.0
Reagan	1973	Adeno plus mixed	16.0
Shingleton	1981	Adeno plus mixed	18.5
Julian	1977	Adeno plus mixed	28.0
Davis	1975	Adeno plus mixed	34.0

to this variance. The inclusion of mixed adenosquamous carcinomas in some series undoubtedly increases the observed frequency in relation to epidermoid cancers.

The relevance of time interval relates to several authors' observations of an increasing incidence, especially over the last two decades (Tasker & Collins 1974, Davis & Moon 1975, Gallup & Abell 1977, Fu et al 1982a). This trend has been explained in terms of a diminishing frequency of squamous carcinoma resulting from screening, although Shingleton et al (1981) could not attribute an increase from 7.2–18.6% over an 11-year period to such an effect, concluding that the rise was actual and not relative. Devesa (1984), reporting on nationwide cervical cancer registration in the United States, also noted an increase in the relative proportion of adenocarcinomas compared with squamous tumours, but could not find evidence to support an actual increase in the glandular neoplasm. Regional variations were quite marked and were assumed to be due to different screening practices. Such an effect may, in part, explain the varying incidences of adenocarcinomas that have been reported.

Age

Many earlier series consistently reported a higher mean age in adenocarcinoma patients than in those with squamous tumours (Gusberg & Corscaden 1951, Abell & Gosling 1962, Bergsjo 1963, Abad et al 1969). A more recent sample does not confirm this earlier finding, the average age at diagnosis varying between 47 and 55 years. Like squamous carcinoma, the majority of cases present in the fourth, fifth and sixth decades; however, unlike its squamous counterpart this disease has been seen in infants and children (Pollack & Taylor 1947, Fawcett et al 1966, Herbst et al 1974). Pollack and Taylor, reviewing cervical carcinoma occurring in the first two decades of life, found 23 out of 31 cases to be adenocarcinomas. Although clear cell adenocarcinoma of the vagina has been recorded as occurring after in-utero exposure to diethyl-stilboestrol, this has not been implicated as a cause for adenocarcinoma of the cervix in infants and adolescents (Kaminski & Maier 1983).

Why earlier studies should find an age discrepancy between the two histological variants might also be explained by the impact of cervical screening. An analysis of mass screening in Finland (Timonen et al 1974) noted that the incidence of cervical cancer in women of reproductive age was decreasing, and a proportionally greater number of women with this disease were over 60 years of age. This apparent shift in age groups was ascribed to large-scale cytological screening programmes directed at the female population of fertile age, the end result being an abolition of the natural age differences between the two histological types of cervical cancer (Korhonen 1980). Naturally this screening effect would not have been apparent in earlier studies.

Race

No relationship with racial origin has been noted in those studies that have analysed this variable (Hurt et al 1977, Shingleton et al 1981, Saigo et al 1986).

Parity

Several authors have commented on the greater frequency of nulligravity and nulliparity in patients with cervical adenocarcinomas; this has ranged from 19–24% (Abell & Gosling 1962, Anderson & Fraser 1976, Korhonen 1980, Milsom & Friberg 1983). This figure is almost twice that recorded for squamous cell cancer (Korhonen 1980, Milsom & Friberg 1983). Others, however (Rombeaut et al 1966, Hurt et al 1977), have not noticed any parity differences from the general population.

Miscellaneous factors

Area of residence has been studied by both Korhonen (1980) and Milsom & Friberg (1983); both found a greater relative frequency of adenocarcinoma in rural dwellers than in city dwellers. This was due to a greater preponderance of the squamous variant in women from an urban background.

Korhonen also found significantly more spinsters amongst adenocarcinoma patients than amongst squamous controls, although there was no difference in the mean age at marriage.

In the same study, no significant differences in the age at menarche or menopause were noted.

There are notable differences in the epidemiology of these two types of cervical cancer. This is a consistent theme in all the reported data, and although cervical adenocarcinoma shares some epidemiological characteristics with endometrial carcinoma, it is seen in relatively younger women.

AETIOLOGICAL FACTORS

Aetiology remains unknown. The epidemiological characteristics suggest that this tumour may have, like endometrial cancer, an endocrinologically dependent component.

Oral contraceptives

Steroid receptors have been described in cervical tissues (Soutter et al 1981), and some epidemiological data have implicated long-term oral contraceptive use with cervical cancer (Harris et al 1980, Vessey et al 1983). The association between combined oral contraceptive use and neoplasia is tenuous, for after controlling for sexual behaviour, Boyce et al (1977) and Swan & Brown (1981) could find no association. These studies have been concerned primarily with squamous malignancies, and it is possible that exogenous hormones may exert a greater effect on steroid responsive glandular tissues as it has been noted that glandular tumours are more responsive to oestrogens than squamous tumours (Hahnel et al 1979).

Microglandular hyperplasia bears certain morphological similarities to dysplastic changes in glandular epithleium, and has been related to progestogenic stimulation (Candy & Abell 1968). Dallenbach-Hellweg (1984) has suggested that this condition is a precursor lesion for cervical adenocarcinoma, and although no other data relating this morphological change to malign transformation have been reported, Qizilbash (1975) and Gallup & Abell (1977) have suggested that the risk of adenocarcinoma is increased if high progesterone preparations are taken for 10 or more years.

Oral contraception has been cited as one possible cause for the increasing incidence of adenocarcinoma of the cervix. Peters et al (1986) observed an increase in cervical adenocarcinoma in young women of higher socioeconomic class averaging 16% per year, and assume that this group would have been most likely to have used oral contraception. Although such an increase was unlikely to have been a chance effect, these data remain inconclusive but worthy of further evaluation.

Pregnancy

Further support for an endocrine aetiology derives from observations by both Cherry & Glucksmann (1961) and Steiner & Friedell (1965). Both reported an increased frequency of the disease occurring during pregnancy or in women who had recently been pregnant. These data have not yet been corroborated.

Clinical profile

Apart from shared epidemiological characteristics with endometrial cancer, similar clinical profiles have also been reported (Korhonen 1980, Milsom & Frieberg 1983, Saigo et al 1986), strengthening the suspicion of a common endocrine aetiological component. These authors all comment on the frequency with which obesity, hypertension and diabetes mellitus occurred in studied populations of adenocarcinoma patients. Saigo (1986) noted that one or more of these characteristics was present in 13% of 136 patients with adenocarcinoma of the cervix, whereas they were seen in only 4–5% of patients with squamous carcinoma.

Hormone replacement therapy

Hormone replacement therapy has not been implicated in the aetiology of this disease in contradistinction to its proposed role in the genesis of endometrial malignancy.

Previous sub-total hysterectomy

Previous sub-total hysterectomy has been reported more frequently in patients developing adenocarcinoma than in those developing squamous cancer (Waddell et al 1962, Rombeaut et al 1966, Gallup & Abell 1977, Korhonen 1980). Gallup and Abell noted that seven of their 30 patients had had a prior sub-total hysterectomy, and Korhonen reported a 6.1% incidence of previous sub-total hysterectomy—four times the incidence seen in the squamous cancer population. Other larger series have not been able to confirm this unusual finding, and it is unlikely that further light will be shed on this situation, bearing in mind how infrequently this operation is now performed.

Viruses

Some limited data have been presented suggesting that herpes simplex (type II) may be one of a group of co-carcinogens implicated in the aetiology of cervical adenocarcinoma (Menczer et al 1981). Sixteen patients with adenocarcinoma were compared with 32 controls. Higher titres of neutralizing antibody were found amongst the study patients. The results were only of borderline significance and in contrast to two previous studies, albeit with even fewer patients, where no association between herpes simplex virus and adenocarcinoma was demonstrated (Rawls et al 1970, Aurelian et al 1973).

Human papilloma virus (HPV) has also been implicated in the aetiology of cervical adenocarcinoma (Smotkin et al 1986). Of nine tumours tested, two were positive for HPV type 16 and four for type 18. The latter were all adenosquamous tumours however. No normal tissue controls were used, which makes this information difficult to interpret, particularly since Cox et al (1986) have documented positive HPV 18 findings in normal tissue.

PATHOLOGY

Glandular neoplasms of the cervix are composed of a heterogeneous group of tumours having complex growth patterns and different cell types. The majority of tumours are made up of cells resembling endocervical cells; others are composed of clear cells or cells like those of endometrial cancers. Some are purely glandular whilst others contain a mixture of glandular and squamous elements.

Recent reviews have dealt with the pathological aspects of adenocarcinoma (Clement & Scully 1982, Anderson 1985). The WHO classification of glandular tumours, established in 1975 (Poulsen et al 1975), is shown in the following list:

Endocervical type
Endometrioid adenocarcinoma
Clear cell (mesonephroid) adenocarcinoma
Adenoid cystic carcinoma

Adenosquamous carcinoma
Undifferentiated carcinoma

A notable exception in this list is adenoma malignum, otherwise known as minimal deviation adenocarcinoma. This is a highly differentiated tumour that is difficult to distinguish from normal endocervical epithelium. This tumour variant has recently been reviewed by Michael et al (1984).

The endocervical carcinoma, where cells resemble those of native cervical columnar epithelium, is generally reported as the most common carcinoma, with the endometrioid or clear cell variants being the second most frequently observed.

Classification has been complicated by an increasing use of special staining techniques. These are now frequently used to identify mucin in undifferentiated tumours and neoplasms previously reported as poorly differentiated squamous lesions. The outcome has been that a proportion of such tumours have been reclassified as glandular lesions. This practice may necessitate a complete re-evaluation of currently accepted databases.

Endometrioid tumours, where the cellular background is similar to that seen in endometrial carcinoma, must be differentiated from tumours of the uterine corpus. The complexity of differentiating corporal from cervical tumours is compounded by the fact that almost half of all adenocarcinomas found in the cervix are endometrial in origin and involve the cervix by extension (Abell & Gosling 1962). Most authors have excluded any case where co-existent endometrial pathology was found, Shingleton (1981) reporting to the extreme of excluding all tumours with an endometrioid pattern. Exclusion of endometrial pathology may pose certain problems if the uterine specimen is not available for inspection (as in cases treated by radiotherapy). Fractional curettage has been employed in an effort to differentiate between the two, but this technique is not without limitations. Korhonen (1978) evaluated fractional curettage in 53 cervical glandular neoplasms. Seventy per cent of the samples contained malignant tissue in both samples, 4% had neoplasm only in the corporal fraction and 26% had neoplasm only in the cervical fraction. When correlated with the hysterectomy specimen, fractional curettage provided an accurate localization of the tumour in only 38% of cases.

Differential staining techniques have been suggested as an alternative approach to identifying corpus tumours. Davis & Moon (1975) have claimed that staining with Alcian blue is helpful, intracellular staining occurring in glandular tissue of endocervical origin but not in endometrial tissue. These authors do not recommend that this technique be used as the sole criterion for excluding endometrial cancers, and it certainly cannot be relied upon, poorly differentiating between these two tumours. Other differentiating features include the increased likelihood of endocervical primary tumours producing intracellular mucin, having a more fibrous stroma, and finding adjacent areas of adenocarcinoma in situ. In addition, the majority of endocervical adenocarcinomas show abundant, diffuse intracellular staining for carcino-embryonic antigen (CEA), whereas in an endometrial primary tumour this is usually focal and restricted to apical surface CEA.

Pomerance & Mackles (1962) and Noda et al (1983) have suggested that endometrioid tumours may arise from ectopic endometrial glands. However, a detailed analysis of the site of origin of glandular carcinomas by Teshima et al (1985) failed to locate any endometrial foci in the lower third of the endocervical canal, yet recognized early endometrioid adenocarcinoma in this area.

Clear cell or mesonephroid tumours are found throughout the genital tract and are thought to arise from remnants of the mesonephric duct.

Adenosquamous tumours contain malign glandular and squamous elements. If the two components are separate they should be recorded as such and not classified as adenosquamous, Shingleton (1981) referring to these tumours as collision tumours. More frequently there is an admixture of malign elements. The glandular component of these mixed tumours may be one of the above mentioned subtypes; indeed, even in pure glandular lesions combinations of different subtypes have been reported. Squamous metaplasia and dysplasia may also be recognized with glandular neoplasms. Mature squamous metaplasia occurring in a glandular tumour is referred to as adenoacanthoma and is comparable to the same situation as seen in corpus cancer. Squamous intra-epithelial neoplasia occurs with a frequency varying from 6% (Korhonen 1978) to 43% (Maier & Norris 1980); even a rate of 6% is higher than one would expect if this were a chance occurrence, suggesting that the two lesions share a common reserve cell (Lauchlan & Penner 1967). Teshima et al (1985), evaluating early cases of glandular carcinoma, also noticed this association and went on to comment that most foci were not in direct contact with adenocarcinoma foci. This observation would not support the theory that such mixed tumours arise from undifferentiated, multipotential subcolumnar cells, although such a theory is attractive when one considers the wide spectrum of tumours seen in the cervix and indeed in the whole genital tract (Burghardt 1973, Ferenczy 1982). LiVolsi et al (1983) and Kaminski & Norris (1984) both report the synchronous occurrence of endocervical and ovarian neoplasia, highlighting the propensity of müllerian epithelium to undergo multicentric neoplasia.

The general consensus supports the view that squamous carcinoma arises as a result of neoplastic transformation occurring in the zone of metaplasia lying between native columnar and native squamous epithelium. A similar mechanism has not been proposed for glandular neoplasms, the whole canal theoretically being a potential site for malign transformation. The question of site of origin was addressed by Teshima et al (1985) who, in a series of 22 early invasive cases, found that malignant glandular patterns were mainly limited to the lower portion of the endocervical canal and transformation zone. Only three cases had malignancy in the upper and middle portions of the endocervical canal. In addition, eight cases of adenocarcinoma in situ were studied (four of endocervical cell type and four of endometrioid cell type). In all cases the lesion was seen in the area just proximal to the squamo-columnar juction.

Adenocarcinoma in situ

Glandular dysplasia, although apparently less common than squamous dysplasia, is almost certainly an underdiagnosed lesion. Many have commented upon the disparity in ratios between pre-invasive and invasive lesions (Qizilbash 1975, Christopherson et al 1979, Boon et al 1981). Our own experience at the Birmingham and Midland Hospital for Women is that 25% of our surgically managed cervical cancers have a glandular component, yet less than 1% of our pre-invasive lesions demonstrate malign glandular elements. One certainly cannot exclude the possibility that adenocarcinoma arises de novo from normal-appearing epithelium without passing through an in situ phase, as suggested by Teshima et al (1985).

DIAGNOSIS

Adenocarcinoma presents in a similar fashion to squamous malignancies, abnormal vaginal bleeding being the most common presenting symptom. This has been reported as occurring even with minimally invasive adenocarcinoma (Qizilbash 1975). Pain, urinary or bowel symptoms generally reflect advanced disease. Seventeen to 29% of patients with cervical glandular neoplasms have no detectable lesion by clinical examination (Abell & Gosling 1962, Korhonen 1978). In these patients histological diagnosis is prompted by abnormal cytological findings.

The recognition of malign glandular cells in Papanicolaou smears has been well documented (Bousfield et al 1980, Betshill & Clark 1986), although this technique was primarily developed to detect squamous abnormalities. In the presence of a smear suggestive of malign glandular tissue, a cone biopsy at least should be performed. This is because the lesions may be small and located high in the endocervical canal, and small punch biopsies have been shown to be unreliable (Luesley et al 1987).

The accuracy of cervical cytology in this condition is somewhat variable, detection rates of 47–92% having been reported (Reagan & Ng 1973, Hurt et al 1977, Korhonen 1978). Those studies reporting high degrees of accuracy have incorporated endocervical aspiration as well as cervical scrapes, implying that endocervical canal sampling improves the detection rate.

The preceding cytological history has equal importance, as the detection of precursor lesions is a major objective of cervical cytology. Unfortunately, such a history is not always easy to obtain. Of 73 patients with glandular neoplasms of the cervix reported by Ireland et al (1985), only 13 gave a history of having had a smear, and eight of these had had a negative smear within 3 years of diagnosis. Hurt et al (1977) reported that 18 out of 43

patients (42%) had negative findings, and Benoit et al (1984), reviewing cytological history in 67 patients with both types of cervical cancer, noted that,
overall, 25 cases had negative smears within 3 years of diagnosis of stage
Ib cervical cancer (37%). Twelve out of 17 (70%) patients developing adenocarcinoma or adenosquamous carcinoma had negative cytology within 3 years
of diagnosis, whereas only 13 out of 50 (26%) developing squamous cancers
had negative smears with 3 years of diagnosis.

Very little data concerning colposcopy in the diagnosis of adenocarcinoma
have been presented. Teshima et al (1985) colposcoped 30 patients with early
adenocarcinoma; six cases had findings strongly suggestive of invasive cancer.
This series included six cases of adenocarcinoma in situ, which is also unrelia-
bly detected by colposcopy (Luesley et al 1987), although it was noted that
in this series of 30 patients with glandular atypia and adenocarcinoma in
situ, several were overdiagnosed as squamous cancers or micro-invasion.

In the absence of overt clinical cancer, any cytological suspicion of glandular
neoplasia requires appropriate histological sampling.

PROGNOSTIC VARIABLES

Several features of adenocarcinoma have been correlated with outcome. These
include clinical stage at presentation, lesion size, depth of penetration and
lymph node metastases. In addition, various pathological aspects of the
tumour have been examined, including histological subtype, degree of differentiation and cellular DNA content. All studies have used retrospective data
and most have not analysed the variables in a multivariate fashion. Inevitably,
this has made interpretation of results difficult.

Clinical stage

Adenocarcinoma of the uterine cervix is staged in the same way as epidermoid
malignancies. The majority of patients present as stage Ib, although quite
wide variation of the incidence of patients in this category are noted between
authors—from 39% (Moberg et al 1986) to 77% (Prempree et al 1985). This
may reflect the referral bias of various institutions but it is important to
keep this variation in mind when treatment options and outcome are considered. All authors have noted a deteriorating outcome with advancing stage
of disease. There are, however, no data suggesting that adenocarcinomas
present more frequently in advanced stage than squamous cancers.

Some have suggested that, stage for stage, adenocarcinoma carries a worse
prognosis than squamous cancer (Milsom & Friberg 1983, Moberg et al 1986).
This has not been confirmed by Shingleton et al (1981) or Ireland et al (1985),
both using matched squamous controls.

Tumour volume

Tumour volume is an important prognostic variable. This is so for squamous
(Mendenhall et al 1984) and glandular lesions (Prempree et al 1985, Berek

et al 1985). To some extent volume and stage are interdependent variables, but as the former is either not measured or, with retrospective studies in mind, is difficult to accurately quantify, stage has assumed the mantle of the most important prognostic indicator (Mikuta & Celebre 1969, Korhonen 1980, Tammimi & Figge 1982, Saigo et al 1986). Several authors (Shingleton et al 1981, Prempree et al 1985, Berek et al 1985, Weiss & Lucas 1986) have commented on the influence of lesion size, with a significantly better outcome seen where lesions are less than 2 cm in diameter. This has generally been found independent of tumour type or grade. It is unfortunate that this variable has not as yet been included in any multivariate analyses so that its importance in relation to other variables can be accurately assessed.

Uterine size

Prempree et al (1985) accounted for this variable in their retrospective analysis of 75 patients with stage I or II primary adenocarcinoma of the cervix. Size was categorized as normal (45 patients), enlarged (equivalent to 4–6 week size uterus) (20 patients) or very enlarged (greater than 6-week size) (10 patients). There was a positive correlation between uterine size and treatment failure rate. The authors postulated that this might reflect extension of the cancer into the lower uterine segment and/or the body of the uterus.

Histological type

As most published series are relatively small, further subdivision into histological categories leads to even smaller comparative groups, rendering the statistical outcome of any analysis rather suspect. Two particular features relating to histological type are common themes in the literature: firstly, that tumours of an endometrioid pattern have a relatively better prognosis (Abel & Gosling 1962, Rombeaut et al 1966, Hurt et al 1977, Fu et al 1982a, Saigo et al 1986) and secondly, that adenosquamous or mixed pattern tumours carry a poor prognosis (Wheeless et al 1970, Tamimmi & Figge 1982, Gallup et al 1985, Saigo et al 1986). The last authors noted a very poor survival, even in small lesions, three out of four patients with occult disease not surviving for 5 years. Data have been presented to contradict these findings (Rutledge et al 1975, Korhonen 1980, Shingleton et al 1981, Milsom & Friberg 1983). One is forced to conclude that while histological subtyping may be of relevance, particularly with regard to the biology of the disease, the inconclusive nature of the data renders it of little use in treatment planning.

Tumour differentiation

As tumours become less well differentiated, a worse prognosis has been reported (Reagan & Ng 1973, Anderson & Fraser 1976, Korhonen 1980, Fu et al 1982a, Berek et al 1985, Weiss & Lucas 1986), although Saigo et al (1986), employing a multivariate analysis, failed to demonstrate any association. This might be explained in part by the elegant studies of Fu et al (1982b), who examined this controversial aspect of the disease in some depth. They concluded that outcome or tumour behaviour was probably a function of stem cell DNA content as measured by flow cytometry rather than by degree of differentiation. In comparing tumours of similar differentiation, poorer prognosis was associated with high ploidy values compared with low ploidy (<3N) values. Since it is not possible to consistently predict ploidy from the histological examination of tissue, the discrepancies in the results of many studies relating differentiation to prognosis might be explained.

Lymph node metastases

The presence of lymph node metastases and tumour emboli in lymph channels have consistently been associated with a poor outcome. Saigo et al (1986) drew attention to lymph channel emboli which, even in the absence of confirmed nodal disease, carried as poor a prognosis as those with documented nodal disease. These authors also noted that lymphatic disease was seen more frequently in association with adenosquamous tumours, although tumour volume was not accounted for in this study, an important omission in the light of Berek et al's data (1985) which positively correlated nodal disease with tumour volume.

The patterns of recurrent disease identified in patients with adenocarcinoma and positive lymph nodes has led to the suggestion that lymph node metastases are indicative of systemic disease and, furthermore, that adenocarcinoma may have a greater propensity for haematogenous spread (Berek et al 1985). A similar hypothesis has been applied to squamous carcinoma where documented nodal disease is associated with a poorer outcome and an increased risk of distant metastases.

Tamimmi & Figge (1982), along with Nogales & Botella-Llusia (1965) have suggested that adenocarcinoma of the cervix has a significantly higher nodal metastasis rate than its squamous counterpart. Ireland et al (1985) in their series utilized matched squamous controls and could find no significant difference in the node metastasis rate or, indeed, in the survival rate between their 73 cases of adenocarcinoma and 158 squamous controls. Webb & Symmonds (1979), Baltzer et al (1979) and Shingleton et al (1981), all with series containing large numbers of patients who had surgical procedures for adenocarcinoma, reached a similar conclusion. This facet of adenocarcinoma is receiving much scrutiny at present and many groups are attempting to reclassify tumours previously reported as undifferentiated. One can only emphasize the need for careful control and analysis of reclassified archive data.

With regard to nodal metastases, another controversial aspect is which component of mixed tumours, i.e. squamous or glandular, is most likely to metastasize? Glucksmann & Cherry (1956) reported that the glandular component was more frequently found in metastases, inferring that this was the more virulent component. Shingleton et al (1981), however, in a larger series of surgically assessed patients, found that in all instances the histological appearance of metastases resembled the primary tumour.

TREATMENT

The management of adenocarcinoma is based on collective experience and has not been formulated as a result of prospective analyses.

As one might expect with malignant pelvic disease, treatment is based on a surgical or radiotherapeutic approach, and often both modalities are employed. Most of the work presented to date concentrates on the treatment of stage I and II disease, being the most common stages for presentation.

The 5-year survivals by stage from nine of the more recent publications are presented in Table 24.2.

Table 24.2 Survival by stage (patient numbers in parentheses)

Principal author	Disease stage				
	IB	IIA	IIB	III	IV
Milsom (1983)	83% (30)	60% (15)	45% (22)	—	—
Moberg (1986)	81% (82)	52% (56)			
Hurt (1979)	53% (15)	33% (6)		0% (9)	
Berek (1985)	83% (41)	43% (10)			
Ireland (1985)	73% (52)	40% (5)	0% (4)	0% (3)	11% (9)
Shingleton* (1981)	84% (92)	50% (19)		0% (7)	
Saigo (1986)	76% (83)	49% (33)		11% (5)	
Weiss (1986)	74% (30)	28% (11)		0% (9)	
Prempree (1985)	77% (31)	64% (44)		18% (22)	

* 3-year follow-up only

Although survival following adenocarcinoma has appeared marginally worse than that associated with squamous tumours, this has not reached levels of significance in those studies using matched controls. There may, of course, be real 'within group' differences that are not apparent because of the small numbers in each group.

It has been suggested the adenocarcinoma is a more radio-resistant tumour than squamous carcinoma of the cervix (Swann & Roddick 1973). There is no substantial data to confirm this; indeed, many have reported excellent results using radiation alone as treatment. Kottmier (1964), in a large series, achieved a 5-year survival rate of 95.5% for stage I disease and a rate of 50% for stage II disease. Gallup & Abell (1977) and Prempree et al (1985) have both commented on the relatively high local recurrence rate following pelvic irradiation. In both of these instances, however, the bulky, less operable lesions were treated primarily with radiotherapy. Tumour volume has been shown to be an important determinant of outcome after radiotherapy, so it is not surprising to find higher relapse rates after radiotherapy if bad prognosis patients are allocated this form of treatment. Waddell et al (1962) noted that two-thirds of hysterectomy specimens taken after completion of pelvic radiotherapy contained histological evidence of adenocarcinoma. They did not conclude that this was evidence for radio-resistance but felt that this occurred because the lesions were often bulky with a tendency to involve the lower part of the myometrium. Such a hypothesis may be possible if one considers that the site of malign transformation is in the less accessible endocervical canal; thus, at the time of presentation such lesions may well be larger and may have involved the lower part of the uterus.

This potential for hidden disease in the uterus has led to the use of post-radiation hysterectomy.

Thus, there are three main approaches to management:

1. Radical hysterectomy $(+/-$ lymphadenectomy),
2. Radical pelvic radiotherapy (intra-cavity, external beam or both, depending on bulk),
3. Pelvic irradiation followed by hysterectomy (simple or radical).

All three approaches have their supporters and critics. Different criteria for patient selection and lack of uniformity of treatment maintain the high level of confusion regarding appropriate management.

Length of survival is generally accepted as the most important measure of success in the management of malignant disease, and therefore the strength of any study depends heavily on the duration of follow-up. Weiss & Lucas (1986) and Saigo et al (1986) have both commented on the number of late recurrences seen in this disease and caution against early evaluation of data. Recurrences have been noted up to 9 years following apparently successful treatment for early adenocarcinoma of the cervix. The mean time to recurrence in Weiss' series was 36 months with all but two of 12 recurrences (all initially stage Ib) presenting at least 3 years after diagnosis. The mean time to recurrence in squamous cancers was 22 months.

MANAGEMENT OF EARLY ADENOCARCINOMA

Invasive adenocarcinoma of less than 2 cm maximum diameter can be treated effectively with radical surgery or by radiotherapy (Kagan et al 1973, Rutledge et al 1975, Mayer et al 1976, Shingleton et al 1981, Prempree et al 1985). For larger lesions, Prempree et al (1985) and Moberg et al (1986) recommend radiotherapy followed by extrafascial hysterectomy, reasoning that occult tumour may persist in the undertreated lower uterine component. Prempree et al (1985) noted a significant improvement in survival using such a combined approach, although patients had not been randomly allocated to treatment type. Shingleton et al's data (1981) contradicts this theory in that excellent control was noted in eight bulky cervical lesions managed by radiotherapy alone. It should, however, be noted that these data only have a 36-month follow-up.

An advantage of a radical surgical approach is that it allows lymph node sampling to be performed. Lymphadenectomy certainly adds an extra prognostic dimension to management, but there is no evidence to support its use in the belief that it will improve survival. The situation is almost identical to that in squamous cancer where poor survival has been associated with lymphatic disease (Kjorstad et al 1984, Gauthier et al 1985), and no survival benefit has been seen to accrue from lymphadenectomy. It is perhaps in lymph node positive patients that adjuvant parenteral therapies should be investigated. Currently, these patients are frequently managed by postoperative pelvic radiotherapy; the outlook remains poor (Berek et al 1985, Ireland et al 1985).

Whether ovarian conservation should be contemplated in these patients is a very debatable point, bearing in mind the presumed aetiological role of steroid hormones in glandular carcinogenesis. It should be remembered that the endocrine background to this disease rests very heavily on the epidemiological similarities with endometrial carcinoma. Milsom & Friberg (1983) report on the use of oestrogen replacement in 13 out of 30 patients with cervical adenocarcinoma. This practice was not shown to influence the 2- or 5-year survival. They went on to suggest that steroid receptor analysis of excised tumours may provide useful guidelines for subsequent therapy. If primary therapy is indeed curative, it would seem unlikely that ovarian preservation will adversely affect long-term outcome. Although the ovary is rarely involved by metastases, the ease with which hormone replacement therapy can be safely administered has prompted most clinicians to remove the ovaries at the time of radical hysterectomy.

MANAGEMENT OF ADVANCED DISEASE

As with node-positive cases, advanced disease carries a poor prognosis, and treatment in these situations is usually palliative. A small number of long-term survivors have been reported following exenterative procedures (Ireland et al 1985) when bladder involvement has been the only evidence of spread beyond the cervix. Clearly this represents a very selected group of patients and emphasizes the need to individualize treatment in such cases. Surgical approaches in advanced disease are mainly confined to palliative procedures such as urinary diversion or colostomies, whereas control of central disease, along with its associated symptomatology of bleeding, pain and discharge, usually falls to the lot of the radiotherapist. Unfortunately, no technique has yet been shown to control reliably advanced glandular malignancy. Again, this could be considered as a suitable area for evaluating more novel techniques such as neoadjuvant chemotherapy, radiosensitizers and other biomodulators. Any such studies will demand widespread co-operation as the numbers of patients seen with advanced adenocarcinoma in any one institution are small.

MANAGEMENT OF ADENOCARCINOMA IN SITU AND MICRO-INVASION

Adenocarcinoma in situ is uncommon and is usually found by chance in a cone biopsy performed for suspicion of squamous disease. Increasing awareness on the part of cytologists, however, is likely to increase the number of conizations performed because of a suspicion of glandular intra-epithelial neoplasia. The lack of accuracy of colposcopically targeted biopsies in this condition (Luesley et al 1988) makes conservative approaches to management unsound, and conization should be performed when there is a suspicion of glandular intra-epithelial neoplasia. Christopherson et al (1979) have recommended that hysterectomy is indicated once a diagnosis of adenocarcinoma in situ has been established, this being based upon the relatively high incidence of residual dysplastic glandular epithelium found in subsequent hysterectomy specimens. Whether these hysterectomies were performed after short diagnostic cones or whether the cones were intended as therapeutic is not clear. A small series from the Birmingham and Midland Hospital for Women has suggested that, based on follow-up criteria of cure (negative cytology), conization is adequate in a proportion of cases, especially if the cone excision margins are not seen to be involved. This area of management is currently being assessed.

The histological definition of micro-invasive adenocarcinoma poses some problems as depth of invasion cannot reliably be used; normal glands can often be found deep within the stromal architecture of the cervix. Nguyen & Jeanot (1984) suggest that the microstructure of the involved gland(s) is of most importance, notably epithelial budding and breakage of the basement membrane. Although one must accept the controversial aspects of histopathological classification, it is neither the place nor the purpose of this account to discuss it. Early adenocarcinoma is a recognized problem but is usually treated with a very favourable outcome (Teshima et al 1985). Whether radical approaches are necessary in these situations is debatable, but one cannot help but feel that radical hysterectomy is probably overtreatment and that current levels of thinking for this disease are as they were for squamous lesions 30 years ago.

SUMMARY OF TREATMENT

Management is currently based on largely uncontrolled, retrospective data. Radical surgery or radiotherapy are both effective in treating small (<2 cm) lesions confined to the cervix, and perhaps the choice of treatment would best be decided by well-designed protocols. Failing that, similar guidelines to those used in the treatment of early squamous cancer should be employed. The bulky lesions are more problematic. Combinations of radiotherapy and surgery might be considered as an alternative to radical hysterectomy, the local availability of expertise and other patient variables being important factors in patient selection. There is no effective treatment for advanced disease.

Super-radical surgery might be considered for a small minority, but generally treatment should be directed towards appropriate palliation.

CONCLUSIONS

1. Adenocarcinoma of the cervix occurs with a frequency ranging from 5–30%. Some individual reports have suggested that the frequency is increasing.
2. Marked epidemiological differences exist between adenocarcinoma of the cervix and its squamous counterpart; it is probable that different aetiological factors are involved. There are epidemiological similarities with adenocarcinoma of the endometrium.
3. The disease behaves in a similar clinical fashion to squamous carcinoma. Tumour stage, lesion volume and lymph node involvement are interdependent prognostic variables. These variables are also important in squamous carcinoma.
4. The histological subtypes of adenocarcinoma are important to recognize and report in a standardized fashion. Subtyping may be of importance in relation to the biology of disease. There is no consensus as to whether clinical outcome is affected.
5. There are no grounds for assuming different treatment approaches to glandular neoplasms than would be applied to squamous neoplasms.

REFERENCES

Abad R S, Kurohara S S, Graham J B 1969 Clinical significance of adenocarcinoma of the cervix. American Journal of Obstetrics and Gynecology 104: 517–522
Abell M R, Gosling J R G 1962 Gland cell carcinoma (adenocarcinoma) of the uterine cervix. American Journal of Obstetrics and Gynecology 83: 729–755
Anderson M C 1985 The pathology of cervical cancer. Clinics in Obstetrics and Gynaecology 12: 87–119
Anderson M C, Fraser A C 1976 Adenocarcinoma of the uterine cervix: a clinical and pathological appraisal. British Journal of Obstetrics and Gynaecology 83: 320–325
Aurelian L, Schumann B, Marcus R L, Davis H J 1973 Antibody to HSV-2 induced tumor specific antigens in serums from patients with cervical carcinoma. Science 181: 161–164
Baltzer J, Kopcke W, Zander J 1979 Das operiente adenokarzinom der cervix uteri. Geburtshilfe und Fraunheilkunde 39: 1011–1017
Benoit A G, Krepart G V, Lotocki R J 1984 Results of prior cytologic screening in patients with a diagnosis of stage I carcinoma of the cervix. American Journal of Obstetrics and Gynecology 148: 690–694
Berek J S, Hacker N F, Fu Y S, Sokale J R, Leuchter R C, Lagasse L D 1985 Adenocarcinoma of the uterine cervix: histologic variables associated with lymph node metastasis and survival. Obstetrics and Gynecology 65: 46–52
Bergsjo P 1963 Adenocarcinoma of the cervicis uteri: a clinical study. Acta Obstetricia et Gynecologica Scandinavica 42: 85–92
Betshill W L, Clark A H 1986 Early endocervical glandular neoplasia. I. Histomorphology and cytomorphology. Acta Cytologica 30(2): 115–126
Boon M E, Baak J P A, Kurver P J H, Overdiep S H, Verdonk G W 1981 Adenocarcinoma in-situ of the cervix: an underdiagnosed lesion. Cancer 48: 768–773

Bousfield L, Pacey F, Young Q, Krumins I, Osborn R 1980 Expanded cytologic criteria for the diagnosis of adenocarcinoma in-situ of the cervix and related lesions. Acta Cytologica 24(4): 283–295.

Boyce J G, Lu T, Nelson J H, Fruchter R G 1977 Oral contraceptives and cervical carcinoma. American Journal of Obstetrics and Gynecology 128: 761–766

Burghardt E 1973 Early histological diagnosis of cervical cancer, W B Saunders, Philadelphia, pp 335–362

Candy J, Abell M R 1968 Progestagen induced adenomatous hyperplasia of the uterine cervix. Journal of the American Medical Association 203: 323–326

Cherry C P, Glucksmann A 1961 Histology of carcinomas of the uterine cervix and survival rates in pregnant and non-pregnant patients. Surgery, Gynecology and Obstetrics 113: 763–776

Christopherson W M, Nealon N, Gray L A 1979 Non-invasive precursor lesions of adenocarcinoma and mixed adenosquamous carcinoma of the cervix uteri. Cancer 44: 975–983

Clement P B, Scully R E 1982 Carcinoma of the cervix: histologic types. Seminars in Oncology 9: 251–264

Cox M F, Meanwell C A, Maitland N J, Blackledge G, Scully C, Jordan J A 1986 Human papillomavirus type-16 homologous DNA in normal human ectocervix. Lancet ii: 157–158

Dallenbach-Hellweg G 1984 On the origin and histological structure of adenocarcinoma of the endocervix in women under 50 years of age. Pathology Research and Practice 179: 38–50

Davis J R, Moon L B 1975 Increased incidence of adenocarcinoma of the uterine cervix. Obstetrics and Gynecology 45: 79–83

Devesa S 1984 Descriptive epidemiology of cancer of the uterine cervix. Obstetrics and Gynecology 63: 605–612

Fawcett K J, Dockerty M B, Hunt A B 1966 Mesonephric carcinoma of the cervix uteri: a clinical and pathologic study. American Journal of Obstetrics and Gynecology 95: 1068–1079

Ferenczy A 1982 Carcinoma and other malignant tumours of the cervix. In: Blaunstein A (ed) Pathology of the female genital tract, 2nd edn, Springer-Verlag, New York, pp 184–222

Fu Y S, Reagan J W, Hsiu J G, Storaasli J P, Wentz W B 1982a Adenocarcinoma and mixed carcinoma of the uterine cervix. I. A clinicopathological study. Cancer 49: 2560–2570

Fu Y S, Reagan J W, Fu A S, Janiga K E 1982b Adenocarcinoma and mixed carcinoma of the uterine cervix. II. Prognostic value of nuclear DNA analysis. Cancer 49: 2571–2577

Gallup D G, Abell M R 1977 Invasive adenocarcinoma of the uterine cervix. Obstetrics and Gynecology 49: 596–603

Gallup D G, Harper R H, Stock R J 1985 Poor prognosis in patients with adenosquamous cell carcinoma of the cervix. Obstetrics and Gynecology 65: 416–422

Gauthier P, Gore I, Shingleton H M, Soong S-J, Orr J W, Hatch K D 1985 Identification of histopathological risk groups in stage Ib squamous carcinoma of the cervix. Obstetrics and Gynecology 66: 559–574

Glucksmann A, Cherry C P 1956 Incidence, histology and response to radiation of mixed carcinomas (adenoacanthomas) of the uterine cervix. Cancer 9: 971–979

Gusberg S B, Corscaden J A 1951 The pathology and treatment of adenocarcinoma of the cervix. Cancer 4: 1066–1072

Hahnel R, Martin J D, Masters A M et al 1979 Estrogen receptors and blood hormone levels in cervical carcinoma and other gynecological tumors. Gynecologic Oncology 8: 226–233

Harris R W, Brinton L A, Cowdell R H et al 1980 Characteristics of women with dysplasia or carcinoma in-situ of the cervix uteri. British Journal of Cancer 42: 359–369

Herbst A L, Robboy S J, Scully R E, Poskanzer D C 1974 Clear cell adenocarcinoma of the vagina and cervix in girls: analysis of 170 registry cases. American Journal of Obstetrics and Gynecology 119: 713–724

Hurt G W, Silverberg S G, Frable W J, Belgrad R, Crooks L D 1977 Adenocarcinoma of the cervix: histopathologic and clinical features. American Journal of Obstetrics and Gynecology 129: 304–313

Ireland D, Hardiman P, Monaghan J M 1985 Adenocarcinoma of the uterine cervix: a study of 73 cases. Obstetrics and Gynecology 65: 82–85

Julian C G, Diakoku N H, Gillespie A 1977 Adenoepidermoid and adenosquamous carcinoma of the uterus: a clinical pathological study of 118 patients. American Journal of Obstetrics and Gynecology 128: 106–115

Kagan A R, Nussbaum H, Chan P Y M, Ziel H K 1973 Adenocarcinoma of the uterine cervix. American Journal of Obstetrics and Gynecology 117: 464–468

Kaminski P F, Maier R C 1983 Clear cell adenocarcinoma of the cervix unrelated to diethylstilboestrol exposure. Obstetrics and Gynecology 62: 720–727

Kaminski P F, Norris H J 1984 Co-existence of ovarian neoplasms and endocervical adenocarcinoma. Obstetrics and Gynecology 64: 553–556

Kjorstad K E, Kolbenstvedt A, Strickert T 1984 The value of complete lymphadenectomy in radical treatment of cancer of the cervix, stage Ib. Cancer 54: 2215–2219

Korhonen M O 1978 Adenocarcinoma of the uterine cervix: an evaluation of the available diagnostic methods. Acta Pathologica et Microbiologica Scandinavica, Section A (suppl 264): 1–54

Korhonen M O 1980 Epidemiological differences between adenocarcinoma and squamous cell carcinoma of the uterine cervix. Gynecologic Oncology 10: 312–317

Kottmier H L 1964 Surgical and radiation treatment of invasive carcinoma of the uterine cervix. Acta Obstetricia et Gynecologica Scandinavica 43 (suppl 2): 1–48

Lauchlan S C, Penner D W 1967 Simultaneous adenocarcinoma in-situ and epidermoid carcinoma in-situ. Cancer 20: 2250–2254

LiVolsi V A, Merino M J, Schwartz P E 1983 Coexistent endocervical adenocarcinoma and mucinous adenocarcinoma of the ovary: a clinicopathologic study of four cases. International Journal of Gynecologic Pathology 1: 391–402

Luesley D M, Jordan J A, Woodman C B J, Watson N, Williams D R, Waddell C 1987 A retrospective review of adenocarcinoma in-situ and glandular atypia of the uterine cervix. British Journal of Obstetrics and Gynaecology (in press)

Maier R C, Norris H J 1980 Coexistence of cervical intraepithelial neoplasia with primary adenocarcinoma of the endocervix. Obstetrics and Gynecology 56: 361–364

Mayer E G, Galindo J, Davis J, Wurzel J, Aristizabal S 1976 Adenocarcinoma of the uterine cervix: incidence and the role of radiation therapy. Radiology 121: 725–729

Menczer J, Yaro-Schiffer O, Leventon-Kriss S, Modan M, Modan B 1981 Herpes virus type 2 in adenocarcinoma of the uterine cervix. Cancer 48: 1497–1499

Mendenhall W M, Thar T L, Bova F J, Marcus R B, Morgan L S, Million R R 1984 Prognostic and treatment factors affecting pelvic control of stage Ib and IIa-b carcinoma of the intact uterine cervix treated with radiation therapy alone. Cancer 53: 2649–2654

Michael H, Grawe L, Kraus F T 1984 Minimal deviation endocervical adenocarcinoma: clinical and histologic features, immunohistological staining for carcinoembryonic antigen and differentiation from confusing benign lesions. International Journal of Gynecologic Pathology 3: 261–276

Mikuta J J, Celebre J A 1969 Adenocarcinoma of the cervix. Obstetrics and Gynecology 33: 753–756

Milsom I, Friberg L G 1983 Primary adenocarcinoma of the uterine cervix. Cancer 52: 942–947

Moberg P J, Einhorn N, Silfversward C, Soderberg G 1986 Adenocarcinoma of the uterine cervix. Cancer 57: 407–410

Noda K, Kimura K, Ikeda M, Teshima K 1983 Studies on the histogenesis of cervical adenocarcinoma. International Journal of Gynecologic Pathology 1: 336–346

Nogales E, Botella-Llusia J 1965 The frequency of invasion of the lymph nodes in cancer of the uterine cervix. American Journal of Obstetrics and Gynecology 93: 91–94

Nguyen G K, Jeannot A R T 1984 Exfoliative cytology of in-situ and microinvasive adenocarcinoma of the uterine cervix. Acta Cytologica 28(4): 461–467

Peters R K, Chao A, Mack T M, Thomas D, Bernstein L, Henderson B E 1986 Increased frequency of adenocarcinoma of the uterine cervix in young women in Los Angeles County. Journal of the National Cancer Institute 76: 423–428

Pollack R S, Taylor H C Jr 1947 Carcinoma of the cervix during the first two decades of life. American Journal of Obstetrics and Gynecology 53: 135–141

Pomerance W, Mackles A 1962 Adenocarcinoma of the cervix. American Journal of Obstetrics and Gynecology 84: 367–374

Poulsen H E, Taylor C W, Sobin L H 1975 Histological typing of female genital tract tumours in histological classification of tumours, No. 13, World Health Organization, Geneva, p 15

Prempree T, Amornmarn R, Wizenberg M J 1985 A therapeutic approach to primary adenocarcinoma of the cervix. Cancer 56: 1264–1268

Qizilbash A H 1975 In-situ and microinvasive adenocarcinoma of the uterine cervix: a clinical, cytologic and histologic study of 14 cases. American Journal of Clinical Pathology 64: 155–170

Rawls W S, Gardner H L, Kaufman R L 1970 Antibodies to genital herpes virus in patients with carcinoma of the cervix. American Journal of Obstetrics and Gynecology 107: 710–716

Reagan J W, Ng A B P 1973 The cells of uterine adenocarcinoma. In: Weid G L (ed) Monographs in clinical cytology, vol 1, 2nd rev edn, S Karger, Basel, pp 96–116

Rombeaut R P, Charles D, Murphy A 1966 Adenocarcinoma of the cervix: a clinicopathologic study of 47 cases. Cancer 19: 891–900

Rutledge F N, Galakatos A E, Wharton J T, Smith J P 1975 Adenocarcinoma of the uterine cervix. American Journal of Obstetrics and Gynecology 122: 236–245

Saigo P E, Cain J M, Kim W S, Gaynor J J, Johnson K, Lewis J L 1986 Prognostic factors in adenocarcinoma of the uterine cervix. Cancer 57: 1584–1593

Shingleton H M, Gore H, Bradley D H, Soong S J 1981 Adenocarcinoma of the cervix. I. Clinical evaluation and pathological features. Obstetrics and Gynecology 139: 799–813

Smotkin D, Berek J S, Fu Y S, Hacker N F, Major F J, Wettstein F O 1986 Human papilloma virus deoxyribonucleic acid in adenocarcinoma and adenosquamous carcinoma of the uterine cervix. Obstetrics and Gynecology 68: 241–244

Soutter W P, Pegoraro R J, Green-Thompson R W et al 1981 Nuclear and cytoplasmic oestrogen receptors in squamous carcinoma of the cervix. British Journal of Cancer 44: 154–159

Steiner G, Friedell G H 1965 Adenosquamous carcinoma in-situ of the cervix. Cancer 18: 807–810

Swan S H, Brown W L 1981 Oral contraceptive use, sexual activity and cervical carcinoma. American Journal of Obstetrics and Gynecology 139: 52–57

Swann D S, Roddick J W 1973 A clinical pathological correlation of cell type classification for cervical cancer. American Journal of Obstetrics and Gynecology 116: 666–670

Tammimi H K, Figge D C 1982 Adenocarcinoma of the uterine cervix. Gynecologic Oncology 13: 335–344

Tasker J T, Collins J A 1974 Adenocarcinoma of the uterine cervix. American Journal of Obstetrics and Gynecology 118: 344–348

Teshima S, Shimosato Y, Kishi K, Kasamatsu T, Ohmi K, Vei Y 1985 Early stage adenocarcinoma of the uterine cervix: histopathologic analysis with consideration of histogenesis. Cancer 56: 167–172

Timonen S, Niemenen V, Kauraniemi T 1974 Mass screening for cervical carcinoma in Finland: organization and effect on morbidity and mortality. Annales Chirurgiae Gynaecologiae Fenniae 63: 104–112

Vessey M P, McPherson K, Lawless M, Yeates D 1983 Neoplasia of the cervix uteri and contraception: a possible adverse effect of the pill. Lancet ii: 930–934

Waddell K E, Decker D G, Welsh J S 1962 Adenocarcinoma of the cervix. American Journal of Obstetrics and Gynecology 83: 1184–1188

Webb M J, Symmonds R E 1979 Wertheim hysterectomy : a reappraisal. Obstetrics and Gynecology 54: 140–145

Weiner S, Wizenberg M J 1975 Treatment of primary adenocarcinoma of the cervix. Cancer 35: 1514–1516

Weiss R J, Lucas W E 1986 Adenocarcinoma of the uterine cervix. Cancer 57: 1996–2001

Wheeless C R Jr, Graham R, Graham J B 1970 Prognosis and treatment of adenoepidermoid carcinoma of the cervix. Obstetrics and Gynecology 35: 928–932

Carcinoma in situ of the vulva— a new disease of young women?

Comyns Berkley and Victor Bonney of the Middlesex Hospital in London described, in 1909, those conditions, mainly types of leukoplakia, thought to lead to the development of carcinoma of the vulva. The name of J. T. Bowen (1912) is frequently applied to in situ vulval carcinoma. More recently, Jeffcoate (1966) introduced the term vulval dystrophy to help describe abnormal vulval epithelium. Considerable efforts have since been made to evaluate the malignant potential of each epithelial abnormality, and the clinical management of the patient has been directed accordingly.

However, in 1971, Donald Woodruff and his colleagues from the Johns Hopkins Hospital, Baltimore, Maryland, reported to the American Association of Obstetricians and Gynecologists (Woodruff et al 1973) their conclusions from an analysis of 44 patients with carcinoma in situ of the vulva. They suggested that, contrary to previous beliefs, the incidence of vulval carcinoma in situ was increasing, especially amongst young women, that the aetiology could involve virus infections and that surgical treatment could, and should, be more conservative than traditional vulvectomy.

Since then, several attempts have been made to offer explanations for and ideas on the management of carcinoma in situ of the vulva in young women— Dr Woodruff's 'contemporary challenge'.

Whereas no study to date has provided the complete answer, certain facts are emerging of which all gynaecologists should be aware. Any discussion of this condition, nevertheless, in our current state of knowledge, is still likely to provide more questions than answers.

The more important questions still to be addressed include the following. Is this a new disease of the young female, distinct from in situ carcinoma of the vulva in older women, with differing disease patterns, malignant potential and therefore treatment? Is the incidence really rising or is the condition just being diagnosed with increasing frequency? Is there any possibility of a causative association with sexually transmitted diseases, particularly those of viral origin? Should a young patient with this condition be observed only or be treated by non-surgical means, conservative surgery or extensive surgery?

GEOGRAPHICAL DISTRIBUTION

Hitherto, reports of vulval carcinoma in situ in young women have been almost exclusively from North America. Scattered reports from other countries have not, as yet, shown significant changes in the incidence of vulval cancer. Menczer et al (1982) reported, for example, from Israel that in contrast to the relatively low incidence of squamous cell carcinoma of the cervix in Israeli Jewish women, the age-specific incidence rates of squamous cell carcinoma of the vulva are similar to those of white women in the United States of America; yet the frequency of vulval carcinoma in situ remained very low in a survey from 1961 to 1973 in Israel. Significantly, reports of vulval carcinoma in situ in young women have been made from data covering the last decade, and more recent surveys are needed in other countries before the true geographical distribution is known.

INCIDENCE

The diagnosis of vulval carcinoma in situ in young women was rarely made at the Middlesex Hospital, London, before 1976. During that year the lesion was diagnosed in a 29-year-old white woman who was 32 weeks pregnant. The lesion did not regress spontaneously and was present in repeat biopsies in 1979. In 1981, a young lady of 20 years had a cervical intra-epithelial neoplasm (CIN)-III lesion of the cervix diagnosed in conjunction with Bowenoid papulosis of the vulva. In 1983, three other women, aged 34, 29 and 26 years, presented with vulval carcinoma in situ. The former woman also had a CIN-III lesion of the cervix and the latter woman presented with a 'warty' appearance of the vulva. Other women with vulval carcinoma in situ diagnosed at the Middlesex Hospital, London, during the past decade, had an average age of 63 years (range: 50–86 years).

Friedrich and his colleagues (1980) from the Medical College of Wisconsin reported that, prior to 1967, the diagnosis of vulval carcinoma in situ had not been made at their institution, but that a 'new awareness' of the entity had led to the diagnosis of 50 cases over the next 10 years.

Whilst recognising the reported increase in vulval carcinoma in situ in parts of North America, there has, for example, been no increase, as yet, in the reported incidence of invasive carcinoma in the state of Connecticut during the past 30 years (Schwartz & Naftolin 1981; see also Japaze et al (1977) in Table 25.1).

AGE AT DIAGNOSIS

The most striking feature of the data emerging from the last decade is the undoubted rising incidence of the disease amongst women under 40 years of age, whilst records before the early 1970s rarely included women who had not reached the menopause (see Table 25.2).

Table 25.1   Diagnosis of in situ and invasive carcinoma of the vulva

Authors	Time band	No. of cases	
		In situ	Invasive
Friedrich et al (1980)	up to 1967	Nil	—
	1967–1977	50	—
Benedet & Murphy (1982)	1970–1974	36	—
	1975–1980	45	—
Kaplan et al (1981)	1966–1976	Nil	—
	1976–1978	10	—
Japaze et al (1977)	1935–1950	7	31
	1951–1965	20	41
	1966–1972	44	49

Table 25.2   Age at diagnosis of in situ carcinoma of the vulva

Authors	No. of patients	Age range (yrs)	Average age (yrs)	% of patients less than:		
				40	50	30 (yrs)
Friedrich at al (1980)	—	14–81	39	—	76	—
Forney et al (1977)	29	19–67	39	—	—	—
Kaplan et al (1981)	10	23–52	39	—	—	—
Bernstein et al (1983)	65	19–72	38	48	—	—
Baggish & Dorsey (1981)	35	20–79	—	43	—	30
Townsend et al (1982)	33	21–75	—	58	—	18
Buscema et al (1980)	106	21–83	47	40	—	—
Japaze et al (1977)	71	21–86	39	—	—	—
Benedet & Murphy (1982)	81	19–87	—	—	—	—
1970–1974	—	—	60	14	—	—
1975–1980	—	—	45	42	—	—

HISTOPATHOLOGY

The International Society for the Study of Vulvar Disease in 1976 defined carcinoma in situ of the vulva as cellular abnormalities extending throughout the full thickness of the epithelium (not including the most superficial keratinized layer), or the presence of intra-epithelial squamous pearls present at the tips of the rete ridges.

By contrast, Paget's disease of the vulva is another, much less common, form of carcinoma in situ. It evolves from a different stem cell and differs in prognosis (Parmley et al 1975).

AETIOLOGY

Josey et al (1976) noticed that patients with in situ carcinoma of the vulva had experienced an increased frequency of sexually transmitted diseases. In Friedrich et al's series (1980), 30 patients (60%) were suffering from, either alone or in combination, condylomata acuminatum (13 patients), herpes simplex (5 patients), gonorrhoea, syphilis (9 patients) and *Haemophilus vaginalis* and *Trichomonas* infection.

Encouraged by the sero-epidemiological (Adam et al 1972) and immunohis-tochemical (Dreesman et al 1980) evidence to suggest an association between herpes virus type 2 with intra-epithelial and invasive cervical neoplasia and the frequent co-existence of cervical and vulval neoplasia, co-workers in America demonstrated the presence of herpes virus type 2 induced non-structural protein antigen in squamous cell carcinoma in situ of the vulva (Kaufman et al 1981, Korhonen et al 1982). All nine patients examined carried serum IgG antibodies to herpes virus type 2, suggesting recent herpes virus type 2 infections. They could not identify structural antigens to the virus, which suggested that the patients did not have acute herpes virus type 2 infections at the time, and only found one virus-like particle. Friedrich (1972) did demonstrate the presence of virus particles in the nuclei of the atypical cells, and positive type 2 herpes virus antibody titres in a 15-year-old girl with vulval carcinoma in situ and classical herpes virus vulvitis.

It is not surprising that patients with carcinoma in situ of the vulva have had exposure to herpes virus type 2; according to Bolognese et al (1976) up to 60% of asymptomatic pregnant women in the 35–44 year age group have been exposed to the virus. However, herpes virus type 2 remains under suspicion as an aetiological agent.

Stein (1980) reported a case of a woman with chronic vulvovaginitis from the age of 20 years who subsequently developed, at the age of 37, vulval carcinoma in situ, 2 years after her husband, who had had penile 'warts' for at least 4 years, had undergone circumcision for penile carcinoma in situ with focal invasion. Stein (1980) also pointed out that there may be similarities between vulval carcinoma in situ in humans and the transmissible venereal, or Stiker, tumour found on the genitalia of both male and female dogs. Like carcinoma in situ in humans, it has been shown to undergo spontaneous regression (Muller & Kirk 1976).

Seski et al (1978), in an in vitro study of lymphocytic transformation in patients with carcinoma in situ of the vulva, found cellular immunity of the delayed type to be diminished when compared with age-matched controls. It is possible that altered cellular immunity compromised by pregnancy may account for lesions appearing during gestation and subsequently undergoing spontaneous regression, as reported by Skinner et al (1973) and in the four cases of Friedrich et al (1980).

In an attempt to investigate the possibility that essentially benign prolife-rations of the vulval epithelium were being incorrectly diagnosed as carcinoma in situ, Fu et al (1981) studied the nuclear DNA content, using Feulgen microspectrophotometry, of 59 patients (51 carcinoma in situ and 8 atypical epithelia). In all cases of carcinoma in situ an aneuploid type was found—evidence clearly against these lesions being benign proliferations. Furthermore, Friedrich et al (1980) confirmed that 92% of 49 vulval carcinoma in situ lesions analysed by microspectrophotometry had an aneuploid DNA pattern which did not correlate with prognosis.

Of doubtful significance is the finding within the series of Friedrich et al (1980) of 50 patients, three of whom had given a history of vulval exposure to Paris green—an arsenical insecticide—related to their childhood experience on potato farms and two of whom were identical twins.

CLINICAL FEATURES

Table 25.3 illustrates the frequency and type of presenting symptoms encountered. The high frequency of those asymptomatic patients mainly discovered

Table 25.3   Symptoms of in situ carcinoma of the vulva

Authors	No. of patients	% with pruritus	% with visible tumour	% asymptomatic
Bernstein et al (1983)	65	60	17	18
Benedet & Murphy (1982)	81	43	30	21
Kaplan et al (1981)	10	40	40	—
Friedrich et al (1980)	50	38	14	48
Forney et al (1977)	29	72	—	28

during routine cervical Papanicolaou screening reflects the heightened awareness of this clinical entity by clinicians in North America. Benedet & Murphy (1982) saw clinical appearances ranging from a red velvety patch to a diffuse multifocal pigmented lesion and occasionally verrucous papular lesions. Some authors have described the multifocal pigmented lesions as 'Bowenoid papulosis' (Wade et al 1979) typically affecting young women, occasionally in association with pregnancy, genital herpes or condylomata acuminatum. Buscema et al (1980) reported that 20% of their patients had lesions which were 'warty' in appearance.

Forney et al (1977) emphasised the value of the colposcope in the diagnosis of these lesions. However, in examining the vulva the patterns of mosaicism and punctation were not usually observed compared with cervical and vaginal intra-epithelial carcinoma; most vulval lesions had a characteristic strongly demarcated, elevated, white plaque. Similarly, contrast was enhanced by the application of 3% acetic acid. Friedrich et al (1980) found that 60% of lesions retained 1% toluidine blue dye applied according to the method of Collins et al (1966), but Bernstein et al (1983), found toluidine blue staining so unreliable that they abandoned its use.

Table 25.4 displays the frequent involvement of structures adjacent to the vulva. In particular, the anus is not only the site for primary disease but also for recurrent, or inadequately excised, disease. The need for multiple biopsies of all suspicious areas, particularly near the anus, is obvious. Forney et al (1977) reported that multifocal lesions were usually more extensive and exhibited a greater tendency to become confluent in younger women (average age 31 years).

Table 25.4 Multifocal disease—the involvement of structures adjacent to the vulva

Author	No. of patients	% with multifocal disease	% with involvement of the: Anus	Vagina	Glans	Meatus
Freidrich et al (1980)	50	70	22	10	18	2
Forney et al (1977)	29	52	17	—	—	—
Bernstein et al (1983)	65:	65	30	—	—	—
	<40 yrs	84	—	—	—	—
	>40 yrs	35	—	—	—	—
Baggish & Dorsey (1981)	35	—	57	—	—	—

ASSOCIATION WITH OTHER CANCERS AND DISEASES

There is a well-known association between carcinoma in situ of the vulva with invasive carcinoma of the cervix and more recently with intra-epithelial cervical carcinoma (Woodruff et al 1973, Jimerson & Merrill 1970). In 1961, Peterka et al put forward the idea of an association between carcinoma in situ of the vulva and the subsequent development of internal cancer; however, this was later denied by Anderson et al (1973).

Benedet & Murphy (1982), in their series of 81 patients, found that of 24 patients under the age of 35 years, 17 (71%) had disease also involving the cervix and/or vagina, as had 14 (25%) of the 57 patients over 35 years of age. They also noted that of patients diagnosed between 1970 and 1974, 25% had multiple site disease and, more recently, between 1975 and 1980, 51% had multiple site disease. In their whole series 1 patient also had chronic leukaemia, 6 had had previous pelvic radiotherapy for cervical cancer, 3 previously had had herpes genitalis and 6 had had condylomata. The possibility that immunocompromised patients are liable to this disease is raised by several authors, as is the possible association with infective agents. Table 25.5 displays the findings of the most recently reported series.

TREATMENT AND RESULTS

No treatment

Skinner et al (1973) have observed spontaneous regression occurring in carcinoma in situ of the vulva. Other authors have reported similar cases in young women, especially where the lesion first appeared during pregnancy. Friedrich et al (1980) observed nine patients without treatment, five of whom underwent spontaneous regression of their lesions. In addition, one patient whose tumour regressed was lost to follow-up, and another showed no change after 2 years. Of the remaining two, one had severe immunosuppression and developed a well-differentiated squamous carcinoma of the vulva, and eventually died with widespread secondary deposits from an undifferentiated tumour of the vagina. The remaining patient developed widespead carcinoma in situ of both the vagina and the vulva, and died later with leukaemia and an astrocytoma. Bernstein et al (1983) observed 13 patients, eight of whom had disease after

Table 25.5   Association between in situ carcinoma of the vulva and other neoplastic conditions

Authors	No. of patients	% with condylomata	% with disease of the:		% with tumours elsewhere
			cervix	vagina	
Buscema et al (1980)	106	—	27	1	2 (ovary)
Townsend et al (1982)	33	—	33	15	—
Baggish & Dorsey (1981)	35	—	46	31	—
Bernstein et al (1983)	65	24	20	—	8 (skin, uterus, breast)
Forney et al (1977)	29	31	→ 31 ←		14 (skin, leukae-mia)
Friedrich et al (1980)	50	—	26	—	—
Benedet & Murphy (1982): 24<35 years			→ 71 ←		—
57>35 years			→ 25 ←		—

an interval of 2–6 months (and were treated with laser). The remaining five patients (aged 23–35 years, none of whom were pregnant) underwent spontaneous regression of their lesions in less than 6 months. One patient who refused any treatment and one patient with persistent disease after treatment with 5-fluorouracil in the series of Benedet & Murphy (1982) developed no change in their disease after 6 and 3 years respectively. Two patients (Buscema et al 1980), who were given no additional therapy after initial biopsy, have been followed for over 5 years without the appearance of a gross lesion.

Development of invasive tumours

According to Benedet & Murphy (1982) they have seen no young patient with an in situ lesion progress to invasive disease; however, three of their older patients progressed after 6, 3 and 2 years following treatment of their in situ lesions. Patients who developed further vulval disease had undergone incomplete surgical excision. Buscema et al (1980) recorded four out of 106 patients who developed invasive cancer; of these four, two were on immunosuppressive therapy, and the other two were aged 75 and 83 years and did not show invasion in their initial biopsies.

Consequences of total vulvectomy

Information concerning the effects of performing total vulvectomy on both young and old women is gradually being accumulated. DiSaia et al (1979) showed that 18 patients treated with widespread local excision for microinvasive vulval cancer maintained their sexual responsiveness in contrast to two total vulvectomy patients who lost orgasmic ability and developed dypareunia. Andersen & Hacker (1983) studied 15 patients who had undergone vulvectomy, including eight patients under the age of 55 years and three patients under the age of 40 years. They found considerable disruption in micturition and sexual function. Many women reported 'persistent and unexpected' numbness, to the extent that on some occasions during intercourse they were unsure when penile penetration occurred. The magnitude of body image disruption after vulvectomy was 'extreme'. The patients felt that the procedure was too intimate to discuss with anyone other than the closest friend or relative; many felt embarrassed, burdened and isolated. Most felt that information regarding sexuality was falsely reassuring.

Skinning vulvectomy

Rutledge & Sinclair (1968) introduced the skinning vulvectomy with split thickness skin grafting, which can be used when the disease is too widespread for local excision. Techniques vary but essentially the skin of the vulva is excised to the depth of the loose fibro-elastic tissue beneath the dermis attaching the vulva to the dartos fascia. The line of excision is continued posteriorly to include all areas of involved anal mucosa (excluding, of course, the structures deep in the anal mucosa) as confirmed by serial frozen section. Careful haemostasis is mandatory. The patient is given an indwelling urinary catheter (and suitable analgesia—the open vulva is painful) for a few days until evidence of epithelialisation is visible. Split thickness skin grafts are taken, e.g. from the thigh, and fashioned to cover the denuded areas. Holes ('pie crusting') are made in the donor skin to allow the drainage of serous fluid collections.

Carbon dioxide laser

Townsend et al (1982) emphasised the advantages of treating a maximum area of 3–4 cm in diameter with the laser and covering all of the affected areas in several outpatient sessions. Of their 33 patients there were only two failures, and only four required repeat treatments for new lesions. The same group felt that carbon dioxide laser treatment was superior to cryosurgery which lacked precision and produced oedema, pain, ulceration, scarring and distortion. Friedrich et al (1980) treated one patient with cryosurgery using a freon unit—there was considerable sloughing. After healing there remained persistent disease that was managed by total vulvectomy. Forney et al (1977) treated four patients without recurrence using cryosurgery. Baggish & Dorsey (1981) treated 35 patients with laser to a depth of 3 mm; only three patients had persistent disease after 1 year. Bernstein et al (1983) treated 18 patients with only one episode of recurrence.

Chemotherapy

Several agents have been evaluated in treating both in situ and invasive vulval and vaginal tumours; recent experience has been reviewed by Barker (1983).

5-Fluorouracil. In the series of Buscema et al (1980), the lesions of three out of 11 patients responded to initial therapy with local 5-fluorouracil applications. Carson et al (1976) reported on a 42-year-old woman with recurrent in situ carcinoma of the vulva who was cleared of the lesion in all but the anal region (this required local excision) using 5% 5-fluorouracil cream in twice daily applications for a month. The patient experienced severe discomfort but it was felt that she had avoided a diverting colostomy. Other reports of 5-fluorouracil application vary from discontinuation of treatment after 2 weeks because of severe irritation and ulceration, to complete eradication of the neoplasia after 3 years of follow-up. Benedet & Murphy (1982) spread treatment with 5-fluorouracil over 6–8 weeks and noted intense pruritus, irritation and discomfort, far in excess of that experienced before treatment. Forney et al (1977) treated six patients who experienced considerable discomfort, all of whom had persistent disease afterwards. Friedrich et al (1980) treated three patients with 5-fluorouracil, which resulted in considerable pain and sloughing. There were no responses and total vulvectomy was performed.

DNCB. Dinitrochlorobenzene (DNCB) elicits a non-specific inflammatory response which is T cell mediated [similar to that of the Bacille Calmette-Guérin (BCG) vaccine]. It is thought that cancer cells are more sensitive to this immune reaction than normal cells. Weintraub & Lagasse (1972) have shown that the production of a hypersensitive response to local DNCB can result in reversing vulvar atypia. Foster & Woodruff (1981) treated six patients (age range 24–63 years) who had recurrent carcinoma in situ of the vulva after surgical excision and/or topical 5-fluorouracil with DNCB challenge, sensitisation and local application. DNCB produced sloughing in all cases after an intense reaction at the area of carcinoma in situ, with only mild erythema of the surrounding skin. Healing resulted in normal or hyperplastic skin in five out of the six patients. The recurrence in the remaining patient was treated by surgical excision.

Bleomycin. Roberts et al (1980), in California, treated 12 patients with topical or intradermal bleomycin. All developed a chemical vulvitis and occasional severe ulceration which, combined with the poor results, led to the authors recommending against its use. Seven patients treated topically with a 5% suspension applied twice daily produced no responses, and only two out of 10 patients treated with intradermal injections of a 1% bleomycin solution showed any improvement at all.

Results of surgery

Table 25.6 displays recent experience using surgical methods to treat in situ carcinoma of the vulva. In the series reported by Friedrich et al (1980), 31 patients had tumour-free margins after initial therapy, and three of these developed recurrent disease. Of six patients with tumour in the margins of resection, three experienced recurrent disease. All recurrences appeared between 10 weeks and 8 years later. Buscema et al (1980) emphasised that 'recurrences' or 'reoccurrences' may appear at any time, the longest interval in their series being 13 years, and that these patients should undergo 'careful and indefinite follow up'.

DISCUSSION

Since the condition of carcinoma in situ of the vulva in young women has only been studied and reported in depth for a relatively short period of time, its true malignant potential over the next 30, 40 or 50 years in these patients cannot be known. It would appear that in the short-term carcinoma in situ of the vulva arising in a young patient seems rarely to eventuate in invasive cancer (Zacur et al 1980), and also that treatment can be conservative initially with the proviso that competetent follow-up is mandatory. On the contrary, the same condition, if indeed it is the same condition, in the postmenopausal patient carries a much higher malignant potential. Similarly, the young patient with any form of long-term immunosuppression, i.e. causes other than pregnancy, must be considered a likely candidate for disease progression in the short term.

Although Zacur et al (1980) caution against premature and unwarranted comparisons of this disease with epithelial neoplasia of the cervix, more aetiological and epidemiological evidence is being acquired to suggest that pre-invasive lesions of the cervix, vagina and vulva share many features in common, and the multicentric nature of carcinoma in situ of the vulva in young women supports the idea of a 'field' change (Henson & Tarone 1977, Singer 1983).

It is not beyond the realms of possibility that a proportion of young women with in situ carcinoma of the vulva will, after a protracted time interval, eventually proceed to invasive cancer. There are, to date, insufficient data to justify withholding therapy in all cases. However, as Bernstein et al (1983) point out from their own experience and the experience of Friedrich (1972) and Skinner et al (1973), observation of up to 6 months to 1 year may be justified in young patients who are pregnant or recovering from a recent herpetic vulvitis. All other patients must be regarded as requiring immediate investigation and treatment.

Colposcopic evaluation and multiple-directed biopsies may identify the surgical target area, but wide excision biopsy and skinning vulvectomy with or without split thickness skin grafting is necessary to obtain histopathological analysis and disease removal. The occasional report of early foci of invasion in older patients, especially in association with intra-epithelial 'pearl' formation, amongst these lesions cannot be dismissed when considering therapy. There seems every justification, however, from our current knowledge, to avoid total vulvectomy with its disastrous psychological morbidity in the young patient.

It is tempting for gynaecologists to ignore the anus and peri-anal skin. The high proportion of involvement of this disease in these structures confirms

Table 25.6 Results of surgical treatment of in situ carcinoma of the vulva

Treatment	Bernstein et al (1983) P	R	Buscema et al (1980) P	R	Benedet & Murphy (1982) P	R	Kaplan et al (1981) P	R	Forney et al (1977) P	R	Friedrich et al (1980) P	R
Total vulvectomy	5	1	28	8	33	14	—	—	3	0	10	1
Partial vulvectomy	5	1	—	—	—	—	—	—	—	—	10	2
Skinning vulvectomy	8	1	—	—	3	2	9	2	8	1	—	—
Local excision	16	2	63	20	42	18	1	0	11	1	17	3

P = number of patients treated, R = number of patients with recurrent disease the importance of regarding the 'field' exposed as the 'anogenital unit' (Franklin & Rutledge, 1972). Wide excision in this area is indicated when involved with disease, as peri-anal recurrence has been frequently reported (Kaplan et al 1981).

There remains a considerable need for further monitoring of this condition, particularly in Europe where experience is not so well recorded as in North America. In the meantime it behoves all gynaecologists encountering this condition in young women to consider very carefully the extent of therapy required and the various treatment options available, and to avoid, in all cases, surgery that is unnecessarily radical.

REFERENCES

Adam E, Rawls W E, Melnick J L 1972 The association of herpes virus type 2 infection and cervical cancer. Preventive Medicine 3: 122

Anderson B L, Hacker N F 1983 Psychosexual adjustment after vulvar surgery. Obstetrics and Gynecology 62(4): 457

Anderson S L, Nielson A, Reymann F 1973 Relationship between Bowen's disease and internal malignant tumours. Archives of Dermatology 108: 367

Baggish M S, Dorsey J H 1981 CO$_2$ laser for the treatment of vulvar carcinoma in situ. Obstetrics and Gynecology 57: 371

Barker G H 1983 Chemotherapy of gynaecological malignancies, Castle House Publications, England, chaps 18 & 19

Benedet J L, Murphy K J 1982 Squamous carcinoma in situ of the vulva. Gynecologic Oncol 14: 213

Berkley C, Bonney V 1909 Leukoplakia vulvae and its relationship to Kraurosis vulvae and carcinoma vulvae. British Medical Journal 2: 1739

Bernstein S G, Kovacs B R, Townsend D E, Morrow C P 1983 Vulvar carcinoma in situ. Obstetrics and Gynecology 61(3): 304

Bolognese R J, Corson S L, Fuccillo D A, Traub R, Moder F, Sever J 1976 Herpes virus hominis type II infections in asymptomatic pregnant women. Obstetrics and Gynecology 48: 507

Bowen J T 1912 Precancerous dermatoses. Journal of Cutaneous Diseases 30: 241

Buscema J, Woodruff J D, Parmley T H, Genadry R 1980 Carcinoma in situ of the vulva. Obstetrics and Gynecology 55(2): 225

Carson T E, Hoskins W J, Wurzell J F 1976 Topical 5 Flurouracil in the treatment of carcinoma in situ of the vulva. Obstetrics and Gynecology 47(1) (suppl) 59S

Collins C G, Hansen L H, Theriot E 1966 A clinical stain for use in selecting biopsy sites in patients with vulvar disease. Obstetrics and Gynecology 28: 158

DiSaia P J, Creasman W T, Rich W M 1979 An alternate approach to early carcinoma of the vulva. American Journal of Obstetrics and Gynecology 133: 825

Dreesman G D, Burek J, Adam J 1980 Expression of herpes virus induced antigens in human cervical cancer. Nature 283: 591

Forney J P, Morrow C P, Townsend D E, DiSaia P J 1977 Management of carcinoma in situ of the vulva. American Journal of Obstetrics and Gynecology 127: 801

Foster D C, Woodruff J D 1981 The use of dinitrochlorobenzene in the treatment of vulvar carcinoma in situ. Gynecologic Oncology 11: 330

Franklin E W, Rutledge F D 1972 Epidemiology of epidermoid carcinoma of the vulva. Obstetrics and Gynecology 39: 165

Friedrich E G 1972 Reversible vulvar atypia. Obstetrics and Gynecology 39: 173

Friedrich E G, Wilkinson E J, Shifu Y 1980 Carcinoma in situ of the vulva: a continuing challenge. American Journal of Obstetrics and Gynecology 136: 830

Fu Y S, Reagan J W, Townsend D E 1981 Nuclear DNA study of vulvar intraepithelial and invasive squamous neoplasms. Obstetrics and Gynecology 57: 643

Henson D, Tarone R 1977 An epidemiologic study of cancer of the cervix, vagina, and vulva based on the Third National Cancer Survey in the United States. American Journal of Obstetrics and Gynecology 129: 525

International Society for the Study of Vulvar Disease 1976 New nomenclature for vulvar disease. Obstetrics and Gynecology 47: 122

Japaze H, Garcia-Bunuel R, Woodruff J D 1977 Primary vulvar neoplasia—a review of in situ and invasive carcinoma 1935–1972. Obstetrics and Gynecology 49(4): 404

Jeffcoate T N A 1966 Chronic vulvar dystrophies. American Journal of Obstetrics and Gynecology 95: 61

Jimerson G K, Merrill J A 1970 Multicentric squamous malignancy involving both cervix and vulva. Cancer 26: 150

Josey W E, Nahmias A J, Naib Z M 1976 Viruses and cancer of the lower genital tract. Cancer 38: 526

Kaplan A L, Kaufman R H, Birken R A, Simkin S 1981 Intraepithelial carcinoma of the vulva with extension to the anal canal. Obstetrics and Gynecology 58: 368

Kaufman R H, Dreesman G D, Burek J 1981 Herpes virus induced antigens in squamous cell carcinoma in situ of the vulva. New England Journal of Medicine 305: 483

Korhonen M O, Kaufman R H, Roberts D, Walker N, Adam E 1982 Carcinoma in situ of the vulva—the search for viral particles. Journal of Reproductive Medicine 27(12): 746

Menczer J, Voliovitch Y, Modan B, Modan M, Steinitz R 1982 Some epidemiologic aspects of carcinoma of the vulva in Israel. American Journal of Obstetrics and Gynecology 143: 893

Muller G H, Kirk R W 1976 Canine transmissable venereal tumor (canine venereal sarcoma). In: Small animal dermatology, 2nd edn, W B Saunders, Philadelphia, chap. 69, pp 600–602

Parmley T, Woodruff J D, Julian C G 1975 Invasive vulvar Paget's disease. Obstetrics and Gynecology 46: 341

Peterka E S, Lynch F W, Goltz R W 1961 An association between Bowen's disease and internal cancer. Archives of Dermatology 84: 139

Roberts J A, Watring W G, Lagasse L D 1980 Treatment of vulvar intraepithelial neoplasia (VIN) with local bleomycin. Clinical Cancer Trials V3(4): 351

Rutledge F, Sinclair M 1968 Treatment of intraepithelial carcinoma of the vulva by skin excision and graft. American Journal of Obstetrics and Gynecology 102: 806

Schwartz P E, Naftolin F 1981 Type 2 Herpes Simplex virus and vulvar carcinoma in situ. New England Journal of Medicine 305(9): 517

Seski J C, Reinhalter E R, Silva J 1978 Abnormalities of lymphocyte transformations in women with intraepithelial carcinoma of the vulva. Obstetrics and Gynecology 52: 332

Singer A 1983 Sex and genital cancer in heterosexual women. Journal of Reproductive Medicine 28(2): 109

Skinner M S, Sternberg W H, Ichinose H, Collins J 1973 Spontaneous regression of Bowenoid atypia of the vulva. Obstetrics and Gynecology 42: 40

Stein D S 1980 Transmissible veneral neoplasia: a case report. American Journal of Obstetrics and Gynecology 137(7): 864

Townsend D E, Levine R U, Richart R M, Crum C P, Petrilli E S 1982 Management of vulvar intraepithelial neoplasia by carbon dioxide laser. Obstetrics and Gynecology 60: 49

Wade T R, Kopk A W, Ackerman A B 1979 Bowenoid papulosis of the genetalia. Archives of Dermatology 115: 306

Weintraub I, Lagasse L D 1972 Reversibility of vulvar atypia by DNCB-induced delayed hypersensitivity. Obstetrics and Gynecology 41(2): 195

Woodruff J D, Puray J C, Mermut T, Katayama P 1973 The contemporary challenge of carcinoma in situ of the vulva. American Journal of Obstetrics and Gynecology 115: 677

Zacur H, Genadry R, Woodruff J D 1980 The patient at risk for development of vulvar disease. Gynecology and Oncology 9: 199

Index